Statistics and research in physical education

Statistics and research in physical education

Jerome C. Weber, Ph.D.

Associate Professor, Department of Physical Education,
University of Oklahoma, Norman, Oklahoma

David R. Lamb, Ph.D.

Associate Professor, Department of Physical Education,
The University of Toledo, Toledo, Ohio

With 17 illustrations

Saint Louis

The C. V. Mosby Company

1970

To our wives

Barbara and Cozette

Preface

This book is designed primarily for use as a supplementary text for undergraduate and graduate courses in statistics and research methods for physical education students. However, we believe the book will also be appropriate as a guide to physical education tests, experimental designs, and statistical methods for those who have completed their formal academic training. The primary emphasis of the book is directed toward statistical methods that are most often encountered in the area of physical education. Our hope is that the material will convey to the student an appreciation of the value of the statistical methods discussed and an understanding of how these methods are used and interpreted by the physical educator. The book is not intended to serve as a substitute for mathematical statistics courses for the advanced graduate student who requires a more detailed understanding of the derivation of statistical methods.

It was our desire to make the book sufficiently flexible to allow the instructor to utilize only those portions that best meet the needs of his students. Certain portions of the book are far more suitable for a graduate level presentation than for an introductory course at the undergraduate level; other portions are too elementary to warrant inclusion in a graduate course. We consider the organization and sequence of chapters to be logical and practical but certainly not the only possible sequence.

Perhaps the most unique feature of the book is the presentation of statistical methods on an intuitive, nonmathematical basis utilizing data and situations that are familiar and meaningful to physical education students. The professional physical educator, whether he is engaged in teaching, coaching, or research, has as great an obligation to be statistically literate as any other professional person. This single assumption has been our primary motivation in the writing of this book. We hope to have contributed to this objective.

We would like to express our sincere appreciation to the literary executor of the late Sir Ronald A. Fisher, to Professor Frank Yates, and to Oliver & Boyd Ltd. for permission to reprint Tables C-1 (squares), C-2 (square roots), C-3 (random numbers), and C-5 (values of the correlation coefficient for different levels of significance) from *Statistical Tables for Biological, Agri-*

cultural, and Medical Research, sixth edition, 1963; to Professor Allen L. Edwards and Holt, Rinehart & Winston for permission to reprint Table C-4 (areas of the normal curve in terms of x/σ) from *Statistical Analysis,* revised edition, 1958; to Professor E. S. Pearson and Professor H. O. Hartley (editors and Cambridge University Press for permission to reprint Tables C-6 (percentage points of the studentized range), C-7 (percentage points of the χ^2 distribution), C-8 (percentage points of the t distribution), and C-9 (the F distribution) from *Biometrika Tables for Statisticians,* third edition, 1966; to Professor Wayne D. Van Huss et al. and Prentice-Hall, Inc., for permission to reprint Table 4-3 (bent-knee sit-ups percentile table) from *Physical Activity in Modern Living,* 1960; and to Professor Edwin A. Fleishman and Prentice-Hall, Inc., for permission to reprint Table A-1 (handgrip norms) from *The Structure and Measurement of Physical Fitness,* 1964.

We would also like to express our gratitude to Professor Wayne D. Van Huss and Professor William W. Heusner of the Department of Health, Physical Education, and Recreation of Michigan State University who provided us with an understanding of the role of quantitative methods in the area of physical education. Our thanks are also extended to the many people, too numerous to mention individually, who helped in various ways in the preparation of this book.

Jerome C. Weber

David R. Lamb

Contents

1 Nature and role of statistics, 1

2 Collecting and presenting data, 7

3 Normal distribution and measures of central tendency, 15

4 Measures of variability, 23

5 Purposes and types of physical education research, 35

6 Hypothesis testing and research design, 45

7 Simple linear correlation, 59

8 Simple linear regression, 73

9 Chi square, 80

10 Other measures of association, 86

11 t tests, 93

12 One-way analysis of variance, 103

13 Randomized blocks analysis of variance, 113

14 Two-way analysis of variance, 123

15 Analysis of covariance, 146

16 Multiple regression and multiple and partial correlation, 158

17 Other statistical methods, 170

18 Typical research paradigms and statistical treatments for physical education, 174

Appendixes

A   Tests and testing in physical education, 181

B   A review of mathematics skills, 188

C   Tables, 197

Statistics and research in physical education

Chapter **1**

Nature and role of statistics

IMPORTANCE OF STATISTICS

Statistics is a subject of increasing importance in every phase of academic and everyday life. To the student preparing for a career in physical education, statistics is a tool that can be of great value in teaching. To the prospective coach a knowledge of statistics is the key that unlocks a great percentage of the current research information dealing with new and improved coaching methods. As a citizen one is constantly exposed to statistics in the form of polls, costs of living, advertising, and so on. Much of what is seen on television is determined, at least in part, by statistical methods. The consumer is informed of "statistically significant improvements" which "prove" that product X is better than product Y. Thus a knowledge of statistics, its procedures and meaning, enables the individual to function more intelligently in many phases of his professional and non-professional life. The reader should now be aware, if he was not previously, that statistical knowledge is vital not only for those who are preparing for a career in research, but also for all of us who meet statistics and therefore are obligated personally and professionally to be able to deal with them.

UNDERSTANDING STATISTICS

Unfortunately many students approach a discussion of statistical methods with much fear and misunderstanding. The fear is based on the presumption that statistics is a subject so difficult to master that anyone who is not a fine mathematician has little chance for success. This misunderstanding is based on the presumption that statistics is a series of abstractions having no realistic basis and therefore is especially difficult to cope with.

Both these premises are false, and the reader should not fall prey to the misapprehension engendered by them. In the first case the reader is correct in assuming that statistical methods are mathematically based and that statistical procedures and formulas are mathematically derived. However, the emphasis in this text is on the ability to apply and understand statistical methods, which does not necessarily presuppose mathematical sophistication. The mathematical processes that will be involved require only a basic understanding of arithmetic and elementary algebra. These processes are reviewed in Appendix B.

The presumption of total abstraction in statistics is also thoroughly unfounded. On the contrary, statistical methods are thoroughly and consistently logical and can be understood on an intuitive basis as well as on a procedural basis.

To master the statistical applications with which we will be dealing, the student will need an understanding of three basic elements. The first is basic mathematics, which we have already mentioned. The second is terminology. Statistics employs many terms that are commonly used. However, statistical terms have precise meanings and are to be used precisely. The student is cautioned against using a statistical term in a way that does not fit the limitations imposed upon it. Finally, symbolic notation is used in any discussion of statistical methods. These symbols might be thought of as a system of shorthand, which, when understood, provides directions concerning the involved procedures.

Unfortunately, statistical symbols are not always constant between texts, but in this presentation an attempt has been made to use notation which is correct, consistent, and most often used in statistics textbooks.

TYPES OF STATISTICS

In general, statistical methods enable us to perform two distinct functions. First, they enable us to describe the characteristics of a set of data in which we are interested. Statistical methods that perform this function are known as descriptive statistics. In this instance a statistic is used to precisely define the point or points about which a distribution of scores centers and the way in which the scores within the distribution vary. Any given set of measures or values of the same thing is known as a distribution. Descriptive statistics concern a group that is of interest and measures drawn from that group. This group may be either a population, which would mean that measures are taken from all members of a group in which there is an interest, or a sample, which would mean that our measures are taken from a subset of a larger group in which there is an interest. The term population in a statistical sense need not imply some vast group, although it often might. For example, the population from which measures are drawn might be a class in gymnastics. If this class contains forty students, this is the population of interest to us. In using descriptive statistics, no attempt is made to extend our conclusions or descriptions beyond the limits of this group.

The second general class of statistics is known as inferential or sampling statistics. In this case there is also a population of interest, but one which is usually so large that it is not feasible to obtain measures from every member. Under these circumstances, a sample is drawn from the larger population, and data are collected only from the sample group. Proper use of inferential statistics allows us to use the data generated from the sample group to make inferences about the entire population. Research problems make extensive use of inferential statistics, since their purpose almost always is to be able to make statements about a total population. For example, our population of interest might be all boys competing in interscholastic wrestling at the high school level in a given state. However, due to considerations of time and money, one may have access to only a segment of that population, such as the high school wrestlers in a given school system.

Of great importance in inferential statistics is the way in which the sample is chosen. If we wish to know the average height and weight of high school wrestlers, we could not simply attend practice sessions at different schools and draw our data from the first 100 wrestlers we meet. There is a chance we would meet only heavyweights in this way, and, obviously, any inferences we would make from this sample would not be representative of all high school wrestlers in the state.

A quantitative characteristic of a population is known as a parameter of the population. A quantitative characteristic of a sample is known as a statistic of the sample. Because we are often unable to obtain data from every member of the population, we estimate the parameters of the population from the statistics of the sample on which we have data. We differentiate these values symbolically by using Greek letters to refer to parameters, and Roman letters to refer to statistics. The mean of a population is referred to as μ, whereas the mean of a sample is referred to as $\bar{X}$. The standard deviation of a population is referred to as σ, whereas the standard deviation of a sample is referred to as S.

It should be obvious to the reader that although the term "sampling" may be broadly used in many contexts, in the statistical sense this word assumes a precise meaning designating specific methods. These methods, which will be dealt with in a later chapter, obligate us to choose our sample in a logical and orderly fashion and enable us to choose a representative sample of the individuals in our population of interest.

USES OF STATISTICS

A common complaint hurled against statistical methods is that they can be used to prove anything. Although it is true that individuals may disguise data or use statistical tricks to make their data show what they want, it should be understood that no statistical method is designed to prove any statement true or false. A proof is a statement of absolute fact and admits of no exception. Statistical methods, by their very organization, are unable to "prove" anything. Statistical methods allow the user to make descriptions, draw inferences, and reject or accept hypotheses within certain limits of confidence. Inherent in statistical methods is the assumption that chance occurrences do happen and must be considered in the process of decision making. Thus a statistical procedure may allow the user to state that training procedure A produces results which are different from those of training procedure B, but he clearly admits to the possibility of having drawn incorrect conclusions because his results may simply be due to chance or error. This admission of possible error demonstrates that absolute proof is not a proper objective in the use of statistical methods.

Let us consider as an example a study in which an investigator is interested in determining if isometric or isotonic training is more effective in increasing the contractile strength of the biceps muscle of the upper arm. The investigator selects twenty subjects for each training method. Group A is trained by isometric methods for a twelve-week experimental period, and group B is trained by isotonic methods for the same period. At the beginning of the experimental period each of the forty subjects is tested for contractile strength of the biceps, using a strain gauge recorder at the same angle of pull. At the end of the experimental period the same testing procedure is used again on each subject. The average strength gain for each of the subjects in group A is then determined as is the average strength gain for each of the subjects in group B. These two averages (means) are then compared.

The problem the investigator now faces is in deciding if these averages are sufficiently different to be considered "real" or "significant," or whether they differ only to the extent that might be expected due to chance occurrences in the selection of his sample or to error in the testing method. The investigator's decision is recorded as "significant differences" or "nonsignificant differences" and is made on the basis of applying the appropriate statistical test to the data. However, the reader should note that such a statistical decision-making process, based on available data, is far from absolute proof that one training method is more effective than another. The reader will find statistical methods more meaningful and understandable if he thinks of them as tools to be used in the decision-making process rather than as definitive methods of proving one course of action superior to another.

If, in the example just discussed, the investigator reports "group B showed a significantly greater average increase in contractile strength of the biceps than group A," he also reports how certain he is that he has made the correct decision. If he reports a 5% level of confidence, he is essentially stating that a 5% risk exists that his decision has been wrong. In other words, the difference between the average of group A and the average of group B is large enough for the investigator to believe that such a difference would probably not arise due to chance but would be more likely to arise as a result of the different training methods used by the two groups. However, the investigator also understands and states the possibility of such a large difference having arisen due to chance or error rather than to differences in training methods. The reader may assume that the investigator is "hedging his bet," but he is simply making a statistical decision rather than attempting to prove one method of training is more effective than another. This is the essential nature and role of statistical methods.

We have considered the use of statistical methods in the process of research, where its importance is obvious. The reader probably is, and should be, concerned with the use of statistical methods even if he is not interested in research. Why bother to learn the methodology and language of statistics if you are interested in teaching physical education classes or coaching?

There are two basic reasons for the teacher and/or coach to be statistically literate. The first reason is that research, whether conducted in a laboratory, a classroom, a swimming pool, or a gymnasium, can be meaningful only if it is reported, read, interpreted, and acted upon. This means that the basic impact of research findings depends as much upon the consumer of research (the reader) as upon the researcher himself. The student must rid himself of the antiquated notion that research is done in an ivory-tower atmosphere by people who are unaware of the real world around them. Most researchers in the area of physical education are people who want to know what happens when circumstances are arranged in a certain way, and why. Their interests may concern physiological, psychological, sociological, historical, or educational methods. The basic questions they ask are the same basic questions any good teacher asks: "How can I be most effective in my teaching?" "How can I insure that my students will derive the maximum benefits from their exposure to me?" "How can I be sure that I am doing the best possible job?" The answers to these questions can be answered only through research and the ability to quantify and analyze data. Therefore, for a teacher to be effective and dynamic he has a distinct obligation to become a consumer of research. This is no less true in physical education than in any other academic area. In this partnership the researcher's obligation is to question, experiment, and report. The teacher's obligation is to read, interpret, and act. Both partners must obviously have the proper tools to fulfill their obligations. Statistical literacy is one of the most important of these tools.

The second reason statistical literacy is essential to the classroom teacher is that it can further enhance his teaching abilities. The ability to analyze data generated by one's classes in a given semester or over a period of years is an obvious advantage to the classroom teacher as an example, this ability enables the teacher to derive norms that are applicable to his students because they are based on data from the same kinds of students. The teacher can make comparisons between different kinds of tests and be more confident and effective in explaining the results of these tests to his students. He can do a more effective job of helping students in choosing appropriate activities if he has more data on which to base his conclusions. He can be more objective in choosing appropriate tests and can have more options available to him in grading, which is obviously beneficial. These examples illustrate that a knowledge of statistical methods provides the teacher with added flexibility, which is to his advantage. This added flexibility can also help to make the teaching process more exciting and dynamic for the teacher as well as for his students.

●　●　●

In conclusion we might examine statistical methods from a more philosophical point of view. While the ability to handle quantities of data has been stressed, we must not forget the perspective from which we deal with data. Many situations exist that cannot be easily quantified. Some situations cannot be quantified at all. How, for instance, do we measure a boy's determination to learn a stunt on the trampoline or to earn a place on the swimming team? The obvious answer is that we cannot. Yet we know that desire enters into any situation in which learning takes place. In many cases we rely heavily on quantitative data to help us make decisions; in other cases we cannot. The teacher who is adept at the use of statistical methods and relies exclusively upon them for all of his decision making will be as poor a teacher as his colleague who totally dismisses them and who relies exclusively upon his subjective feelings about a situation. Data analysis, experience awareness, and teaching methodology are all part of the total skill that a teacher brings to a given teaching situation. It is foolish to either entirely depend upon or entirely dismiss statistical procedures in the teaching situation. They are tools to be used when appropriate. The better teacher has the better tools.

Problems

1. Discuss the accuracy of the predictions made about the outcome of the last presidential election and the kinds of statistics used in making these predictions.
2. Find examples of "statistics" used in advertising.
3. Read some articles in the *Research Quarterly* that report significant differences between treatment groups.
4. List some government agencies that make extensive use of statistics, and explain how these statistics are obtained.
5. What kinds of statistics are used by pollsters such as Gallup and Harris?
6. How does the television industry make extensive use of statistical procedures?
7. Discuss how your admission to college was affected by statistical procedures.
8. Discuss the various kinds of statistical procedures that are used in sports situations.
9. Find examples of statistics in such magazines as *Time, Newsweek, U. S. News & World Report, Fortune, Life,* and *Look.*
10. Read and report on *How to Lie With Statistics* by Darryl Huff.

Chapter **2**

Collecting and presenting data

DISCRETE AND CONTINUOUS SCORES

In our materially oriented society there is a pronounced effort to quantify whenever possible. In the province of the physical educator this is certainly possible. The items with which we deal, such as height, weight, push-ups, running times, and test scores, all lend themselves to quantification. Scores may be classified as either discrete or continuous. This classification depends upon the procedure used in generating the scores. *Discrete scores* are those counted in whole units. If the intramural department wishes to know how many students use the tennis courts on a given week-end, the procedure is simply to count the number of students. Obviously this score is exact and is determined by counting in whole units.

Continuous scores are those that, at least theoretically, are capable of any degree of subdivision. If we wish to measure a student's height, the procedure is to measure, using a ruler of some type. A height of 70 inches may represent any height between 69.5 and 70.4 inches. If our measuring instrument is sufficiently accurate, we may determine the student's height to be 70.31 inches. However, even this is only an approximation that represents any height between 70.305 and 70.314 inches. Thus, in summary, we may state that a procedure of counting will yield discrete scores, whereas a procedure of measuring on some scale will yield continuous scores.

SCALES OF MEASUREMENT

It is also possible to classify the type of scale used for a particular measurement. The four types are nominal, ordinal, interval, and ratio scales.

A *nominal* (category) scale is one that contains mutually exclusive categories. A nominal scale may contain as few as two categories (e.g., male or female), or it may contain many categories (e.g., position played on a football team). In the latter case we would be dealing with an eleven-category nominal scale. The term "mutually exclusive" precludes the possibility of an individual being placed in more than one category. A nominal scale should also be complete in that it includes all possible categories of a particular type. Other examples of data that might be measured on a nominal scale are the choice of a path taken through an experimental maze by a rat or the college that a student attends. The reader should note that the categories in a nominal scale are not used to differentiate in a quantitative sense. Inclusion in one category is not better than, worse than, larger than, or smaller than inclusion in another category; it is simply different.

An _ordinal_ (rank) scale is used when we wish to provide some information about the order or rank of a set of objects in regard to some specific characteristic. For example, we might have the members of a class line up in order of height. We are now dealing with height as an ordinal scale. The order of finish in a race or the standing of teams in a tournament are other examples of ordinal scales. Note that the use of an ordinal scale does not allow any statements more precise than those concerned with rank. In the example of height we can state that the first boy in line is taller than the second, that the second boy is taller than the third, and so on. However, we have no way of determining how much taller the first boy is than the second or how much taller the second boy is than the third. In addition, we cannot make any determination of the relative differences from rank to rank. In the example of tournament standing the difference between teams 1 and 2 is not related to the difference between teams 2 and 3.

An _interval_ scale is one that has equal units of measurement. In this case we can state not only that A is larger than B, but also we can state how much larger. For example, if we measure the I.Q.'s of a class of students, we can specifically state how much higher one score is than another. The distance from a score of 50 to a score of 100 is precisely the same as the distance from a score of 100 to a score of 150. Another example of an interval scale might be temperature as measured by either a Fahrenheit or centigrade scale. The use of an interval scale does not allow statements as to the proportionate value of scores. For example, a temperature of 80° F. is not exactly twice as hot as a temperature of 40° F. Likewise, a boy with an I.Q. of 160 is not exactly twice as smart as a boy with an I.Q. of 80.

A _ratio_ scale possesses all the characteristics of an interval scale and also has an absolute zero point. This allows the kind of proportional comparisons that cannot be made with any other kind of measurement scale. For example, if we measure the height of children in a class with some type of ruler, we are dealing with a scale that possesses some absolute zero point. There is such a thing as zero in height even though the value zero itself is not approached in any actual measurement. Thus a boy who is 78 inches tall is precisely twice as tall as his younger brother who is only 39 inches tall. Temperature can also be measured on a ratio scale using the Kelvin or absolute scale. Absolute zero in this scale is the point at which all kinetic motion ceases. On this scale a temperature of 80° represents twice as much kinetic motion or heat as a temperature of 40°. The vast majority of ratio measures are those that involve time and distance.

FREQUENCY DISTRIBUTIONS

Many times, because of large numbers of scores, it is quite difficult to work with data unless they are arranged in a more convenient form. A frequency distribution, or frequency table, is a means of summarizing or grouping data. A group of raw scores, such as 2-3-7-6-4-5-2-8-6-7-1-5-1-4-6-3-8-4-2-5-3-5-6-10-7-3-9-4-0-4-8-6-7-5-5-9, could be represented in the frequency distribution shown in Table 2-1.

Table 2-1

Score	Frequency (f)
10	1
9	2
8	3
7	4
6	5
5	6
4	5
3	4
2	3
1	2
0	1
	36 = N

A frequency distribution is simply a table that presents raw scores and the frequencies with which each raw score occurs. The sum of the numbers in the f column is the total number of raw scores and is symbolized as N. In Table 2-1 the scores range only from 0 to 10, and there is no reason not to use each of the scores in the first column. However, in many instances the range of scores from highest to lowest will be so large that using each score in the range will make the table cumbersome to work with. Also, there may be large gaps in the range where no scores occur, and it is again inconvenient to use each score. In such cases it is more convenient to represent scores within intervals or groups rather than individually.

Choosing a step interval for a frequency distribution

In choosing a step interval for use in a frequency distribution it must be understood that using grouped data is a less accurate means of computation than using the individual raw scores. However, the resulting ease of operation is justifiable if the step interval is chosen carefully so that no great loss of accuracy is suffered.

In general, if the size of the interval (symbolized as i) is approximately equal to one fourth the standard deviation, less than 1% of the meaning of the data will be lost. Also, as the number of cases (N) increases, the range (R) of the data will also increase. The terms "standard deviation" and "range" will both be discussed in detail in later chapters. For random samples chosen from normal populations, Table 2-2 indicates approximate values of the range divided by the standard deviation, where range $= R =$ (high score $-$ low score) $+ 1$ and standard deviation $=$ Greek letter σ (sigma).

In determining i, i should $= \frac{1}{4}\sigma$, or $\sigma = 4i$. This is based on the previous statement that if i is approximately equal to one fourth the standard deviation, less than 1% of the meaning of the data will be lost.

Table 2-2

N	R/σ
100	5.00
200	5.50
300	5.75
400	5.95
500	6.00

Example: Given a distribution of 200 scores with a high score of 267 and a low score of 158, what size interval should be used in setting up a frequency distribution?

Step 1. Find the range.

$$R = (\text{high-low}) + 1$$
$$R = (267 - 158) + 1$$
$$R = 109 + 1 = 110$$

Step 2. For a distribution of $N = 200$, the value of R/σ is approximately 5.5 (from Table 2-2). Therefore:

$$R/\sigma = 5.5$$

Step 3. Substituting 110 for R and $4i$ for σ:

$$\frac{110}{4i} = 5.5$$

$$22i = 110$$

$$i = 5 \text{ (the size of the interval)}$$

Table 2-3

Interval	f	X
265-269	3	267
260-264	5	262
255-259	5	257
250-254	6	252
245-249	7	247
240-244	9	242
235-239	9	237
230-234	10	232
225-229	12	227
220-224	14	222
215-219	14	217
210-214	12	212
205-209	14	207
200-204	14	202
195-199	12	197
190-194	10	192
185-189	9	187
180-184	9	182
175-179	7	177
170-174	6	172
165-169	5	167
160-164	5	162
155-159	3	157
	200 = N	

Table 2-4. Weights of seventh-grade boys

Interval	Midpoint	Frequency	Cumulative frequency
129-131	130	2	100
126-128	127	3	98
123-125	124	3	95
120-122	121	4	92
117-119	118	2	88
114-116	115	4	86
111-113	112	10	82
108-110	109	10	72
105-107	106	14	62
102-104	103	9	48
99-101	100	8	39
96-98	97	4	31
93-95	94	5	27
90-92	91	5	22
87-89	88	5	17
84-86	85	4	12
81-83	82	4	8
78-80	79	3	4
75-77	76	1	1

The resulting frequency distribution is shown in Table 2-3. Note that each interval contains five scores, that there is no gap in the table so that each score between the low of 158 and the high of 267 can be represented in the table, and that the bottom score in the lowest interval (155) is a multiple of the interval used. Table 2-3 represents a complete group frequency distribution in which each interval may be represented by a single score, which is the midpoint of that interval. The individual score representing each interval is symbolically represented by the capital letter X.

The reader should now note that Table 2-4 also represents a frequency distribution. In this case the interval used is 3. Also notice that all the scores in each of the intervals are represented by a single score, which is the midpoint of that interval. For example, in Table 2-4 all the scores in the interval 114-116 are represented by a score of 115. The midpoint is chosen as the single most representative score in an interval.

GRAPHIC PRESENTATION

Data are often presented in picture or graphic form. This is valuable because it enables the reader to easily determine a distribution without the necessity of reading through all the raw data. There are many different types of graphs, but we will consider only a few that are commonly used to present physical education data.

Let us graph the data in Table 2-4, which represents the weight, in pounds, of 100 seventh-grade boys (Fig. 2-1). This particular type of bar graph, known as a histogram, uses vertically drawn bars. As in most other types of graphs, the abscissa (X or horizontal axis) is used to represent the scores, and the ordinate (Y or vertical axis) is used to represent the number

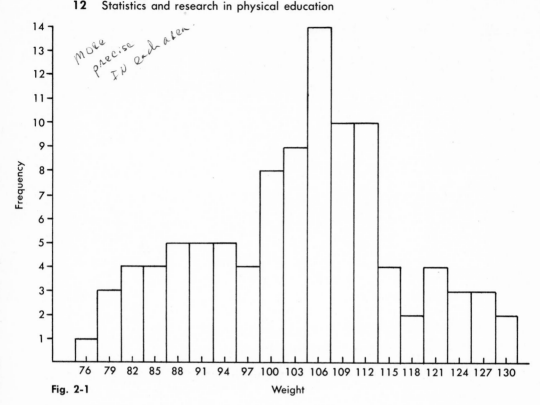

Fig. 2-1

of times each score occurs (frequency). Along the abscissa the midpoint of each interval is used to represent that interval. In essence, each bar will run from the lower limit (lowest score) of the interval to the upper limit (highest score) of that interval.

The reader can now see from the graph that the interval represented by a score of 106 occurs most frequently in the distribution of weights given in Table 2-4. It is easy to see how often the scores in each interval occur and thus gain an immediate understanding of the way the scores are distributed.

Another commonly used graph is a particular type of line graph known as a frequency polygon. The abscissa is again used to represent scores, and the ordinate is used to represent frequency. In this case the frequency in an interval is indicated by a point drawn above the midpoint of that interval. When all the successive points are drawn, they are connected by straight lines. The frequency polygon for the data in Table 2-4 is shown in Fig. 2-2.

A third type of graph presents information to the reader in terms of cumulative frequency up through each interval rather than in terms of the number of scores in each interval. This type of graph is known as an ogive and is shown in Fig. 2-3. The abscissa again represents scores, and the ordinate represents cumulative frequency.

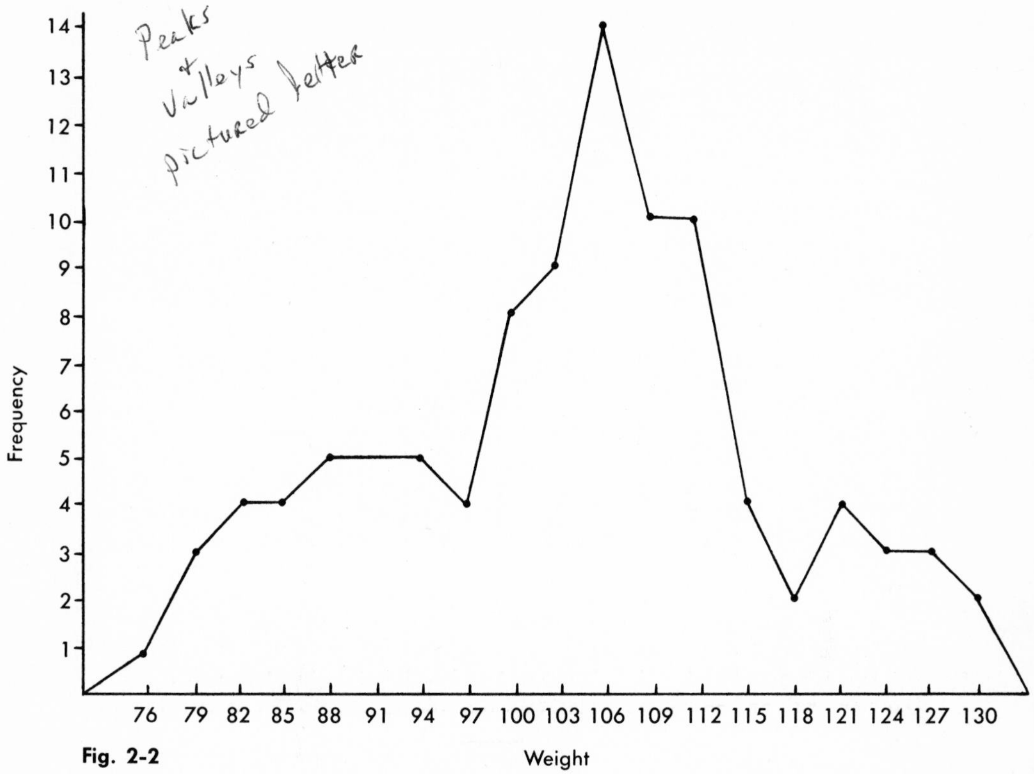
Peaks
&
Valleys
pictured better
Frequency
14
13
12
11
10
9
8
7
6
5
4
3
2
1
76 79 82 85 88 91 94 97 100 103 106 109 112 115 118 121 124 127 130
Weight

Fig. 2-2

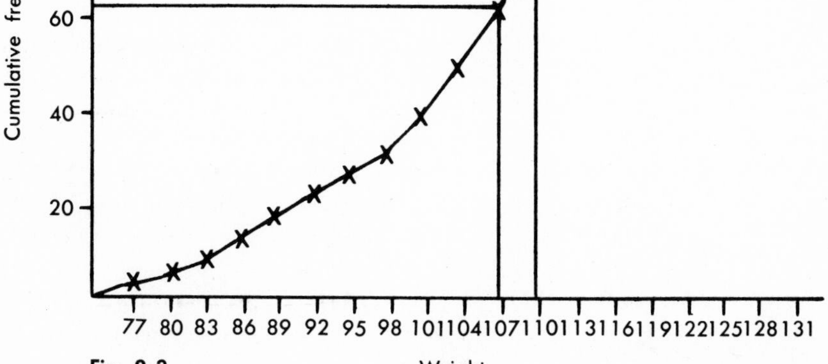
OGIVE.
Cumulative frequency
100
80
60
40
20
77 80 83 86 89 92 95 98 101104107110113116119122125128131
Weight

Fig. 2-3

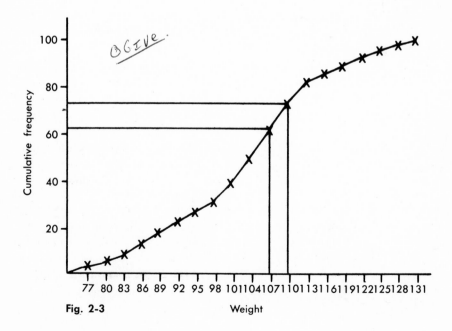

It may be noted that the frequency within any interval may be determined from an ogive merely by subtracting the cumulative frequencies in successive intervals. For example, the cumulative frequency through 107 is 62, and the cumulative frequency through 110 is 72. Therefore the interval 108-110 contains ten scores. Also notice that the abscissa is labeled with the upper limit of each interval rather than with the midpoint, since the purpose of an ogive is to show how many scores there are up to and including the upper limit of each interval.

Problems

1. Name five continuous variables and five discrete variables that a teacher of physical education might encounter in his work.
2. The number of push-ups thirty students in a class do are 19, 20, 26, 21, 20, 12, 17, 8, 11, 16, 13, 17, 21, 21, 4, 14, 20, 11, 17, 13, 11, 18, 36, 20, 18, 6, 21, 22, 23, 24. Construct a grouped frequency distribution for these scores and draw a histogram and frequency polygon from the frequency distribution.
3. The weights of forty men on a football team are 183, 187, 212, 218, 206, 224, 163, 214, 200, 196, 174, 205, 218, 180, 172, 178, 194, 186, 206, 215, 221, 237, 236, 246, 196, 185, 167, 174, 180, 175, 213, 218, 226, 204, 206, 211, 197, 184, 174, 200. What size step interval should you use to construct a frequency distribution? Draw an ogive from the frequency distribution. histogram
4. Construct a frequency distribution, histogram, frequency polygon, and ogive for the following numbers: 18, 23, 16, 21, 20, 19, 17, 13, 14, 26, 23, 19, 18, 17, 16, 20, 22, 34, 28, 16, 22, 15, 19, 17, 17, 20, 21, 16, 13, 19, 22, 21, 23, 18, 20, 21, 21, 19, 20, 22.
5. Draw a histogram and frequency polygon for the data in problem 3.
6. Draw an ogive for the data in problem 2.
7. What size step interval would you use in constructing a frequency table for a distribution of 500 scores with a high score of 362 and a low score of 219?
8. Given a distribution of 100 scores with a high score of 87 and a low score of 28, what size step interval would you use to set up a frequency table?

Chapter **3**

Normal distribution and measures of central tendency

IMPORTANCE OF THE NORMAL DISTRIBUTION

Most of the statistical methods commonly used in both descriptive and inferential statistics are based upon the assumption that a distribution is normal. This is a common term in both statistical and everyday language, and it is well worth consideration at this point. The normal distribution is graphically represented by the normal curve shown in Fig. 3-1.

Essentially, the normal distribution is theoretical in that few distributions ever exactly fit all the requirements of normality. However, from a practical point of view, if the distribution is based on a sufficiently large number of scores, items of interest to the physical educator will constitute a distribution closely approximating the normal distribution. This may be precisely defined by a mathematical formula, but a knowledge of calculus is essential to its understanding and is therefore beyond the scope of this text.

MEASURES THAT FIT THE NORMAL CURVE

As mentioned previously, the types of data collected by the physical educator are generally assumed to fit the shape of the normal curve. This assumption is based on the central limit theorem, which states that if we draw a sufficiently great number of random samples, all of the same relative size, from an infinitely large population and compute the sum of each sample, the distribution formed by these sums will be normal. It should be noted that no assumption is made concerning the shape of the distribution from which the samples are drawn.

As an illustration, let us consider the number of push-ups that adult males are able to do. We would expect that this distribution would be normal for the following reasons. First, we might consider that the score on a push-up test is a measure of the strength of the extensors of the elbow joint (i.e., triceps and anconeus), but further consideration indicates that the score on a push-up test is really the sum of a number of factors. For example, the score may have been influenced by such factors as the type of surface on which the test was taken, the time of day, heredity, tempera-

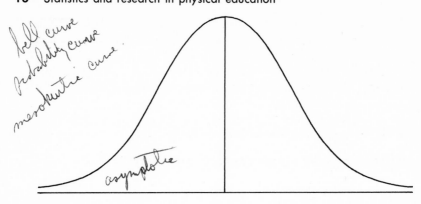

bell curve
probability curve
mesokurtic curve

asymptotic

Fig. 3-1

ture, altitude, familiarity with the test, rate at which the push-ups were done, interest, cross-sectional area of the involved muscles, amount of activity the day before, nutritional state, weight, present occupation, and psychological state.

Each of these factors contributes in some way to the number of push-ups an individual can do, and thus each individual's score is the sum of a definite number of factors. Let us arbitrarily say that there are forty factors which contribute to the score obtained on a push-up test. These forty factors contribute to every individual's score, although they may contribute differently in each case. Thus the number of push-ups done by different men is really the sum of a large number of equally sized samples. Therefore, according to the central limit theorem, it is to be expected that a distribution composed of scores on a push-up test will be normal.

CHARACTERISTICS OF THE NORMAL DISTRIBUTION

The normal distribution possesses certain characteristics that will define it sufficiently for our purposes.

1. The normal distribution can be represented by a bell-shaped curve as shown in Fig. 3-1.
2. The normal distribution curve remains unchanged regardless of the number of terms within that distribution.
3. The normal curve possesses absolute symmetry about the central (vertical) axis; that is, the same percentage of the distribution lies to the right of the vertical axis as to the left (i.e., 50%). Further, the same percentage of the distribution lies between the vertical axis and any distance to the right as between the vertical axis and the same distance to the left.
4. The greatest number of scores in a normal distribution will lie at the vertical axis, and there will be fewer and fewer terms as you move toward the ends of the distribution.
5. There is no upper or lower limit to the normal distribution. As terms move further and further from the vertical axis, they become more

and more rare. Beyond a certain distance from the vertical axis in either direction, the terms become so rare that they are usually ignored. However, the normal curve is drawn so that it is not brought completely down to the base line at either end. This graphically indicates that terms of any magnitude may theoretically exist.

6. All measures of central tendency (i.e., mean, median, and mode) lie at the same point, which is indicated by the vertical axis. These measures are treated fully in the following discussion.

7. See Below

IMPORTANCE OF MEASURES OF CENTRAL TENDENCY

Since the physical educator will generally be concerned with measures that tend to be normal in their distribution, these distributions will have a strong tendency to cluster about the center. Therefore the first descriptive statistics with which we shall be concerned are those which provide information about how a distribution is centered and which are called measures of central tendency. These include the mean, median, and mode.

The mean

The most commonly used measure of central tendency is the mean, which is simply the arithmetic average of a distribution of scores. The mean is the most sensitive measure of central tendency. This sensitivity is both its greatest strength and greatest weakness. On the positive side, the mean will respond to changes in the magnitude of scores in a distribution and will thus always reflect any change within a distribution of scores. On the negative side, if one score in a distribution is highly deviant in either direction, the mean will be pulled greatly in that direction and may give an unfair picture of that distribution. For example, if we have a bowling team that scores 125, 127, 136, 128, and 124, respectively, their team average is 128, which gives us a fair picture of the way the team scores cluster. However, if the next week the scores are 116, 109, 103, 107, and 300, the team average is 147. Obviously the average score is higher than all but one of the individual scores and does not truly reflect the bowling ability of the five team members. One highly deviant score (i.e., 300) pulled the team average very far in its direction.

For computational purposes we shall discuss two formulas for the mean. The first formula is for ungrouped data that is not in a frequency distribution. The following are the basic symbols we will use:

$\bar{X}$ = the mean of a distribution of scores
Σ (Greek capital Sigma) = "the sum of"
X = each of the individual scores in a distribution
N = the number of scores in a distribution

Therefore:

$$\bar{X} = \frac{\Sigma X}{N}$$

states that the mean of a distribution of scores is equal to the sum of the individual scores divided by the number of scores in that distribution.

7. St. Dev. is approx $\frac{1}{6}$ of the range.

Thus, in finding the mean for ungrouped data we simply add up all the individual scores and divide that sum by the number of scores we have.

The formula for grouped data in a frequency distribution is

$$\bar{X} = \frac{\Sigma fX}{N}$$

which states that the mean of a distribution of scores is equal to the sum of the products of the midpoint of each interval and the frequency in that interval, divided by the number of scores in the distribution.

Example: Find the mean of the following grouped data.

Interval	f
24-26	3
21-23	4
18-20	7
15-17	9
12-14	7
9-11	4
6-8	3

We first represent each interval by a single number, which will be the midpoint of that interval and which we call X. The resulting frequency distribution and the solution for the mean are as follows:

Interval	f	X	fX
24-26	3	25	75
21-23	4	22	88
18-20	7	19	133
15-17	9	16	144
12-14	7	13	91
9-11	4	10	40
6-8	3	7	21
	37 = N		592

$$\bar{X} = \frac{\Sigma fX}{N}$$

$$\bar{X} = \frac{592}{37}$$

$$\bar{X} = 16$$

It is worth noting at this point that it is possible to subject one set of data to these two methods of determining the mean and to get two answers that are not precisely the same. For example, the following distribution: 15, 15, 14, 13, 13, 11, 11, 11, 10, 9, 9, 9, 9, 8, 7, 5, 5, 3, 3, 1.

1. Ungrouped:

$$\Sigma X = 181 \qquad N = 20$$

$$\bar{X} = \frac{\Sigma X}{N}$$

$$\bar{X} = \frac{181}{20}$$

$$\bar{X} = 9.05$$

2. Grouped:

Interval	f	X	fX
14-15	3	14.5	43.5
12-13	2	12.5	25.0
10-11	4	10.5	42.0
8-9	5	8.5	42.5
6-7	1	6.5	6.5
4-5	2	4.5	9.0
2-3	2	2.5	5.0
0-1	1	0.5	0.5
	20		174.0

$$\bar{X} = \frac{\Sigma fX}{N}$$

$$\bar{X} = \frac{174.0}{20}$$

$$\bar{X} = 8.70$$

The reason for this discrepancy is that when data are put into a frequency distribution, it is assumed that the scores within any given interval are distributed normally. This assumption allows us to represent an interval by the midpoint (i.e., the mean). However, in some cases this will not be true. The five scores in the interval 8-9 are represented by a single score of 8.5. Going back to the original distribution, we can see that there are four scores of 9 and one score of 8. The mean of these scores is really 8.8, not 8.5. In most cases such discrepancies within given intervals balance out over the whole distribution, but, as we have seen, this is not always true. In essence, the "true" mean is given by the ungrouped method.

The median

The median is another measure of central tendency and is defined as that point in a distribution of scores above and below which 50% of the measurements lie. The median has two primary advantages. First, the value of the median is not affected by extreme scores and therefore is a more representative measure of central tendency than is the mean in distributions containing extreme values. Second, the median is basically a measure of position and is affected primarily by the number of scores in a distribution rather than by the size of the scores. Thus the median is an applicable statistic for truncated distributions (i.e., those cut off at one end). For example, if we were to record the weights of adult males in a given state, we might find ten men who weigh 300 pounds and over. We would not be able to find the mean for this distribution without knowing each of these ten weights, but we could find the median.

To calculate the median for ungrouped data, simply arrange the scores according to magnitude. If the distribution has an odd number of scores, the median is the middle value. For example, in a distribution of thirty-five scores the median is the eighteenth score from the bottom or the top when the scores are arranged according to magnitude (i.e., seventeen scores on either side). If the distribution has an even number of scores, the median is the arithmetic mean of the two middle scores. For example, in a distribution of twenty-eight scores the median is the mean of the fourteenth and fifteenth score from the bottom or the top according to magnitude (i.e., fourteen and one-half scores on either side).

To calculate the median for grouped data we make use of a simple formula

$$Mdn = L + \left(\frac{\frac{N}{2} - \Sigma f_b}{fw} \right) i$$

where Mdn = the median, L = the lower limit of the interval containing the median, Σfb = the sum of the frequencies below the interval containing the median, fw = the frequency within the interval containing the median, and i = the size interval.

Example: Find the median of the following grouped data.

Interval	f		Interval	f	
85-89	2	50	65-69	8	24
80-84	5	48	60-64	8	16
75-79	9	43	55-59	7	8
70-74	10	34	50-54	1	1

Summing the f column we find that there are fifty scores in this distribution. We therefore must find the twenty-fifth and twenty-sixth scores from the botton, the mean of which will be the median. Addition of the frequencies in each interval, starting at the bottom interval, indicates that there are twenty-four scores up to and including the interval 65-69. Since there are eleven scores in the interval 70-74, we know that the twenty-fifth and twenty-sixth scores (i.e., the median) lie in this interval. This observation is necessary to locate the interval containing the median. Once this interval is located, we can easily find the median using the formula just given.

$$Mdn = L + \left(\frac{\frac{N}{2} - \Sigma f_b}{fw} \right) i$$

$$Mdn = 69.5 + \left(\frac{\frac{50}{2} - 24}{10} \right) 5$$

$$Mdn = 69.5 + .5$$

$$Mdn = 70$$

The student should note that the lower limit of the interval 70-74 is 69.5. Any score between the values of 69.5 and 74.4 would fall in this interval. Generally the lower limit is expressed in one decimal place more than the interval itself is written.

The mode

The mode is simply defined as that score in a distribution which occurs most frequently. This is determined by observation for both grouped and ungrouped data. For grouped data the midpoint of the interval with the greatest frequency is the mode. The mode is the least often used measure of central tendency. The student should also be aware that it is possible for a distribution to have no mode or more than one mode. The mode would be a good statistic to use if you were a football coach who had to order helmets for next season's team. The mean and median might be misleading, but if you knew the size helmet most frequently worn, you would have valuable information for your purposes.

POSITION OF THE MEAN, MEDIAN, AND MODE IN DISTRIBUTIONS

As mentioned previously, the mean, median, and mode will all fall at the same point in a normal distribution, as shown in Fig. 3-2.

However, not every distribution will be normal. A curve that lacks symmetry with respect to its vertical axis is called a skewed curve. A distribution may be skewed positively (to the right) or negatively (to the left). The direction of skewness is toward the side of the curve having the longer tail. The distribution in Fig. 3-3 is positively skewed.

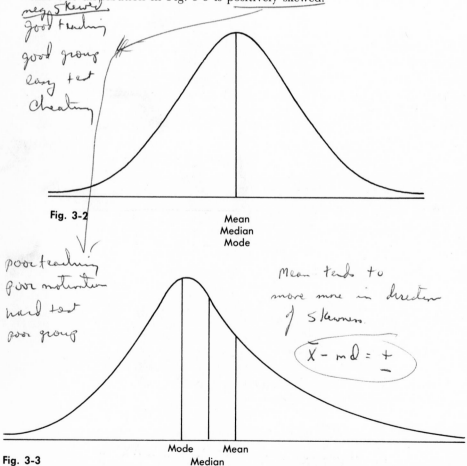

nego skewed
good teaching
good group
easy test
Cheating

Fig. 3-2

Mean
Median
Mode

poor teaching
poor motivation
hard test
poor group

Mean tends to move more in direction of skewness.

$X - md = +$ / $-$

Fig. 3-3

Mode   Mean
Median

Since there are still more scores occurring at the point indicated by the highest point on the curve, the mode remains at that point. The median and the mean both move in the direction of skewness as shown above, and the mean moves further in the direction of skewness than the median. This occurs because the mean, as pointed out previously, is a more sensitive measure than the median.

Problems

1. Find the mean, median, and mode for each of the following distributions:
    a. 3, 6, 8, 17, 17, 11, 13, 10, 14, 10, 9, 7, 18, 23, 22, 21, 21, 11, 11, 19, 17
    b. 4, 8, 8, 9, 9, 9, 9, 9, 10, 11, 11, 12, 14
    c. 1, 2, 3, 4, 5
    d. 170, 170, 150, 155, 165, 160, 170, 175, 155, 160, 180, 180, 155, 170, 155, 170
    e. 1, 1, 1, 1, 1, 1, 3, 3, 3, 3, 3, 3, 5, 5, 5, 5, 5, 5, 7, 7, 7, 7, 7, 7, 9, 9, 9, 9, 9, 9, 9
    f. 13, 15, 17, 16, 17, 14, 12, 13, 18, 16, 19, 20, 17, 16, 15, 14, 15, 12, 15, 11, 15
    g. 118, 176, 194, 158, 163, 176, 191, 147, 111, 203, 111, 111, 197, 153, 164
    h. 36, 36, 36, 37, 38, 39, 39, 40, 40, 41, 45, 45, 48, 51, 51, 57, 58, 64, 64, 66
    i. 74, 71, 73, 70, 71, 72, 75, 76, 74, 73, 72, 79, 77, 75, 73, 74, 76, 77, 71, 73, 70
    j. 3, 67, 19, 42, 36, 78, 45, 19, 11, 39, 84, 80, 71, 65, 54, 90, 93, 17, 47, 55

2. Find the mean, median, and mode for each of the following frequency distributions:

a. Interval	f		b. Interval	f
30-32	3		117-125	6
27-29	4		108-116	8
24-26	17		99-107	10
21-23	19		90-98	7
18-20	4		81-89	4
15-17	3			

c. Interval	f		d. Interval	f
50-54	3		18-19	4
45-49	6		16-17	7
40-44	9		14-15	6
35-39	12		12-13	5
30-34	10		10-11	8
25-29	9		8-9	4
20-24	6		6-7	3
15-19	3		4-5	2
			2-3	3

Chapter **4**

Measures of variability

WHY MEASURE VARIABILITY?

In any distribution it is totally unrealistic to expect that every score will have the same value. Rather, within any given distribution, the scores will be spread out to some greater or lesser degree. If, in addition to being able to describe the central tendencies of a distribution, we were also able to describe the extent to which the scores are spread, we would have a great deal of meaningful information about the distribution. The statistics used to describe this spread are called measures of variability.

The importance of having a measure of variability can be demonstrated by referring to two distributions, each with a mean of 25. This measure places the arithmetic average of both distributions but gives us no further information as to the way these distributions compare. For example, let us suppose that each distribution contains five terms ($N=5$) and that they are as follows:

$$\text{Distribution A:} \quad 15, 19, 25, 27, 39 \qquad \bar{X}=25$$
$$\text{Distribution B:} \quad 7, 13, 18, 23, 64 \qquad \bar{X}=25$$

In this example it is obvious that the terms in distribution B are more spread apart than those in distribution A. We may therefore conclude that distribution B has greater variability than distribution A. However, it will not always be possible to compare the variability of distributions in such cursory fashion. Further, even though we can see that distribution B has greater variability than distribution A, we are not able to state how much greater the variability is. The measures of variability that we will consider, particularly the standard deviation, will enable us to make such statements in precise terms.

THE RANGE

The simplest measure of variability is the range. We have already discussed this in relation to choosing a step interval. Basically the range serves the function of telling us over how great an area our scores are spread. The range is rather limited in its usefulness since it gives us no information about how the scores are distributed within this given area. For example, the distribution 8, 15, 22, 31, 40, 45 has a range of 38. The distribution 26,

26, 27, 27, 28, 63 also has a range of 38. These two distributions certainly do not have the same degree of variability, yet this is not indicated by the range.

AVERAGE DEVIATION

The concept of deviations is one that is easily understood. Let us consider the mean as being representative of all the scores in a distribution. It is obvious that some terms will have a larger value than the mean, and other terms will have a smaller value. A deviation, then, is the distance a given score lies from the mean of its distribution. Those scores larger than the mean will deviate positively, and those scores smaller than the mean will deviate negatively. We will represent the deviation of a score by d. We may now mathematically define the deviation of a score as follows:

$$d = X - \bar{X}$$

which states that the deviation of any observed score is equal to that score minus the mean of the distribution from which that score was drawn.

Average deviation is simply the arithmetic average of the deviations of each score in a distribution. The distribution 2, 5, 5, 6, 6, 7, 8, 8, 9, 9, 12 has a mean of 7. These scores and their deviations can be tabled as in Table 4-1.

Table 4-1

X	d
12	5
9	2
9	2
8	1
8	1
7	0
6	-1
6	-1
5	-2
5	-2
2	-5

If we were to sum the deviations and divide by 11 (the number of scores), we would find the true average deviation is zero, since the sum of the deviations is zero. This will occur in any distribution, since the mean represents the arithmetic average, and the sum of the deviations from the mean will always be zero. Therefore the value for the true average deviation will always be zero and will be quite meaningless in giving us any information concerning the distribution. In practice, the deviations in a distribution are summed with no regard to sign and then divided by N. The value of a term with no regard to its sign is called its absolute value. The formula for average deviation may now be written:

$$A.D. = \frac{\Sigma |d|}{N}$$

where *A.D.* = average deviation, $\Sigma|d|$ = the sum of the absolute values of *d,* and *N* = the number of scores in the distribution. We may now find the average deviation for the data in Table 4-1 as follows:

$$A.D. = 22/11$$
$$A.D. = 2$$

The average deviation is a simple statistic to compute and gives us more information than the range, since it takes all the scores in a distribution into account. In addition, average deviation has other values for the beginning student of statistical methods.

First, it serves as a logical and simple introduction to the concept of deviation that should help the beginning student understand other measures of variability such as the standard deviation.

Second, we are now prepared to make statements about the spread of data when we compute average deviation. We may state that if a distribution is normal, the scores that fall between a value of the mean minus one average deviation and the value of the mean plus one average deviation will contain approximately 58% of the total distribution. For example, if we have a normal distribution of weights with a mean of 163 and an average deviation of 12, approximately 58% of the distribution will fall between the values of 151 and 175.

Finally, we may also use average deviation as a means of determining the accuracy of a measuring technique by the addition of one simple step—to find percent error. For example, suppose that you are using a pair of fat calipers to measure the amount of abdominal fat (in millimeters) of your high school students. Since the calipers are new and the technique is not one you are familiar with, you wish to determine your accuracy in taking these measures. Using one subject, you repeat the measure several times, determine the average deviation for the measures, and then divide the product of the average deviation and 100 by the mean of your measurements to determine percent error. Thus the formula for percent error is as follows:

$$\% \text{ error} = \frac{100 \ (A.D.)}{\bar{X}}$$

Assuming that the six measures of abdominal fat shown below had been taken on the same subject, the calculations are as follows:

X	d
9.8	−0.2
10.0	0.0
10.1	0.1
9.6	−0.4
10.5	0.5
10.0	0.0
$\Sigma X = 60.0$	$\Sigma|d| = 1.2$
$N = 6$	$N = 6$
$\bar{X} = 10.0$	$A.D. = .2$

also known as precision coefficient.

$$\% \text{ error} = \frac{100 \ (A.D.)}{\bar{X}}$$

$$\% \text{ error} = \frac{100 \ (.2)}{10}$$

$$\% \text{ error} = 2$$

Generally a technique that has a value of 3% or less for percent error is considered to have acceptable accuracy. Therefore the abdominal fat measurement discussed above is an acceptable technique.

STANDARD DEVIATION

Standard deviation is the most commonly used measure of variability. The Greek small letter sigma (σ) is used to indicate standard deviation when we are dealing with population values. Since we will generally deal with population samples rather than with whole populations, we will use S to denote sample standard deviation. It might be pointed out that variance is another common measure of variability and is simply the square of the standard deviation. The population variance is usually represented as σ^2, whereas the variance of a sample is S^2.

Once the basic concept of the deviation is understood, calculation of the standard deviation is quite simple. We shall introduce three formulas for the standard deviation. These formulas are equivalent, and the choice of formula depends upon the form of the data and the availability of a calculator. These formulas are as follows:

1. Where the data are ungrouped:

$$S = \sqrt{\frac{\Sigma d^2}{N-1}}$$

2. Where the data are grouped:

$$S = \left(\sqrt{\frac{\Sigma f d^2}{N-1}}\right)(i)$$

3. Where a calculator is available:

$$S = \sqrt{\frac{N\Sigma X^2 - (\Sigma X)^2}{N(N-1)}}$$

The student should notice that in the first two formulas the mean of the distribution must be determined before the value for the deviation of each term or interval can be found.

We will now take a distribution and compute the standard deviation each of three ways so that the procedure for each method will be understood and the equivalence of the formulas will be demonstrated. For our example let us choose a distribution of number of push-ups done in a physical education class of twenty-one boys. The scores obtained on the push-up test are 2, 4, 5, 7, 8, 8, 9, 9, 10, 10, 10, 10, 10, 11, 11, 12, 12, 13, 15, 16, 18.

6 std dev. include 99.9% of cases
(3 each way)

1. For ungrouped data:

X	d	d²
18	8	64
16	6	36
15	5	25
13	3	9
12	2	4
12	2	4
11	1	1
11	1	1
10	0	0
10	0	0
10	0	0
10	0	0
10	0	0
9	−1	1
9	−1	1
8	−2	4
8	−2	4
7	−3	9
5	−5	25
4	−6	36
2	−8	64

$\Sigma X = 210$
$N = 21$
$\bar{X} = 10$

$\Sigma d^2 = 288$

$$S = \sqrt{\dfrac{\Sigma x^2}{N} - \bar{X}^2}$$

$$S = \sqrt{\dfrac{\Sigma d^2}{N-1}}$$

$$S = \sqrt{\dfrac{288}{20}}$$

$$S = \sqrt{14.4}$$

$$S = 3.8$$

2. For grouped data:

= # of intervals away from mean

X	f	fX	d	d²	fd²
18	1	18	8	64	64
17	0	0	7	49	0
16	1	16	6	36	36
15	1	15	5	25	25
14	0	0	4	16	0
13	1	13	3	9	9
12	2	24	2	4	8
11	2	22	1	1	2
10	5	50	0	0	0
9	2	18	−1	1	2
8	2	16	−2	4	8
7	1	7	−3	9	9
6	0	0	−4	16	0
5	1	5	−5	25	25
4	1	4	−6	36	36
3	0	0	−7	49	0
2	1	2	−8	64	64

$N = 21$ $\Sigma fX = 210$
$\bar{X} = 10$

$\Sigma fd^2 = 288$

$$S = \sqrt{\dfrac{\Sigma fd^2}{N-1}}$$

$$S = \sqrt{\dfrac{288}{20}}$$

$$S = \sqrt{14.4}$$

$$S = 3.8$$

VARIANCE = S^2

3. With a calculator:

X	X²
18	324
16	256
15	225
13	169
12	144
12	144
11	121
11	121
10	100
10	100
10	100
10	100
10	100
9	81
9	81
8	64
8	64
7	49
5	25
4	16
2	4
ΣX = 210	ΣX² = 2,388

$$S = \sqrt{\frac{N\Sigma X^2 - (\Sigma X)^2}{N(N-1)}}$$

$$S = \sqrt{\frac{21(2,388) - (210)^2}{21(20)}}$$

$$S = \sqrt{\frac{50,148 - 44,100}{420}}$$

$$S = \sqrt{\frac{6,048}{420}}$$

$$S = \sqrt{14.4}$$

$$S = 3.8$$

The standard deviation in each of the examples just given has the same value, showing the equivalence of the formulas. The standard deviation gives us a quantitative measure of variability, which is easily computed in a number of ways, which increases as the variability of a distribution increases, which is not affected by the number of terms in a distribution, and which takes every term into account.

z SCORES

It is now possible to talk about the variability of a normal distribution of scores with great precision if we know the mean and standard deviation of that distribution. For any score in the distribution we may determine the corresponding z score, which is as follows:

$$z = \frac{X - \bar{X}}{S}$$

The z score corresponding to a particular score is that particular score minus the mean of the distribution, divided by the standard deviation of the distribution. For example, what is the z score corresponding to a score of 100 in a distribution with a mean of 80 and a standard deviation of 10?

Standard Scores are Raw Scores converted to a certain scale.

$$z = \frac{X - \bar{X}}{S}$$

$$z = \frac{100 - 80}{10}$$

$$z = 2$$

Range is generally ±3

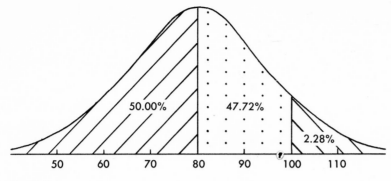

50.00%   47.72%   2.28%

50   60   70   80   90   100   110

Fig. 4-1

If we now look at Table C-4, Appendix C, we find that 47.72% of the total area of the normal curve lies between the mean and 2.00 standard deviations (i.e., between the mean and a score with a corresponding z score of 2.00). This is true for any normal distribution, regardless of the size of the terms or the number of terms. Since we know the normal curve is symmetrical about the vertical axis, we present only the right half of the curve. However, if a z score were -2.00, 47.72% of the normal curve would again fall between it and the mean, except that now it would be to the left of the mean. Remember also that 50% of the normal curve lies on either side of the mean. Thus we may picture our distribution with a mean of 80 and standard deviation of 10 as in Fig. 4-1.

Since a score of 100 has a z score of 2.00, it falls two standard deviations to the right of the mean. Also, half the distribution lies to the left of the mean and half the distribution lies to the right of the mean. Therefore 97.72% of the distribution (i.e., 47.72% + 50%) lies below (to the left of) a score of 100 (i.e., a z score of 2.00) and 2.28% of the distribution (i.e., 50.00% − 47.72%) lies above (to the right of) a score of 100.

The same procedure may be followed to determine what percentage of scores lies above or below any point in a normal distribution. We may also find the exact number of scores rather than percentage simply by multiplying the percentage by N. We may therefore use the same procedure and logic to determine the following:

1. Percentage of scores below any given score
2. Number of scores below any given score
3. Percentage of scores above any given score
4. Number of scores above any given score
5. Percentage of scores between any two scores
6. Number of scores between any two scores

Essentially we may think of z scores as a particular type of derived score taken from the original or raw scores. In this case the original distribution is transformed to a derived or second distribution in which the mean is zero and the standard deviation is 1. This allows us to compare scores from distributions with different means and standard deviations.

For example, suppose that Tom received a grade of 57 on a test with a mean of 50 and a standard deviation of 3.5 and John received a 100 on a test with a mean of 80 and a standard deviation of 20. Tom's z score is 2.00 and John's z score is 1.00. Therefore Tom did relatively better on his test than John did on his. In general, we may state that scores from tests with large standard deviations will have more effect on an average of test scores than will scores from tests with small standard deviations. Therefore it is sometimes fairer to mark on the basis of z scores than raw scores. The method a teacher uses in grading will depend on a large number of factors but most of all on his philosophy of teaching and grading.

Let us take the following case in which Tom and John have each taken the same five tests. Table 4-2 shows their raw scores, z scores, mean, and standard deviation for each of the tests and the average raw score points and z score points.

Table 4-2

Test	$\bar{X}$	S	Raw (John)	Raw (Tom)	z (John)	z (Tom)
1	50	3.5	50	57	0.00	+2.00
2	80	20	100	85	+1.00	+0.25
3	100	18	127	109	+1.50	+0.50
4	76	6	70	85	−1.00	+1.50
5	144	25	194	169	+2.00	+1.00
Average			108.2	101	0.70	1.05

Thus we see that John's average is higher in raw scores, but Tom's average is higher in z scores. John did his best on tests 2, 3, and 5, which had large standard deviations, and Tom did his best on tests 1 and 4, which had small standard deviations. To whom would you assign the higher grade? Why?

STANDARD ERROR OF THE MEAN

When dealing with sample statistics, we are often interested in estimating the parameters of the population from which the sample is drawn. Suppose that we are interested in the height of males over 21 years of age in the United States. It is obviously possible to draw many samples from this population and compute the mean and standard deviation for each sample. If we were to draw 1,000 samples, each containing fifty subjects, we would have 1,000 means and standard deviations. The distribution of these 1,000 means would be normal and is called a sampling distribution. The mean of these 1,000 means would be a good estimate of the population mean. However, it is obvious that there would be variability within this sampling distribution. This variability is measured by the standard error of the mean, which is simply the standard deviation of the distribution of means.

The standard error of the mean can be estimated from a single sample by

$$S_{\bar{x}} = \frac{S}{\sqrt{N-1}}$$

where $S_{\bar{x}}$ = standard error of the mean (estimated), S = standard deviation of a given sample, and N = number of subjects in the sample.

Let us assume that we have actually drawn one sample of fifty adult males and have found that the mean and standard deviation of this sample of height (in inches) are 70 and 10.5, respectively. If the sample has been properly drawn, this sample mean will be an unbiased estimate of the population mean. The standard error of the mean is estimated as follows:

$$S_{\bar{x}} = \frac{S}{\sqrt{N-1}}$$

$$S_{\bar{x}} = \frac{10.5}{\sqrt{50-1}}$$

$$S_{\bar{x}} = \frac{10.5}{\sqrt{49}}$$

$$S_{\bar{x}} = 1.5$$

Since the mean of our sample is one of many constituting a theoretically normal sampling distribution, and since our sample mean estimates the population mean, by knowing the estimated standard error of the mean (i.e., the standard deviation of the sampling distribution), we may now use this information just as in the case of z scores. With a sample mean of 70 and standard error of the mean of 1.5, we would expect that the scores between the mean minus one standard error and the mean plus one standard error should encompass 68.26% of the sampling distribution of means. Another way of saying this is that we would expect 68.26% of the sample means in our sampling distribution to be between the mean minus one standard error and the mean plus one standard error (i.e., between 68.5 and 71.5).

PERCENTILES

Percentiles are commonly used to describe the position of a score in a distribution. Their most common and most valuable use lies in the construction of norms that may be used in evaluating performance. Is a bowling average of 120 for a term of bowling good, bad, or average? How do you rate a score of 10 chin-ups or 120 pounds on a grip strength test? Obviously these scores are impossible to evaluate without some basis for comparison. The construction and use of percentile tables allows such comparisons to be made. The percentile rank of a score may be defined as the percent of the total distribution falling below that score. Thus a score with a percentile rank of 80 (P_{80}) is one in which 80% of the distribution falls below that score and 20% of the distribution falls above that score. A percentile table gives the teacher much information about evaluating performance. For example, we might note that for college freshmen a score of 120 pounds on a grip-strength test falls at the 55th percentile. We then know that our student scored better than 55% of the group used to construct the table.

Computation of percentiles is a simple procedure and one that we have actually done already in a different form. The basic formula is the median formula, which is adapted as follows:

$$P_X = L + \left(\frac{\frac{X\,(N)}{100} - \Sigma fb}{fw} \right) i$$

where P_X = the particular percentile score desired, L = the lower limit of the interval containing the percentile score, X = the percentile, N = the number of terms in the distribution, Σfb = the total frequency below the interval containing the percentile score, fw = the frequency within the interval containing the percentile score, and i = the size interval.

Note that the interval containing the percentile score is determined by inspection as in the case of the median. For example, if we wished to find P_{90} in a distribution of forty scores, we would need to locate the interval containing the thirty-sixth score from the bottom.

Example: Given the following frequency distribution, find P_{60}.

Interval	f	Interval	f
33-35	3	21-23	8
30-32	4	18-20	6
27-29	5	15-17	5
24-26	6	12-14	3
			40 = N

Step 1. Locate the interval containing the desired percentile score. Since $N = 40$, we wish to locate the interval containing the twenty-fourth score from the bottom of the distribution. This would be the interval 24-26.

Step 2. Substitute the appropriate values in the formula just given:

$$P_X = L + \left(\frac{\frac{X\,(N)}{100} - \Sigma fb}{fw} \right) i$$

$$P_{60} = 23.5 + \left(\frac{\frac{60(40)}{100} - 22}{6} \right) 3$$

$$P_{60} = 23.5 + \left(\frac{2}{6} \right) 3$$

$$P_{60} = 23.5 + 1$$

$$P_{60} = 24.5$$

The major drawback of percentile tables is that they tend to exaggerate differences in the center of the distribution as opposed to the ends. A look at Table 4-3 will illustrate this point. Bent-knee sit-ups were scored for 152 male college freshmen and the results are presented in percentile form. Note that from P_{25} to P_{15} the differences between succeeding percentiles is 2 or 3 units. However, as the ends of the percentile table are approached, the differences increase to 4, 5, 6, and 7 units between succeeding percentiles. This is the form usually taken by percentile tables.

Table 4-3*

Percentile	Bent-knee sit-ups
100	81
95	75
90	68
85	63
80	58
75	54
70	51
65	48
60	45
55	43
50	40
45	38
40	36
35	33
30	30
25	27
20	23
15	18
10	13
5	6
0	0

*From Van Huss, Wayne D., et al.: Physical activity in modern living, Englewood Cliffs, N. J., 1960, Prentice-Hall, Inc., p. 95; by permission of the publisher.

OTHER MEASURES

In addition to the median that divides a distribution into two parts and percentiles that divide a distribution into 100 parts, two other measures are often used. Quartiles are used to divide a distribution into four parts. The first quartile (Q_1) is the same as P_{25}, and so on. Deciles are used to divide a distribution into ten parts. The first decile (D_1) is the same as P_{10}, and so on. It may be seen that the median $= P_{50} = Q_2 = D_5$.

Problems

1. Find the variance and standard deviation for each of the distributions in question 2, Chapter 3.
2. Find the percent error of your measuring technique in cases giving the following measures:
   a. 76, 76, 72, 74, 78, 74
   b. 97, 97, 99, 99, 101, 101
   c. 50, 51, 52, 54, 50, 48, 45
   d. 126, 126, 123, 125, 124, 128, 125, 123
   e. 8, 10, 18, 12, 11, 13, 8, 9, 9, 10
   f. 16, 16, 17, 18, 19, 20, 19, 18, 19
3. Given the following values for $\overline{X}$ and S, find the z score corresponding to X:
   a. $\overline{X} = 65$, $S = 5$, $X = 75$
   b. $\overline{X} = 16$, $S = 2$, $X = 21$
   c. $\overline{X} = 75$, $S = 7$, $X = 61$
   d. $\overline{X} = 53$, $S = 8$, $X = 61$
   e. $\overline{X} = 80$, $S = 4$, $X = 75$
   f. $\overline{X} = 10$, $S = 2$, $X = 13$

4. Given the following values for $\bar{X}$, S, and N, determine the following:
   a. $\bar{X}=70$, $S=4$, $N=100$, how many scores are above a value of 76?
   b. $\bar{X}=45$, $S=5$, $N=150$, how many scores are above a value of 45?
   c. $\bar{X}=63$, $S=3$, $N=120$, how many scores are below a value of 60?
   d. $\bar{X}=81$, $S=6$, $N=160$, how many scores are below a value of 84?
   e. $\bar{X}=50$, $S=8$, $N=100$, how many scores are between 46 and 54?
   f. $\bar{X}=25$, $S=4$, $N=136$, how many scores are between 20 and 27?
5. For each of the following distributions find P_{10}, P_{50}, and P_{75}:

a.

X	f
30-35	4
25-29	6
20-24	8
15-19	10
10-14	8
5-9	6
0-4	4

b.

X	f
30-32	3
27-29	4
24-26	5
21-23	7
18-20	8
15-17	7
12-14	5
9-11	4
6-8	3

c.

X	f
20-21	4
18-19	7
16-17	10
14-15	10
12-13	8
10-11	3

d.

X	f
75-77	7
72-74	11
69-71	21
66-68	36
63-65	50
60-62	36
57-59	21
54-56	11
51-53	7

Chapter **5**

Purposes and types of physical education research

PURPOSES OF PHYSICAL EDUCATION RESEARCH

There are many reasons why persons undertake research in physical education, foremost of which is probably the meeting of thesis requirements for an advanced degree! At other times research is done to provide persuasive information to the local school board so that it will continue to support physical education and athletics in the school program, to provide a "scientific" basis for one's belief in the value of a particular type of weight training, to show evidence that physically fit individuals do better in the classroom than do the unfit, or for a multitude of similar reasons.

Notice that all the above examples have a common denominator of "practicality." In each instance the investigator hopes that his studies will show a need for more physical education or a different type of physical education. The researcher hopes his research will make a specific change in the physical education or athletic programs of his and other schools.

Although all these reasons for doing research may be seen as admirable from one viewpoint, they should not be confused with the *scientific purpose of physical education research, which is to explain the natural phenomena underlying man's movement and exercise and his sports and game participation.* It is always pleasant to know that one's research has a definite, practical application, but practicality is not a scientific requisite of research. "Impractical," "theoretical" research should not be looked upon with disdain, since one theoretical research study may in the long run have far more "practical" value than several hundred, so-called practical studies. For example, a study that experimentally develops a theory explaining why the heart responds differently to various types of physical training would be extremely practical in the long run because the theory could be used to predict the best type of physical training for improvement of cardiac function. On the other hand, it would take several hundred practical trial-and-error studies of the effects of one or another types of training on heart function to finally arrive at the best of all possible methods.

Unfortunately very few research studies actually develop significant

35

theories. Before a theory can be developed, a certain body of known facts must be available on which to base the theory. In physical education the body of known facts is extremely limited; therefore much physical education research is done simply to describe the present state of affairs so that others following later may use these facts to develop theory. For example, one wishing to develop a theory explaining precisely the way in which awkward gait patterns develop in children would first like to know when such abnormal patterns develop so that he might associate with gait some of the other factors (e.g., upright posture and unilateral muscular development) occurring at the same time. Since only a few studies of gait development in children can be found in the literature, the investigator wishing to develop a theory of gait development may spend the first three years of his work simply describing gait patterns in children of different age groups.

Even after a certain body of facts has been developed, there is another reason why few studies actually develop a significant theory to explain natural phenomena. The reason is that a significant theory must explain a phenomenon that occurs in many different types of exercises, movements, or games, and the investigator usually does not have the financial or technical resources to study more than one situation at a time. Since evidence for a theory should come from more than one experimental situation, the investigator usually ends up studying several situations before he can express confidence in a general theory. For instance, the investigator attempting to develop a theory explaining awkward gait development should not be content with studying only the gait of children 2 years of age if some children do not acquire the awkward gait until they are 5 years of age. Before one can have a great degree of confidence in a general theory, it should be shown that the theory holds for most, if not for all, cases.

It should be apparent to the reader by now that many practical research studies of limited scope are important because they help provide the body of facts and experimental evidence that can be used to develop theory and theory can in turn be used to predict the outcomes of most other experimental situations. Therefore neither the practical nor the theoretical researcher need apologize for his work, since the practical researcher supplies needed information to the theoretical researcher and the theoretical researcher often provides theories having practical values. However, research that provides theories explaining natural phenomena is usually considered of greater ultimate value than most research of a practical nature only.

TYPES OF RESEARCH IN PHYSICAL EDUCATION

We will classify physical education research into four categories—descriptive research, retrospective research, nonexperimental hypothesis testing, and experimental research. Next we will define, illustrate, and comment on each type in turn.

Descriptive research or descriptive investigation

Descriptive research for our purposes is the careful collection of facts about a population or populations with no structured attempt made to discover relationships between variables or to control one or more variables. This type of research is exemplified by the following:

1. A physical education supervisor conducts a survey to see how many schools in the state offer tennis instruction.
2. An administrator sends out a questionnaire to determine the teacher to pupil ratio in physical education classes throughout the country.
3. A football coach polls his colleagues to determine which offensive formations are most popular.
4. A teacher tests all the male students of his high school to find out how many push-ups and sit-ups they can do.

These examples of descriptive research should illustrate three important features of this category: first, no attempt was made to control any variables or to discover any relationships between variables; second, this research is largely a matter of compiling facts accurately; and third, it may have very practical applications. The first two of these features are obvious, and the third takes only a little imagination to illustrate. If the physical education supervisor can show that 90% of the high schools in his state offer tennis instruction, he has some facts that may convince the local school board to initiate tennis instruction in the local schools too. The administrator in the second example may get some evidence that will help convince the school board to provide funds for more physical education teachers so that class sizes can be reduced and instruction improved.

The use of the word "research" to describe this kind of routine fact gathering is somewhat misleading. *True scientific research is a controlled investigation of hypothetical propositions about relationships among natural phenomena.* Since the type of work outlined above is not controlled and is not meant to investigate any particular hypothesis, it does not qualify as scientific research and should instead probably be called "descriptive investigation," since it merely describes some characteristics of a given population.

Although descriptive investigations are the least sophisticated research efforts, the facts gathered by such investigations may be essential before more sophisticated types of research can be carried out. For example, before testing a hypothesis about the influence of "vigorous" daily running on the cardiovascular health of school children, one should first have data that will tell him what "vigorous running" is for children of different ages. If it turns out that less than 50% of an age group can run for 30 minutes at 5 miles per hour, it would be foolhardy to use that speed and duration in a study. On the other hand, if the descriptive investigation shows that most children in an age group can run at 4 miles per hour for 20 minutes and that less than 10% of the group can run at that speed longer than 25 minutes, then such an exercise bout could factually be called vigorous for that group. Descriptive investigations such as these are often used as small group "pilot" studies to gain information prior to a more sophisticated experiment.

Retrospective research

Retrospective research is an attempt to find relationships between phenomena by observing and recording outcomes and then looking in retrospect at other factors or variables that may have influenced those outcomes.

Studies of this type may be viewed as somewhat more sophisticated than descriptive investigations, since some attempt is made to discover causal relationships among variables. However, they still are not true scientific studies because (1) hypotheses about relationships are not made before the data are gathered and (2) there exists no control over the independent variables involved.

Examples of retrospective research include the following:

1. Mr. Kootz measured the maximum oxygen consumption capacity of seventy-five high school seniors in the local university's physical performance laboratory. After observing a wide variability in the scores, he questioned all participants on the type of diet they consumed. He discovered that all those who ate bacon and eggs for breakfast had high oxygen consumption scores, and he concluded that high protein breakfasts were important for achieving high oxygen consumption values.

    Mr. Kootz obviously had no hypothesis in mind about the relationship between oxygen consumption and type of breakfast before he collected his data. Therefore he also did not provide for any control of variables such as fitness level and body composition of his subjects. Both of these variables were undoubtedly more important contributors to the variance in oxygen consumption scores than the type of breakfast eaten.

2. A college professor hypothesized that blind children who had been trained to find their way in an artificial maze would be better able to walk in a straight path than untrained blind children. The results of the professor's well-designed experiment showed the opposite effect —the trained children did not walk as straight as the untrained. Disturbed by this turn of affairs, the investigator searched for other factors that could have caused this and noted that a majority of the untrained group was left handed. He concluded that there was a relationship between hand dominance and ability to walk a straight line.

    The professor obviously had no preexperimental hypothesis about the relation between the two variables, hand dominance and ability to walk a straight line, and also had no control over the variable of hand dominance. If he had found a high correlation between hair length and ability to walk a straight path, he probably would have rejected the relationship as absurd; but since hand dominance seemed to be a factor that might possibly influence the ability to walk straight, the professor could not resist making his conclusion. In actuality the differences between his groups may have been one of motivation. The trained subjects may have been bored by all the training procedures, whereas the untrained subjects concentrated harder on a novel task.

These two examples illustrate a type of research discovery that should never be considered complete in itself. The relationship between breakfast and oxygen consumption in the first example and hand dominance and ability to walk a straight line in the second should only be considered as weak evidence that may suggest a hypothesis worthy of testing. If, after observing such a relationship retrospectively, the investigator believes that the results were not accidental, he should then proceed to test an exact hypothesis about that relationship by carrying out a research project in which some control is exerted over the independent variable (i.e., type of breakfast or hand dominance).

Nonexperimental hypothesis testing

A third type of research often undertaken in physical education is one in which an experiment is designed to test a hypothesis, but in which little or no control of independent variables is attempted or, in some cases, in which control of such variables is impossible. Such experiments might be classified as nonexperimental hypothesis testing.

Many historical and sociological studies can be classified as nonexperimental hypothesis testing. For example, one might wish to test the hypothesis that the existence or threat of war has a direct bearing on national interest in physical fitness. To test this hypothesis, one might randomly select fifty school systems throughout the country and compare the ratio of physical education instructors to total number of teachers in wartime with the ratio in similar periods during peacetime. The assumption behind such a research project would be that the national interest in physical fitness is reflected by the relative number of teachers hired as physical educators.

Even if this assumption were valid, the investigator would have no way of knowing whether it was the existence of war that caused any significant difference in the measured ratios or whether a difference might in fact be due to some of the many other variables that the investigator could not possibly control. Perhaps, for instance, the number of physical educators hired varies with the financial support of school systems, and this support may be changed in a war economy.

Another hypothesis often tested with no control of many independent variables is that regular physical activity will help one avoid coronary heart disease in later life. By comparing the coronary heart disease mortality rates of active and sedentary populations (e.g., bus conductors and drivers) one discovers that relatively fewer individuals die from heart disease in the active populations. Although the tendency for most believers in the value of physical fitness has been to conclude that it is exercise which protects one from heart disease, there are many other uncontrolled variables that may be the causal factors involved. It may be that the physically active are protected simply because they are generally less obese; perhaps strict diet control would be more effective than exercise to remove strain on the heart caused by excess body weight.

Several comments about nonexperimental hypothesis testing are in order. First, a relatively high degree of confidence can be placed in the results of such studies only if two conditions are met: first, similar results should be forthcoming in many repetitions of similar studies, and, second, alternative hypotheses should also be tested and rejected. In the case of activity and heart disease, such studies have been reported so many times with similar results that very few experts doubt the value of exercise in helping to combat coronary heart disease. Studies in which diet has been controlled have also been conducted to determine the influence of diet on coronary heart disease mortality. Although diet, serum cholesterol levels, body weight, and smoking are also related to heart disease mortality, there is little question after many years of research that exercise is one of the important factors influencing that mortality.

A second precaution regarding interpretation of the results of non-experimental hypothesis testing is that conclusions should be presented as statements about the degree of relationship found between independent and dependent variables, not as statements of causal relationship. It is proper, for example, to say that there is a significant relationship between amount of regular exercise and mortality due to coronary heart disease, but it is not acceptable to conclude that a lack of exercise *causes* heart disease or that regular exercise prevents heart disease. A cause-and-effect relationship can be concluded only when all independent variables have either been controlled or manipulated by the investigator in a true scientific experiment or when all other alternative hypotheses have been tested and found wanting.

Finally, it should be pointed out that nonexperimental hypothesis testing is a useful and important type of research because it is the only type that can be used to test hypotheses about the relationships between intelligence, creativity, social class, and other variables that are important in everyday life but that defy experimental control and manipulation. In fact, many such studies are far more meaningful than exquisitely controlled laboratory experiments in which completely artificial methods are used to control variables. If the results of nonexperimental hypothesis-testing research are interpreted with caution, they may have a great deal of significance because those results were obtained in "real life" situations.

Experimental research

A true experimental study is one in which the investigator observes the effects of his manipulation of one or more independent variables on one or more dependent variables and in which the investigator can assign subjects to experimental groups or experimental groups to subjects. Typical experimental studies in physical education are those in which an experimenter manipulates the amount or type of training or exercise and observes the effect of the training or exercise on a dependent variable such as strength, skill, performance, or body weight. The experimenter should be able to assign experimental treatments (types of training or exercise) to the subjects in any way he chooses. If he cannot assign treatments at will, there is a possibility that some extraneous variable will influence the results of his experiment.

An informative example of a study in which an extraneous variable could have influenced experimental results is a study done to assess the effects of two different types of body conditioning programs on the body fat of college males. The investigator knew that two voluntary conditioning classes were being taught on his campus and that the two instructors involved had markedly different views on the nature of the exercise that should be included in such a program. One instructor emphasized heavy weight-lifting activities, whereas the other utilized a running and stretching program almost exclusively. The investigator hypothesized that the running and stretching class would lose more body fat than the weight-lifting class, so he measured body fat by several methods before and after the 10 weeks of the school term.

At first glance this may seem like a straightforward, well-designed experiment. But, although the investigator could control the exercise program, he did not have the power to assign individuals to exercise programs or exercise programs to individuals. Therefore the investigator could not disregard the possibility that some factor which determined whether a subject volunteered for the running group or the weight-lifting group was the actual cause of any changes shown. For instance, those who chose the running group may have done so precisely because they wanted to lose weight; those who chose the weight-lifting group may have wanted to gain weight, and both groups may have controlled their diets accordingly; that is, the running group ate less and the weight-lifting group more. In this circumstance the running group probably would have reduced their body fat with no exercise at all. Much more confidence in the results of such a study could be attained if the subjects were randomly assigned to the two exercise treatments so that no self-selection factor could have been designed into the study. Also, a third group of subjects who did not participate in an exercise program would be important to rule out extraneous variables. Perhaps fat was lost simply because the experiment was undertaken in the fall semester after a lazy summer of good eating. Most students probably lose some body fat after the summer months.

Another example of an experimental research project is one in which the investigator believed that the psychological stress of being observed for grading purposes inhibits students from executing motor skills with their optimum proficiency. The investigator was teaching several gymnastics classes at the time and had worked a great deal with his students on performance of a handstand on the parallel bars. To test his hypothesis that the psychological stress of grading would be detrimental to performance of this stunt, the instructor performed the following experiment.

First, he secretly evaluated the students' performance on a 10-point rating scale and then matched the students in pairs, with the two best performers as the first pair, the next two best performers as the second pair, and so on until the two worst performers formed the last pair. Next, he randomly assigned one member of each pair to a stress or nonstress group and the remaining pair member to the other group so that an equal number of highly skilled and unskilled performers were assigned to each group. Then he asked three expert judges to rate the students on handstand performance, again on a 10-point scale. The students in the stress group were asked to perform the stunt for a grade in front of the three judges, whereas the nonstress subjects were told to make their best executions in preparation for grading during the next week. Unknown to these subjects they were observed by the judges through a one-way viewing window. In an attempt to eliminate bias on the part of the judges, the judges were told that this was an experiment to see if performance rating reliability would be reduced by viewing performers through the window.

Note that all conditions for a good experiment were met: the investigator controlled and manipulated an independent variable (grading stress), observed its effect on a dependent variable (skill execution), and assigned subjects to experimental groups in a manner designed to control variables (level of skill) of secondary importance.

CONFIDENCE IN THE RESULTS OF DIFFERENT TYPES OF RESEARCH

The tightly controlled experimental type of research is the most rigorous method man can use to obtain knowledge. If an experiment has been well conducted, the investigator can have a great deal of confidence that any observed effects were due to his manipulation of independent variables and not to some extraneous variable unknown to him. However, with varying degrees of deviation from a well-designed experiment, the experimenter must be resigned to placing less and less confidence in his results.

In nonexperimental hypothesis testing, the researcher can have confidence that some kind of relationship exists between his independent and dependent variables, but he can have very little confidence in a cause-and-effect relationship until his results have been confirmed several times and alternative cause-and-effect relationships have been investigated and rejected.

The retrospective investigator can have little confidence in any relationship at all that his data may seem to support. To gain such confidence, he must test the hypothesis he has arrived at retrospectively, by an experiment preferably, or at least by a nonexperimental test of a hypothesis if an experiment is impractical.

Finally, the investigator who collects data simply to describe a phenomenon can have much confidence in his facts if he has done a good job of collecting. Of course, he has tested no hypothesis so there are no conclusions about relationships that require confidence judgements.

CHOOSING A GOOD RESEARCH PROBLEM

One of the most troublesome academic hurdles for most graduate students is choosing a good research problem. Once the first research study is completed, good problems are seemingly infinite in number, but the first trial at problem selection can be miserable. The typical physical education graduate student chose that major so that he could become qualified to coach his favorite sport. Therefore his first inclination is to do his research on some aspect of that sport. Typical problems presented by first-year physical education graduate students are the following:

1. Effect of weight training on sprinting speed
2. Effect of a 3-minute wrestling bout on heart rate
3. New method for teaching the golf swing

4. Effect of weight training on pitching velocity
5. Relationship between grip strength and batting power

Too often such studies, although well motivated, are wastes of time and effort. This is not to say that they are always "bad" research because good research problems can be built from just such studies when they are properly designed. Even though few professors can agree on what makes a research problem a "good" problem, we will attempt to give a few guidelines in the form of questions one should ask of a proposed study. These questions are as follows:

1. *Has the problem already been thoroughly investigated?* Most professors agree that an aggravating characteristic of enthusiastic students is their readiness to undertake a time-consuming research study without first having made a careful review of the scientific literature to determine whether this novel and unique type of study has already been reported once or several times previously. If the problem has already been thoroughly researched, the student should either use the previous research as a springboard for a more comprehensive problem or should find a new problem area. He should not simply alter one small step in the procedure (e.g., weight training 5 days a week instead of 4) and repeat someone's work unless the previous research was very poorly designed.

2. *Is the problem important?* This is probably the most difficult question to answer about a research study. Perhaps this question might be better stated: Will the study explain or at least clarify one or more of the natural phenomena of exercise, movement, games, sport, or physical education programs? An example of an unimportant research study might be a collection of psychological testing data to determine whether female physical education majors are more aggressive than non-physical education majors. The answer to the question implied by this study is unimportant scientifically because the hypothesis behind the study is unimportant. Whether female physical education majors are more aggressive than other majors is of no importance unless connected to some broader hypothesis that may help explain an exercise or sports phenomenon. The same data could be very useful, for instance, in testing some hypothesis about the sociopsychological forces that motivate one to participate in physical activity.

A corollary question to the question of importance is: Can the study be conducted so that it has broader scope? A hypothesis about the aggressiveness of physical education majors versus other majors is of very limited scope, whereas one about the forces that motivate persons to exercise is of much broader scope and is therefore of much more importance.

3. *Will the data collected answer the problem?* Sometimes researchers have very important problems at the base of their studies but then proceed to collect data that do not really impinge on the problem. Consider the case of Major Psoas who believed that a reduced supply of oxygen to the tissues (i.e., hypoxia) was responsible for the cardiovascular

effects of physical training. To test his theory, Major Psoas put ten subjects in a hypobaric (low-pressure) chamber at reduced oxygen concentrations for 30 minutes every day for 3 weeks and compared before and after resting heart rates of the subjects. Notice that the Major had an important problem which might help explain why regular exercise improves cardiovascular function, but the data collected did not include exercise as a variable. The only question the data could answer was: Does hypoxic conditioning change resting heart rates? To answer his original problem the Major should have included exercised normal and exercised hypoxic groups in his design.

4. *Can the study be conducted at a more sophisticated level?* If a problem can be attacked experimentally, the investigators should make every attempt to perform an experiment with rigid controls. If an experiment is impractical, a nonexperimental study can be undertaken to test a hypothesis. In most cases of academic research a descriptive investigation is acceptable only when higher levels of sophistication are impossible and when the problem is nonetheless deemed important.

5. *Is the research scope too broad and therefore impractical?* An excellent problem for a medical student is to discover the cause of cancer, but if his degree depended on solution of the problem, the poor student would likely be an old man before he could begin practice. Most investigators have limited time and limited financial resources with which to conduct a study. A student in particular should have a clear agreement with his thesis director as to the limitations on the student's responsibility for a research project. Sometimes students want to give up on a problem before putting up a battle, and at other times professors forget that students have obligations other than research.

If these five questions can be answered satisfactorily, one can be quite certain that he has a good research problem. If not, a little work and thought can usually effect a salvage job for the initial problem. If the salvage fails, it is then time to think about a new problem.

Problems

1. List five examples of unexplained natural phenomena that should eventually be explained by physical education researchers.

2. List two examples of each of the four categories of research. It may be helpful to review issues of the physical education research journals for examples.

3. Using one of the examples of unexplained phenomena you listed in response to question 1, develop a theory based on what you already know that might explain the phenomenon and then give examples of studies that you could conduct to lend credence to your theory. The "correctness" of your theory is not as important for this problem as the logic used to undertake research that might support the theory. At this stage you will need to be very general in your statements of how the research is conducted.

Chapter **6**

Hypothesis testing and research design

Before the actual data collection of a research study is begun, the investigator must know three things if he is to have a successful study. First, he must know precisely what hypothesis he wants to test by his research; second, he must know how to plan or design his study so that his hypothesis is tested in the best possible manner; and, third, he must know what instrumentation he will use in data collection and how valid and reliable that instrumentation is. In this chapter, hypothesis testing and research design will be discussed. Methods of testing the validity and objectivity of instrumentation are outlined in Appendix A.

HYPOTHESIS TESTING

Before conducting an investigation a researcher should have two types of hypotheses—*scientific* and *statistical*. These two types of hypotheses can be illustrated by examining closely the manner in which Charlie Equus conducted his research project. He noticed that after two months of hard training for the steeplechase his heart seemed to beat much more slowly at rest than it had before training. In fact, his resting heart rate was about 70 before training and had dropped to 50 after training. The more Charlie thought about it, the more he was convinced that regular exercise caused a reduction in heart rate. This was his crude scientific hypothesis, that regular exercise reduces resting heart rate. After some review of the literature available in his hometown library, he found that most isometric exercises were ineffective in reducing heart rate; therefore he modified his first hypothesis and was now quite certain that vigorous *dynamic* exercise for at least 15 minutes every other day would lower one's resting heart rate.

Charlie had taken a statistics class in college and knew that one way to test his scientific hypothesis was to randomly select subjects from some population and compare their heart rates before and after a training program he would devise. Since he worked at an aircraft factory that had gymnasium facilities available for the workers, Charlie decided to select subjects from the male population of his factory. This in effect again

45

changed the scientific hypothesis he would be able to test. Now his hypothesis was that vigorous exercise for 15 minutes every other day would lower resting heart rates in male workers at the B. Arn aircraft plant. If Charlie believed that the Arn aircraft workers were representative of the population of all adult males, he might be willing to extrapolate his results to that population, but his limited choice of subjects restricts the scientifically acceptable conclusions to the Arn worker population.

The *scientific hypothesis* is the belief the investigator holds regarding the relationship between the two or more variables he has chosen to investigate. Charlie believed that the dependent variable, heart rate, would be lowered by the independent variable, exercise, which he would manipulate. Examples of other scientific hypotheses in physical education research are as follows: participation in vigorous sports reduces emotional tension; success in combative sports is related to social class; dehydration through severe weight reduction is harmful to performance in wrestling; the learning of motor skills is influenced positively by mental practice; weight lifting has no effect on cardiovascular endurance.

The next step in Charlie's study was for him to transpose his scientific hypothesis into a statistical hypothesis which he could test experimentally so that he would be able to express statistical confidence in his results. If he were simply to say that most of the men decreased their heart rates with training, critics would suggest that his results could have been due to chance, or that the decreases were too small to be significantly different from pretraining values. But, let him instead test a statistical hypothesis such as "the mean heart rate of trained men is less than the mean heart rate of those men before training." Then, if he finds a consistent difference, he can conclude precisely that differences as great as he observed could be due to chance only once or five times in a hundred. Others could then accept or reject Charlie's hypothesis at that level. If they require that similar results occur in all experiments, they will never have confidence in any experimental results. For most people, 95% to 99% confidence is sufficient.

Notice that the *statistical hypothesis* is a mathematical statement about a population parameter. In mathematical terms, Charlie's statistical hypothesis was $\mu_t < \mu_u$, where μ_t is the mean heart rate of men after training and μ_u the mean heart rate of the untrained men.

Most statistical hypotheses in physical education are statements about one or more population means, variances, covariances, or correlation and regression coefficients. There is an infinite number of hypotheses about these parameters. Hypotheses about the means of two populations (e.g., trained and untrained) may be stated in many ways, including the following:

$$\mu_t - \mu_u = 0$$
$$\mu_t - \mu_u > 0$$
$$\mu_t - \mu_u < 0$$

$$\mu_t = \tfrac{1}{3}\mu_u$$
$$\mu_t - \mu_u = 8$$
$$\mu_t \neq \mu_u$$

Statistical hypotheses should always be tested against alternative hypotheses. In Charlie's case, $\mu_t < \mu_u$ should be tested against the alternative that $\mu_t \geq \mu_u$, and the statistical test used will help him choose with some degree of confidence one or the other hypothesis as representing the true state of affairs.

Statistical tests

A statistical test is a decision-making rule invoked to help the researcher decide which of two alternative hypotheses represents the true state of affairs. In Charlie's case a rule was needed to help him decide between the hypothesis that the mean heart rate of males after training is lower than the pretraining mean ($\mu_t < \mu_u$) and the alternative that the mean post-training rate is greater than or equal to the pretraining mean ($\mu_t \geq \mu_u$). Examples of other hypotheses and their alternatives are as follows:

H_0 – Null hypothesis

$$\mu_1 - \mu_2 = 0 \qquad \sigma_1^2 = \sigma_2^2 \qquad \mu_1 - \mu_2 \geq 8$$
$$\mu_1 - \mu_2 \neq 0 \qquad \sigma_1^2 \neq \sigma_2^2 \qquad \mu_1 - \mu_2 < 8$$

$$P_{xy} = 0 \qquad P_{xy} > .50 \qquad \frac{\mu_1 + \mu_2}{3} = \frac{\mu_3 + \mu_4}{2}$$

$$P_{xy} \neq 0 \qquad P_{xy} \leq .50 \qquad \frac{\mu_1 + \mu_2}{3} \neq \frac{\mu_3 + \mu_4}{2}$$

Although statistical tests help one decide which of two hypotheses he should have confidence in, such tests in practice are applied only to one of the hypotheses at a time. If a statistical test of the hypothesis $\mu_1 - \mu_2 = 0$ gives no evidence that the hypothesis is false, the investigator may then accept that hypothesis as plausible and reject its alternative, $\mu_1 - \mu_2 \neq 0$. On the other hand, if the statistical test presents evidence that $\mu_1 - \mu_2 = 0$ is not correct, then the investigator rejects that hypothesis and accepts the alternative as being correct.

The statistical tests or decision-making rules for most research problems in physical education will be the subject matter of succeeding chapters. For now, let it suffice to say that the decision rule is a rule which says that if the best estimate of the parameter(s) of interest does not fall within a predetermined range of values, but instead falls in a critical region of rejection, then the tested hypothesis will be rejected and the alternative assumed correct. On the other hand, if the best estimate falls within the acceptance range, then no evidence favors the alternative hypothesis. The best estimate of population parameters, μ and σ^2, for instance, are $\bar{X}$ and S^2, respectively.

Before an experimenter tests alternative hypotheses he must decide which of the alternatives should be subjected to the statistical test. Should Charlie, for instance, test his statistical hypothesis $\mu_t < \mu_u$ or should he test its alternative, $\mu_t \geq \mu_u$? This decision is not always easy to make but should be based upon the relative consequences of making false conclusions about the alternative hypotheses. With statistical tests the probability of making certain types of false conclusions can be limited to a narrow range, whereas the probability of making other false conclusions may be great or even unknown. To make his decision on which hypothesis to test, the researcher must not only know the *relative consequences* of making false conclusions about the alternative hypotheses, but he should also know the *probabilities* of making various false conclusions, or statistical errors.

Types of statistical error

In testing the hypothesis H_1: $\mu_1 = \mu_2$ there are two possible types of statistical error one may commit—type I (α) and type II (β). Since the statistical test is based only on the data obtained from a small sample of the two populations in question, there is a certain probability that we will reject H_1 when, in fact, it is true. This is known as the probability of committing a type I or an alpha (α) error. There is also a certain probability that we will accept H_1 when it is false. This is the probability of committing of type II or beta (β) error. *A type I error is the error of rejecting a tested hypothesis when it is true, and a type II error is the error of accepting a tested hypothesis when it is false.*

The probability of committing a type I error can and should be easily and precisely determined before any data collection begins. All the investigator need do is decide how much he is willing to risk the rejection of the test hypothesis when it is true and then select the proper rule according to that decision. By convention, many workers decide to set the probability of committing a type I or α error at the .05 or 5% level. This means that five times out of one hundred a true hypothesis will be rejected by chance when using the particular decision rule or statistical test. Other investigators prefer to take a smaller risk of rejecting a true hypothesis and set the α level at .01 or even .001. There is no statistical or mathematical decision involved in how low one sets the probability of committing a statistical error. It is purely a matter of the risk of error one is willing to take.

The probability of committing a type II error is more difficult to set and is usually much larger than the probability of making a type I error. As a general rule, the probability of a β error increases as the probability of an α error decreases. The best way to reduce the probability of committing a β error is to increase the size of the sample, that is, number of subjects. Methods for estimating the β error risk are beyond the scope of this text but can be found elsewhere.*

Selecting the test hypothesis and the alternative hypothesis

Now let us return to the problem of deciding which of two hypotheses should be put to statistical test. A good rule of thumb is the following: *One usually tests the hypothesis that he hopes the data will disprove.* In most cases, when dealing with trained and untrained subjects, physical educators would like to disprove the hypothesis that training produces no change or produces an adverse change. Charlie then would want to use $\mu_t \geq \mu_u$ as a test hypothesis and $\mu_t < \mu_u$ as an alternate hypothesis. If one rejects the hypothesis he hopes the data will disprove, he can be quite certain that the alternative hypothesis is true, since the probability of rejecting the test hypothesis incorrectly is usually set at .05 or .01. If, on the other hand, one tests the hypothesis he wishes to prove, he can usually have little confidence in his conclusion because the probability of accepting a test hypothesis when it is false is either unknown or much higher than .05 or .01.

---

*For estimating the β error risk in t tests and analysis of variance tests, see Guenther, W. C.: Analysis of variance, Englewood Cliffs, N. J., 1964, Prentice-Hall, Inc.

In physical education research the alternative hypotheses are often of the form $\mu_1 = \mu_2$ and $\mu_1 \neq \mu_2$. In this situation the hypothesis of no differences, the null hypothesis, is usually the test hypothesis:

$$H_o: \mu_1 = \mu_2 \qquad\qquad H_o: \mu_1 - \mu_2 = 0$$
$$\text{or}$$
$$H_A: \mu_1 \neq \mu_2 \qquad\qquad H_A: \mu_1 - \mu_2 \neq 0$$

With this notation, H_o symbolizes the null hypothesis and H_A the alternative hypothesis.

An example follows to again make the point that the investigator should subject to statistical test the hypothesis he would like to disprove and also to point out a common error of interpretation of statistical results.

Miss Smith was a great believer in the athletic potential of females and refused to admit that women could not be at least as proficient in track and field events as men if they would only train as hard. To prove her thesis she selected six female disciples to train for two years in the shot put event and compared their best puts at the end of the period with those of six males who trained in a similar fashion. Miss Smith chose to test the hypothesis $\mu_F \geq \mu_M$ against the alternative that $\mu_F < \mu_M$, where $\mu_F =$ the average of the best shot puts of females and $\mu_M =$ the average of the best puts for males. Data were as follows:

Female subject	Best put (feet)	Male subject	Best put (feet)
1	17	1	47
2	43	2	40
3	20	3	38
4	49	4	49
5	40	5	33
6	29	6	45
Total 6	198	6	252
Average	33		42

By using the appropriate test of statistical significance, Miss Smith found that she could not reject her test hypothesis, $\mu_F - \mu_M \geq 0$, at the 1% level. Therefore she accepted that hypothesis as representing the true state of affairs and told all her associates that she had just completed a research experiment proving that females are as good as or better than males in putting the shot if both sexes train equally hard.

To the statistically naive, this conclusion may seem reasonable, but most of us would suspect that Miss Smith has committed a type II error by accepting a false test hypothesis. Even though she set the probability of committing a type I error at .01 (which sounds scientifically respectable), Miss Smith failed to realize that with only six subjects per group and with a large variance in her data she had a very large (greater than 80%) chance of committing a type II error.

Similar misinterpretations of research results are common among graduate students who have little statistical background but have spent a great deal of time and effort on a research project or master's thesis with small numbers of subjects. Rather than report the results as having provided no evidence to reject the test hypothesis, they choose to take the fatal step into the unknown void and conclude that the test hypothesis is true. Remember:

A failure to reject a tested hypothesis gives the researcher little confidence that the tested hypothesis is therefore true. Only when the probability of committing a type II error has been limited to a narrow range (usually by testing large numbers of subjects) does a failure to reject have much meaning. Only rarely can type II error risk be held to such low levels.

Let us examine the consequences Miss Smith suffered by not testing the hypothesis she wished to disprove, $\mu_F < \mu_M$. Since she now believed she had proof of female equality, if not superiority, in the shot put, she told all her professors and a television sportscaster about her findings. Her professors (Miss Smith was a physical education major) immediately pointed out her error, directed her to twenty publications that contradicted her results, and dismissed her as an aphid brain. The sports announcer told a nationwide audience of her study, and so much adverse publicity came to her and her school that no one, including Miss Smith, could get a job after graduating from that physical education department. However, if she had tested the alternative hypothesis, $\mu_F < \mu_M$, and again failed to reject it, little harm could result in her claiming to have proved that males are better shot-putters than females—everyone already knows that!

In most physical education studies such dire consequences as Miss Smith suffered by testing the wrong hypothesis do not exist. In all cases the researcher can have great confidence in his results if he tests the hypothesis he would like to disprove and produces statistical evidence to reject that hypothesis. If he fails to reject the hypothesis, the investigator can make no important conclusions unless he has restricted the risk of a type II error to a low value (i.e., 20% or less), generally by using many subjects.

Summary of hypothesis testing

The first step in performing a research study is to arrive at a *scientific hypothesis,* which is a succinct statement of the belief one holds regarding the relationship between two or more variables of interest. Next the investigator must transpose this belief into a *statistical hypothesis*—a mathematical statement about population parameters that can be accepted or rejected on the basis of *statistical tests* or decision rules. The statistical hypothesis is not always the one put to test. For every hypothesis there is an alternative, and under most circumstances the *test hypothesis* is that alternative which the investigator hopes to disprove. The investigator should know the approximate probabilities of committing type I or II statistical errors when making decisions regarding the correctness of the test hypothesis. In particular, he should remember that a failure to reject the test hypothesis usually gives one little assurance that the test hypothesis represents reality, since the probability of accepting the test hypothesis when the alternative is true is usually very great.

RESEARCH DESIGN

It is most difficult to isolate an analysis of research design from a discussion of hypothesis testing and statistical methods because the research design is the way in which a study will be conducted to determine the probabilistic accuracy of a hypothesis. Therefore the design must be such that the method of collecting data does not violate the mathematical assumptions upon which the statistical techniques for determining probabilistic accuracy are based. At this point our discussion must necessarily deal with general principles and leave many of the nuances of research design for later discussions on specific statistical methods and for more advanced texts.

Characteristics of a good research design

There are many important characteristics of good research designs, but we shall discuss only two broad characteristics and some of the features implied by them. The two characteristics are (1) a good research design provides a method of answering, at least in part, the question posed by the scientific hypothesis and (2) a good design maximizes the variance due to manipulation of independent variables and minimizes the variance due to variables of little or no interest.

Answering the question posed by the scientific hypothesis. The most important characteristic of a good research design is that it provides a method of answering, if only partially, the question proposed by the scientific hypothesis. If the scientific hypothesis is that isometric strength training is more effective than isotonic methods, a good research design properly carried out will answer the question of isometric versus isotonic at least for a given population and under the given experimental conditions. An inadequate research design will not only provide no answer to the hypothetical question but may even confuse the issue by providing error-ridden data. For example, if one were to study strength gains with isometric and isotonic training routines, using the isometric method on untrained subjects and the isotonic method on trained weight lifters, he would undoubtedly find that the isometric routine was better because the untrained would naturally respond with greater strength increments than the trained weight lifters. If the investigator were not made aware of his poor research design and fallacious conclusions, he might publicize his findings widely and multiply the possibly erroneous outcomes of his research design.

A few guidelines can be used to help one determine whether a research design will answer the question proposed by the scientific hypothesis. These are presented as a guide only and may not apply in some cases.

1. *Make certain that the hypothesis is testable.* There is no research available that can answer some questions, for example, whether regular exercise gives one a better personality. Since a "better personality" means different things to different people, and since it would be impossible to isolate the effects of regular exercise from all the other variables that influence personality, such a hypothesis is untestable. Make certain that all terms in the hypothesis can be readily defined and can be measured with some accuracy. Such a hypothesis might be that daily participation in tackle football reduces aggressive tendencies as measured by the Minnesota Multiphasic Personality Inventory.
2. *Make certain that the research design is practical.* If a research project requires too much money or time or too many subjects or testing

personnel, the project will not be completed, and the hypothesis will remain untested. Therefore, if only a complex, impractical design can test a hypothesis, the investigator had better narrow the scope of his problem. Inexperienced researchers usually bite off more than they can chew on their first few experiments. It is far better to get an answer to a question of narrow scope than to have no answer at all to a very broad question.

3. *Make certain that the research project is designed to answer the question of primary interest.* Often when a research project is completed many answers are provided to problems of only secondary interest. If one were interested in the effects of regular exercise on basal metabolic rate (BMR), he would be foolish to attempt to simultaneously measure the effects of exercise on maximal oxygen consumption. Completion of vigorous exercise before recording the basal metabolism would elevate the metabolic rate as would anticipation of exercise if the BMR were recorded prior to maximal oxygen consumption. In this case the investigator might well discover the effects of exercise on maximal oxygen consumption but would not be able to determine changes in BMR, since any such change would have been obscured by the exercise or anticipatory elevation of the metabolic rate. Although it sometimes seems wise to take as many measures as possible on subjects, the results obtained from multimeasure studies are often obscured by interactions among measures. It is better to make one test accurately than to make many tests with reduced accuracy.

4. *When possible, control groups should be included in the research design.* It is important to have some evidence that an experimental outcome (e.g., an increased maximal oxygen consumption with regular exercise) is not the result of attention paid to subjects, body weight gain over time, or some other unexamined variable. Therefore, whenever possible, a control group of subjects should be treated exactly the same as the experimental group except for the one variable of interest, that is, exercise. This is particularly important when an experiment is conducted over a long period of time with young subjects, and pretest versus posttest scores are of interest. Since maturation alone can cause marked changes in many measures, the investigator must compare the scores of the experimental group with those of a control group to be sure that he is answering a question about the effects of exercise or activity and not the effects of maturation.

5. *Determine whether the research design will help provide answers to questions about the population of interest and whether the sampling from that population has been done in a random fashion.* In most instances, physical educators are interested in how and why physical activity affects human beings. This implies that all physical education research should be performed on random samples of all human beings. Of course this is impossible, and the investigator is limited in his sampling to those subjects he has at his disposal or who can be easily reached, for example, through the mail for a questionnaire study. In fact, most of the sampling done

for physical education research is from narrowly restricted populations of one age group of one sex from one school or school system. In some cases of physiological research, animals must be used because human blood or tissue samples are not readily obtained.

Whatever the restrictions on the population studied, the investigator must recognize those restrictions. If a research design implies so many restrictions that the population under study is no longer of interest to the investigator, he should revise the design and/or the problem to be studied so that a question of interest to him can be answered.

Once having been satisfied that the population implied by the research design is still of interest, the researcher should do all in his power to design the project so that random samples are drawn from that population for the experimental and control groups.* A random sample is selected from a population in such a fashion that all members of the population have an equal chance of being selected for the sample. This is usually done by assigning a number to each member of the population and then drawing the required number of subjects from a table of random numbers (Table C-3, Appendix C). For example, if one were to study the attitudes of Podunk State College students toward regular exercise, he might obtain a student directory from the campus, assign a number to each student listed, and begin drawing a sample of 200 numbers from a table of random numbers. In this manner the investigator would soon have a random sample of 200 Podunk State College students that he might then interview.

Unfortunately many experimenters cannot hope to approach this high degree of randomization in sampling procedures. Often the population studied may not be the 27,000 students of a university but the twenty middle-distance runners on the varsity track team. Assuming that a student wanted to study the effects of "pep" pills on performance in the 800-meter run, and that he had time only to test six subjects on pep pills and six on placebos, he might draw twelve subjects randomly from the twenty track men, every other subject being assigned to the experimental group of six. However, since a man once picked as an experimental subject then had no chance of being picked as a control subject, the selection was not truly random. A truly randomized selection requires that sampling be done with replacement; that is, once a number or subject is picked, it must be replaced in the population so that it has a chance of being selected again. If the population is large and the sample size is fairly small, say less than one fifth of the population size, then sampling without replacement usually has little effect on the random nature of that sample. However, in most instances scientists in physical education do not have such large populations to draw upon and there is often a serious question as to the randomness of the selected sample. Although little can be done to alleviate this problem, the investigator must keep in the back of his mind the fact that most

---

*Sampling procedures other than random sampling are sometimes used, particularly in sociological types of research. See Blalock, H. M., Jr.: Social statistics, New York, 1960, McGraw-Hill Book Co., chap. 22.

statistical methods assume random sampling, and deviations from that assumption, particularly when small populations are sampled, may erroneously influence the statistical results. When random sampling is not possible, it is a good rule to withhold judgement on the results until the experiment has been repeated with other samples and similar results have occurred.

To summarize, a research design that does not include random sampling may not answer research questions because statistical interpretations may be invalid due to the violation of statistical randomness assumptions.

6. *If the research design does not include provisions for random selection of samples, it should at least provide for random assignment of subjects to groups, or treatments to groups.* If one wished to study the effects of an exercise program on food consumption, he would not select the ten largest subjects of his sample as the experimental exercise group and the ten smallest as the nonexercised control group because larger subjects would generally eat more than smaller subjects regardless of the effects of the exercise program.

To avoid the possibility that some known or unknown variable might affect the criterion or dependent variable (food consumption), the research design should call for randomness in the assignment of subjects to groups. For example, names of the twenty available subjects might be thrown into a hat and a naive observer asked to select one name alternately for the two or more groups involved. A better method would be to use a table of random numbers (Table C-3, Appendix C).

In some cases the investigator may not have the power to assign subjects to groups but may have groups (e.g., classrooms, schools, gym classes) available for experimentation. In this case the research design should provide for the random assignment of treatments (i.e., exercise regimens and control regimens) to the groups of subjects so that the personal bias of the researcher does not cause, for instance, the selection of the brightest class for his pet treatment or the dullest class as the sedentary control group.

In summary of this discussion, a research design will usually be adequate to answer the question posed by a scientific hypothesis if the hypothesis is, in fact, testable, if the research design is practical with respect to time, money, and personnel, if the project is designed to answer the question of primary interest and not chiefly those of secondary interest, if control groups have been included in the research design, if the population of interest has been randomly sampled, and if the design provides for random assignment of subjects to groups, or treatments to groups.

Many of these criteria cannot be satisfied in physical education research projects. In large-group, sociological or psychological types of research, it is particularly difficult to obtain control groups and to provide for random assignment of subjects to groups. Such excursions from the ideal should not cause one to reject all such research but to beware of possible errors arising from these excursions. Before assuming a great deal of confidence in the results of nonexperimental studies not meeting the criteria of adequacy, one should demand replication and the testing of alternative hypotheses.

Variance control. Another characteristic of a good research design is that it maximizes the variance due to experimental manipulation of independent variables and minimizes or controls the variance due to variables of little or no interest. If a swimming coach wished to study the relative effectiveness of an interval training program and a continuous swim program, for example, he would like to maximize differences due to the two types of training and control or minimize the variability within the two groups due to differences in variables such as age, weight, experience, and pretraining swim times. The coach should also minimize the variance due to inaccurate timing of work and rest intervals, record keeping, and other sources of technical error that may tend to obscure any significant differences in performance due to the two training methods.

There are many ways to accomplish this maximizing of between-groups variances and controlling or minimizing of variance due to variables of little or no interest. The techniques to be discussed are the following: (1) maximum manipulation of the independent variables, (2) elimination of identifiable interfering variables, (3) control of identifiable interfering variables by including them as independent variables or using them as matching variables, (4) randomization of interfering variables, and (5) minimization of nonidentifiable variance by the use of reliable measurement techniques under standard conditions and by the completion of pilot studies.

Maximum manipulation of independent variables. To maximize the variance due to the independent variables (i.e., exercise vs. sedentary, isometric vs. isotonic, continuous vs. interval, middle class vs. upper class, high I.Q. vs. low I.Q.) one should manipulate those variables to the maximum in most cases so that great differences between independent variable classifications do occur. For example, to study the difference between the effects of exercise and sedentary conditions on body weight, one would not select one push-up per day as an exercise regimen because any slight changes in body weight due to this exercise would surely be masked by the variation in body weight due to food consumption, water consumption, sweating, and many other nonidentifiable sources of variance. Instead, the investigator would choose a vigorous exercise regimen so that changes would not be masked by interfering variables. In other words, the independent variables or experimental conditions must be sufficiently different so that the variance of the dependent variable (e.g., body weight) caused by the experimental conditions has a chance to be greater than error variance from uncontrolled variables.

A word of caution should be inserted here so that the reader is not led to rely so heavily on the principle of maximizing differences between experimental conditions that he forgets certain practical considerations. For instance, it would seem ridiculous to study the effects of a daily 8-hour treadmill run on body weight if the purpose of the research was to develop an exercise regimen that could be used by the general population to control weight. Even if the exercise routine effectively removed 100 pounds in two weeks, its proponents would doubtlessly be limited to the mentally deranged! It would be more realistic in this case to limit the exercise routine to less than 30 minutes per day, since few Americans will subject themselves to longer exercise periods.

Elimination of identifiable interfering variables. When a variable other than the independent variable of interest is suspected of having an influence on the variance of the dependent variable, the investigator may effectively erase that influence by eliminating the interfering variable. In physical education research, most studies are conducted on only one sex to help minimize the variance due to interfering variables. It would be more difficult, for instance, to assess the effects of an exercise program on the iron content of the blood in a group of males and females than in a group of males alone because the monthly blood loss of females would introduce greater variability into the iron measurements. Other examples of variables that are often controlled by partial elimination are age, intelligence, race, species (in animal research), social class, educational background, athletic background, and state of physical training.

Control of identifiable interfering variables by including them as independent or matching variables. Another way to control identifiable interfering variables is to let them serve as independent variables. Rather than eliminating sex as a variable from a research design, one might separate from the overall dependent variable variance that portion of the variance due to sex by studying sex as another independent variable. If this can realistically be accomplished, the added information derived (i.e., knowledge of the influence of sex on the dependent variable) may be very helpful and thus make such a design better than the one that eliminated sex as a factor.

Sometimes this same effect of including an interfering variable as an independent variable can be done by matching subjects or taking repeat measures on the same subjects. If one were to study the effects of three different training methods on the performance of a complex motor skill, he might control the influence of I.Q., for example, by organizing his sample into matched trios, with the first trio having the three highest I.Q.'s, the second trio having the next three highest I.Q.'s, down to the last trio having the three lowest I.Q.'s, and then randomly assigning one member of each trio to a different training method. This method of matching could then be used to isolate the variance in motor skill performance due to intelligence and give added information to the experimenter.

By taking repeat measurements (e.g., pretest and posttest) on the same subjects and then analyzing the differences between tests, investigators are sometimes able to eliminate most interfering variance and to study only the remaining variance, presumably due to the treatment (e.g., exercise program), that occurred in the interval between pretest and posttest. It is necessary, of course, to have control groups in such designs to evaluate the effects of other variables, such as maturation, that may also have occurred in the interval between tests.

Matching procedures can be valuable if there is a high degree of relationship between the matching variable (sex, intelligence, body weight) and the dependent variable (blood iron, motor performance, food intake). If a high correlation (>.50) does not exist, matching is a waste of time. It may be very difficult and time consuming to find enough subjects matched on one variable, let alone more than one.

Randomization of interfering variables. In most cases the best method of controlling extraneous variance is to randomize the assignment of subjects to groups and groups to conditions. When one matches on a single variable, he cannot be certain that the effects of other variables (e.g., age, strength, preexperimental training) are equally distributed among groups. With a reasonable degree of randomization, however, the investigator can have a great degree of confidence that any significant differences exhibited between groups are due to his manipulation of the independent variable(s) (e.g., exercise) and not to an extraneous variable. However, if an investigator has prior knowledge that the dependent variable is almost wholly dependent on another variable, he should not hesitate to resort to matching techniques to subtract that source of variance from the overall variance of the dependent variable.

Use of reliable measurement techniques. The last but by no means the least important technique for controlling variance due to extraneous variables is that of minimizing measurement error by using reliable methods of measurement under standardized conditions and by performing small sample pilot studies to reduce operator error. Since the methods of determining reliability of measurement are discussed in Appendix A, we will not pursue it further here. However, one way to improve measurement reliability is to employ experienced testers or technicians, and one of the best ways to get such experience is through completion of pilot studies that require the exact measurements to be employed in later large-scale experiments. Most novice investigators fail to recognize the importance of the pilot study until their large-scale experiment is over and they realize their efforts have largely been wasted because of poor measurement reliability due to a lack of experience with measurement techniques.

When possible, all measurements should be made under similar conditions for all groups of subjects. This principle is most important for physiological research where variability in temperature, time of day, humidity, diet, time of year, and surroundings can cause marked variation in such measures as heart rate, basal metabolism, endurance, strength, and ventilation. It is well known that similar factors as well as tester personality, method of giving instructions, and mental fatigue can influence investigations that utilize psychological or sociological measures. Although obvious in importance, this principle is often overlooked by those overly eager to compile data.

Problems

1. List two *scientific* hypotheses of interest to you and see if you can develop *statistical* hypotheses that might be used to support or reject your scientific hypotheses when adequately tested.

2. Using the statistical hypotheses developed in problem 1, show how type I and type II errors might be made when conclusions are based on sample data.

3. Design an experiment to test one of the hypotheses of problem 1 and then determine whether your design satisfies the criteria of a good experimental design as presented in this chapter.

4. List three examples of experiments when the control of an identifiable interfering variable by including it as a matching variable might be helpful in minimizing unwanted variance. Try to use examples with which you are familiar and avoid contriving unlikely experiments.

Chapter **7**

Simple linear correlation

MEANING OF CORRELATION

The topics considered in Chapters 2 and 3 enabled us to precisely describe a given distribution. However, in many cases it is highly useful to be able to determine the relationship, if any, that exists between two or more distributions. The coefficient of correlation (r) is a statistic used to express this type of relationship.

In Chapter 3 we discussed the central limit theorem, which explains why the types of measures we use in physical education are usually normally distributed. In this discussion we saw that any measure is really the end product of a large number of contributing factors. If we simply keep this in mind, we can see that any two distinct measures (e.g., push-ups and pull-ups) are each the sum of a number of different factors. Therefore some of the factors that contribute to one of these measures might be the same as some of the factors that contribute to the second measure. In our example of push-ups and pull-ups the primary factor being measured in each case is different. In the case of push-ups we are measuring the strength of the elbow extensors and in the case of pull-ups we are measuring the strength of the flexors. However, some of the other contributing factors such as general physical condition, nutritional level, and motivational level may be the same in both measures. Essentially, if most of the factors contributing to the first measure are the same as those contributing to the second measure, we would reasonably expect these two measures to be highly correlated. In its most basic sense the coefficient of correlation tells us the degree to which the factors contributing to two variables are associated.

REPRESENTING CORRELATION

The measurement of correlation requires not only a magnitude but also a direction. The value of a coefficient of correlation may lie anywhere between 0 and 1. Any value between these points would be a positive correlation. In addition, a coefficient of correlation may lie between 0 and -1. Any value between these points would be a negative correlation.

In the case of positive correlation an increase in the first variable corresponds to an increase in the second variable. In a negative correlation the opposite is true; as one variable increases, the second variable decreases. This can best be illustrated by Tables 7-1 and 7-2. In Table 7-1, eight subjects were measured on tests of push-ups and pull-ups. It can be seen that as each score on the push-up test goes up, the corresponding score on the pull-up test also goes up. This would then be a positive correlation.

In Table 7-2, eight different subjects were measured on these same tests, and in this case it can be seen that as the scores for individuals on the

Table 7-1

Subject	Push-ups (X)	Pull-ups (Y)
A	2	3
B	4	6
C	6	9
D	8	12
E	10	15
F	12	18
G	14	21
H	16	24

Table 7-2

Subject	Push-ups (X)	Pull-ups (Y)
I	1	14
J	3	13
K	5	12
L	7	11
M	9	10
N	11	9
O	13	8
P	15	7

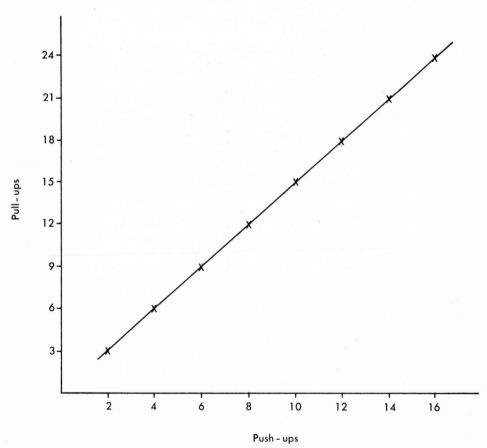

Fig. 7-1

push-up test go up, the corresponding scores on the pull-up test go down. This illustrates a negative correlation.

Having observed these relationships in Tables 7-1 and 7-2, which concern the direction of the correlations, we may now also make observations concerning the magnitude of these correlations. In Table 7-1, each increase in value of 2 units on the push-up test corresponds to an increase of 3 units on the pull-up test. This holds true throughout the table. For the data in Table 7-2, each increase in value of 2 units on the push-up test corresponds to a decrease of 1 unit on the pull-up test. Both of these correlations are called perfect correlations. Table 7-1 represents a perfect positive correlation, and Table 7-2 represents a perfect negative correlation.

If we were to construct a graph of the scores in Table 7-1 with the push-up scores on the X axis (abscissa) and the pull-up scores on the Y axis (ordinate), we could then draw a single straight line that connects all the points and rises as it moves to the right. The resulting graph is pictured in Fig. 7-1.

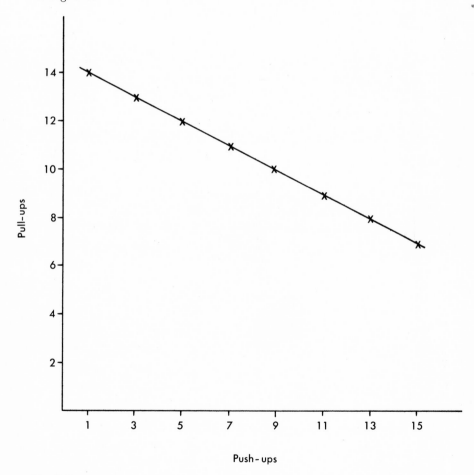

Push-ups

Fig. 7-2

If the same procedure were followed for the data in Table 7-2, the resulting graph would look like Fig. 7-2. Again, all the coordinates can be connected by a single straight line. In this case the line drops as it moves toward the right.

Thus, for a perfect linear correlation, either positive or negative in direction, a single straight line will intercept all the coordinates of the two variables. Of course, in actuality very few variables correlate perfectly, and we might imagine that any possible correlation (between −1.0 and 1.0)

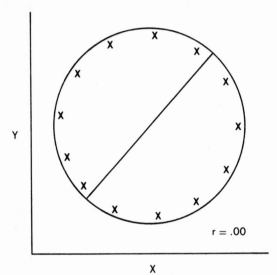

r = .00

Fig. 7-3

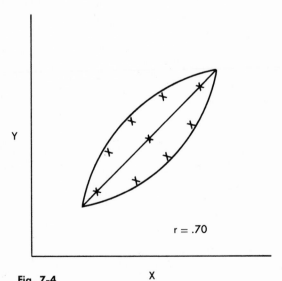

r = .70

Fig. 7-4

can be graphed in a fashion similar to those in Figs. 7-1 and 7-2. Perfect correlations will have every intercept lie on the line of best fit shown in the graphs. As a correlation becomes less than perfect (i.e., as the value of r moves from -1.0 or 1.0 toward 0), a smaller and smaller percentage of the intercepts will lie along this line. If we imagine an envelope enclosing these points, we see that as r approaches 0 (no correlation), this envelope will resemble a circle with the intercepts not fitting any single line (Fig. 7-3). Correspondingly, as r approaches 1.0 or -1.0 (Fig. 7-4), this envelope will become flatter until it collapses on the line when $r = 1.0$ or -1.0.

INTERPRETING r

The coefficient of correlation is, like other statistical terms, of little value unless it can be adequately interpreted. The first and least meaningful interpretation is simply to label the value of r. This labeling system is shown below:

$$0 \ \ r \le .19\text{—a slight correlation}$$
$$.20 \le r \le .39\text{—a low correlation}$$
$$.40 \le r \le .69\text{—a modest correlation}$$
$$.70 \le r \le .89\text{—a high correlation}$$
$$.90 \le r \le 1.00\text{—a very high correlation}$$

Obviously, merely describing a correlation as modest or high cannot truly be termed an interpretation of the correlation. To fully interpret r we must again think of the central limit theorem. Since any variables we may wish to correlate are the sum of a large number of contributing factors, it would be highly advantageous to be able to determine what percentage of the factors contributing to two variables are associated.

The coefficients of determination and nondetermination are used to more fully interpret r. Let us take an example of a correlation between height (X) and weight (Y) of men. Let us hypothetically assume that in this case $r = .80$. The coefficient of determination is obtained by squaring r, and the coefficient of nondetermination is simply $1 - r^2$. In our example the coefficient of determination is $.80^2 = .64$, and the coefficient of nondetermination is $1 - .64 = .36$. This is interpreted to mean that 64% of the variance in Y is related to the variance in X and that 36% of the variance in Y is not related to the variance in X.

In correlation problems one variable is called the dependent or Y variable, and the other is called the independent or X variable. The use of r^2 and $1 - r^2$ obviously gives us far more information about the degree of relationship existing between two variables than does the labeling procedure just described. Note that the coefficients of determination and nondetermination are not affected by the sign that precedes r (i.e., whether the correlation is positive or negative), since the value is squared. Thus two variables with $r = -.80$ would have precisely the same relationship as in the previous example.

Another method often used to interpret r is known as the predictive index (P.I.). The predictive index tells us how much better we would be in predicting Y if X were known than if X were unknown, and our prediction were based purely on chance. Following is the formula for the predictive index:

$$P.I. = 1 - \sqrt{1 - r^2}$$

$$\frac{PI}{2} + 50 = at\ \%$$

The values of the predictive index for selected values of r are shown in Table 7-3.

Table 7-3

r	P.I.	not ratio	r	P.I.
.05	.002		.55	.165
.10	.005		.60	.200
.15	.012		.65	.240
.20	.020		.70	.286
.25	.032		.75	.338
.30	.046		.80	.400
.35	.064		.85	.474
.40	.083		.90	.564
.45	.107		.95	.668
.50	.134		1.00	1.000

Table 7-3 also lets us make another observation about r. A glance at the table shows us that there is not a linear relationship between the value of r and its predictive index. For example, an r of .90 is not merely three times as good as an r of .30 as a predictive measure, but is more than twelve times as good. However, an r of .30 is still 4.6% better than chance as a predictive measure, whereas an r of .90 is 56.4% better than guessing.

Finally, there is the statistical criterion of significance, which was discussed in Chapter 6. It is important to understand that it is possible to obtain a value of r other than 0 even when *no* correlation actually exists. This may come about due to chance alone, and there are tables available that tell us what value of r must be obtained before we can assume that some linear correlation actually does exist between two variables. See Table C-5 in Appendix C. The first column refers to the degrees of freedom, which equal $N-2$. For example, if we had twenty-seven *pairs* of scores we would have 25 degrees of freedom (d.f.). We can now see from Table C-5 that it would be necessary to have $r=.381$ or higher if we wished to assume that some linear correlation truly existed between twenty-seven pairs of scores if we are using the .05 level of significance. Likewise, if we are using the .01 level of confidence in a case where there are eighty-two pairs of scores, we would have to have $r=.283$ or higher to assume that the correlation is not merely due to chance. We may also note from the table that as the value of N increases (i.e., as the sample size increases), the value of r needed for significance at a given level decreases.

COMPUTING r

The computation of r will be presented in two different forms. First, we shall use the straight formula method, and then we shall proceed by what is known as the scattergram method. We shall use the data in Table

7-4 as an illustration of both methods. These are scores on a push-up test (X) and a sit-up test (Y) for high school boys.

Table 7-4

X	Y	X	Y	X	Y	X	Y
9	25	15	17	15	33	11	36
12	38	10	13	10	31	18	58
2	23	5	26	3	13	14	29
11	38	18	47	12	27	10	20
8	33	6	35	16	28	7	18
7	16	15	46	21	47	7	17
11	27	2	2	19	32	9	29
10	45	17	49	12	14	16	14
13	26	9	37	13	32	4	24
1	6	12	31	4	30	17	20
14	40	5	8	17	32	6	23
10	24	13	23	8	41		
7	13	8	13	16	41		

Following is the formula used to determine r:

$$r = \sqrt{\frac{[N\Sigma XY - (\Sigma X)(\Sigma Y)]^2}{[N\Sigma X^2 - (\Sigma X)^2][N\Sigma Y^2 - (\Sigma Y)^2]}}$$

Although this may seem like a rather frightening formula at first, we see that there are only six values needed to compute r. These six values are N, ΣX, ΣX^2, ΣY, ΣY^2 and ΣXY. Each of these values is easily obtained if we set our data up as shown in Table 7-5. We compute N simply by counting the number of pairs of scores. In the present example, $N = 50$.

The computation of r is as follows:

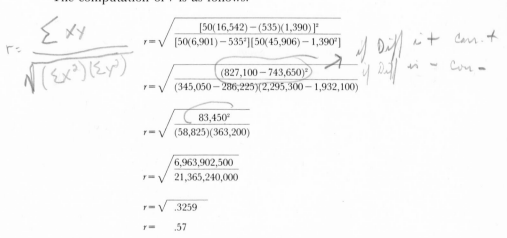

$$r = \sqrt{\frac{[50(16,542) - (535)(1,390)]^2}{[50(6,901) - 535^2][50(45,906) - 1,390^2]}}$$

$$r = \sqrt{\frac{(827,100 - 743,650)^2}{(345,050 - 286,225)(2,295,300 - 1,932,100)}}$$

$$r = \sqrt{\frac{83,450^2}{(58,825)(363,200)}}$$

$$r = \sqrt{\frac{6,963,902,500}{21,365,240,000}}$$

$$r = \sqrt{.3259}$$

$$r = .57$$

This method of computing r will serve in all cases, but it is quite obvious that it is most suitable when a desk calculator is available. On some calculators it is possible to obtain all six values needed for the formula by one entry of data into the machine. Many colleges and universities have a statistics laboratory and instruction in the use of desk calculators available

Table 7-5

X	Y	X^2	Y^2	XY
9	25	81	625	225
12	38	144	1,444	456
2	23	4	529	46
11	38	121	1,444	418
8	33	64	1,089	264
7	16	49	256	112
11	27	121	729	297
10	45	100	2,025	450
13	26	169	676	338
1	6	1	36	6
14	40	196	1,600	560
10	24	100	576	240
7	13	49	169	91
15	17	225	289	255
10	13	100	169	130
5	26	25	676	130
18	47	324	2,209	846
6	35	36	1,225	210
15	46	225	2,136	690
2	2	4	4	4
17	49	289	2,401	833
9	37	81	1,369	333
12	31	144	961	372
5	8	25	64	40
13	23	169	529	299
8	13	64	169	104
15	33	225	1,089	495
10	31	100	961	310
3	13	9	169	39
12	27	144	729	324
16	28	256	784	448
21	47	441	2,209	987
19	32	361	1,024	608
12	14	144	196	168
13	32	169	1,024	416
4	30	16	900	120
17	32	289	1,024	544
8	41	64	1,681	328
16	41	256	1,681	656
11	36	121	1,296	396
18	58	324	3,364	1,044
14	29	196	841	406
10	20	100	400	200
7	18	49	324	126
7	17	49	289	119
9	29	81	841	261
16	14	256	196	224
4	24	16	576	96
17	20	289	400	340
6	23	36	529	138
$\Sigma X = 535$	$\Sigma Y = 1,390$	$\Sigma X^2 = 6,901$	$\Sigma Y^2 = 45,906$	$\Sigma XY = 16,542$

to students on a nonfee basis, and the student is advised to learn about and make use of this facility.

When a desk calculator is not available and the data are extensive, the scattergram method may be used to compute r. We shall again use the data presented in Table 7-4 for our example.

1. Our first step is to choose appropriate step intervals for the X and Y data. In this case we shall use intervals of 2 and 5, respectively. The data are then entered as shown in Table 7-6. There is *one* tally mark entered in the table for each coordinate of scores. For example, the first pair of scores is 9 (X) and 25 (Y), and this is entered in the intersecting box of 8-9 along the top (X) and 25-29 along the left (Y). Each pair of scores is tallied in similar fashion. The total number of tally marks in the table is equal to N and equal to the number of pairs of scores.

2. We next complete the table by heading the last columns across the top f, y', fy', fy'^2, and $\Sigma fx'y'$. This last column is further subdivided into a column headed $+$ and another headed $-$. The same is done along the left-hand column, with x in place of y.

3. Fill in the f (frequency) column for X and Y by adding the number of tally marks down and across, respectively. The sum of the column equals the sum of the row and is N.

4. Guess a mean for the X variable and another for the Y variable. It is generally easiest to guess the means over the column and row that have the greatest frequency. We will guess 25-29 (i.e., 27) and 10-11 (i.e., 10.5) as our X and Y means. Rule off this column and row again to separate it visually from the others.

5. The value for x' is determined by starting at the interval containing the guessed mean and labeling it 0. Each successive interval to the right increases by $+1$ and each successive interval to the left increases by -1. Thus x' is the value of the deviation of the variable X in terms of the number of intervals from the guessed mean, regardless of the size of the interval. The same is done for the y' column, and in this case we increase by $+1$ as we go up the column and by -1 as we go down the column.

6. The fx' row is completed by multiplying the value of f by the corresponding value of x'. Sum this row to find $\Sigma fx'$. Do the same to find $\Sigma fy'$.

7. The fx'^2 row is completed by multiplying the value of fx' by the corresponding value of x'. Sum this row to find $\Sigma fx'^2$. Do the same to find $\Sigma fy'^2$.

8. Find $\Sigma fx'y'$ in the following manner:
   a. For each box, multiply the value of x' by the corresponding value of y' and enter this figure in the upper left-hand corner of the box. Notice that all the values in the upper right and lower left quadrants are positive and all the values in the upper left and lower right quadrants are negative. Also notice that the column and row over the guessed means have no value.

Table 7-6

Y \ X	0-1	2-3	4-5	6-7	8-9	10-11	12-13	14-15	16-17	18-19	20-21	f	y'	fy'	fy'²	Σfx'y' (+)	Σfx'y' (−)
55-59	-30	-24	-18	-12	-6		6	12	18	24 ⌒1	30 ⌒1 (20)	1	6	6	36	24	—
50-54	-25	-20	-15	-10	-5		5	10	15	20 ⌒(24)	25	0	5	0	0	0	0
45-49	-20	-16	-12	-8	-4	1	4	8 ⌒1	12 ⌒1	16 ⌒1	20 ⌒1 (20)	5	4	20	80	56	0
40-44	-15	-12	-9	-6	-3 ⌒1(-3)	1 1	3	6 ⌒1	9 ⌒1(9)	12 ⌒1(16)	15	3	3	9	27	15	0
35-39	-10	-8	-6	-4	-2 ⌒1(-2)	1	2	4 ⌒1(6)	6 ⌒1	8	10	5	2	10	20	2	-3
30-34	-5	-4	-3 ⌒1(-3)	-2 ⌒1(-4)	-1 ⌒1(-1)	1	1 1	2 ⌒1(2)	3 ⌒1	4 ⌒1(4)	5	8	1	8	8	11	-6
25-29	0	0	0	0	1 1	1 1	1 1	1	1			8	0	0	0	0	-4
20-24	5	4	3 ⌒1	2 1	1		-1 ⌒1(-1)	-2	-3 ⌒1(-3)	-4	-5	7	-1	-7	7	9	0
15-19	10	8	6	4 111(12)	2		-2	-4 1 ⌒(-4)	-6	-8	-10	4	-2	-8	16	12	-4

X \ Y	0-1	2-3	4-5	6-7	8-9	10-11	12-13	14-15	16-17	18-19	20-21	f	y'	fy'	fy'^2	$\Sigma fx'y'$ +	$\Sigma fx'y'$ −
10-14	15	2 / 12	9	6	3	1	-3	-6	-9	-12	-15	6	-3	-18	54	21	-12
5-9	20 / 1	16	12 / 1	8 / 1 6	4 / 1 3	1	1 / -3	-8	1 / -9 -12	-16	-20	2	-4	-8	32	32	0
0-4	25 / 1	20 / 1 20	15 / 1 12	10	5		-5	-10	-15	-20	-25	1	-5	-5	25	20	0
f	1	3	4	6	6	8	7	5	6	3	1	$\Sigma = 50 = N$		$\Sigma = 7$	$\Sigma = 305$	$\Sigma = 202$	$\Sigma = -33$
x'	-5	-4	-3	-2	-1	0	1	2	3	4	5						
fx'	-5	-12	-12	-12	-6	0	7	10	18	12	5	$\Sigma = 5$					
fx'^2	25	48	36	24	6	0	7	20	54	48	25	$\Sigma = 293$					
+	20	36	15	20	3	0	4	16	24	44	20	$\Sigma = 202$					
−	0	0	-3	-4	-6	0	-4	-4	-12	0	0	$\Sigma = -33$					

$\Sigma fx'y'$

b. For each box containing tally marks, multiply the number in the upper left-hand corner of the box by the number of tallies and set this value in the lower right-hand corner of the box. Be sure the sign ($+$ or $-$) is correct. It is wise to set off this number by placing a quarter circle around it.

c. For the $+$ column, place the total number in each box reading across the page. Do the same for the $-$ column. Sum each of these. The difference is $\Sigma fx'y'$. There is no real need to do this for the $+$ and $-$ rows, but, since the value of $\Sigma fx'y'$ must be the same both ways, it serves as a check. In this case $\Sigma fx'y' = 202 - 33 = 169$.

9. We now have all necessary values and are ready to use the formula

$$r = \frac{\dfrac{\Sigma fx'y'}{N} - Cx'Cy'}{Sx'Sy'}$$

where

$$Cx' = \frac{\Sigma fx'}{N} \qquad\qquad Sx' = \sqrt{\frac{\Sigma fx'^2}{N} - Cx'^2}$$

$$Cy' = \frac{\Sigma fy'}{N} \qquad\qquad Sy' = \sqrt{\frac{\Sigma fy'^2}{N} - Cy'^2}$$

10. The calculations in our example are

$$Cx' = \frac{5}{50} = .1 \qquad\qquad Sx' = \sqrt{\frac{293}{50} - (.1)^2} = \sqrt{5.85} = 2.42$$

$$Cy' = \frac{7}{50} = .14 \qquad\qquad Sy' = \sqrt{\frac{305}{50} - (.14)^2} = \sqrt{6.08} = 2.47$$

and substituting these values in our formula we get the following:

$$r = \frac{\dfrac{169}{50} - (.1)(.14)}{(2.42)(2.47)}$$

$$r = \frac{3.37}{5.98}$$

$$r = .56$$

It is worth noting at this point that the value of r obtained by the two methods is not precisely the same. Theoretically they should be, but in using the scattergram method we used the midpoint of each interval for X and Y as representative of all the scores in that interval. In reality, this may not be precisely correct, and the resulting discrepancy in scores thus occurs. Therefore the straight formula method is most accurate and is to be preferred when a calculator is available or the data are not too extensive.

Problems

1. Use the machine formula to find the coefficient of correlation for the following X (sit-up) and Y (push-up) data.

X	Y	X	Y
44	28	36	22
16	10	32	26
22	16	18	13
21	18	39	21
28	19	34	30

2. The following X (height) and Y (weight) data were obtained from twenty high school boys. Use the scattergram method to find the coefficient of correlation for these data.

X	Y	X	Y
60	124	68	180
73	200	61	120
65	140	60	141
67	185	68	166
72	208	74	187
70	165	67	182
70	173	72	190
71	197	63	145
62	135	75	208
69	163	70	190

3. The following X (basketball season scoring average) and Y (average number of turnovers) data were obtained from the eight members of a college conference. Use the machine formula to determine the coefficient of correlation.

X	Y	X	Y
78	16.5	60	11
82	14	63	15.5
75	18	81	21
90	12	67	16.3.5

4. Use the scattergram method to determine the coefficient of correlation between the following X (average number of yards penalized per game) and Y (average number of yards gained per game) data obtained from the eighteen members of two college conferences.

X	Y	X	Y
70	243	78	318
45	158	85	287
65	162	101	262
110	188	109	305
86	197	94	209
94	200	89	218
120	182	100	230
103	290	87	255
90	365	112	246

5. Describe in your own words the meaning of coefficient of correlation, coefficient of determination, and predictive index.

6. Interpret in as many ways as possible the following coefficients of correlation:

a.	.80	f.	1.00
b.	.66	g.	.72
c.	−.50	h.	−.21
d.	.42	i.	.90
e.	−.13	j.	−1.00

7. Determine if the following coefficients of correlation, with the associated N, are significant at the .01 and .05 levels:

a.	.61, $N=16$	f.	−.87, $N=7$
b.	−.36, $N=25$	g.	−.25, $N=50$
c.	.90, $N=6$	h.	.58, $N=18$
d.	.43, $N=32$	i.	.12, $N=100$
e.	.24, $N=50$	j.	−.79, $N=12$

Chapter **8**

Simple linear regression

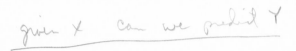

given X   can we predict Y

To begin our discussion of simple linear regression let us look at the data in Table 8-1. We can see that each Y value is 1.5 times the corresponding value of X. We can state this in a general equation

$$Y = bX$$

where $b = 1.5$ is a constant multiplying each value of X to determine the corresponding value of Y.

Table 8-1

Subject	Push-ups (X)	Pull-ups (Y)
A	2	3
B	4	6
C	6	9
D	8	12
E	10	15
F	12	18
G	14	21
H	16	24

The values of X and Y are not so obviously related in the data of Table 8-2. The general equation relating each value of X to its corresponding value of Y can be stated

$$Y = a + bX$$

where b is some constant multiplying each value of X, and a is also some constant that we add to the product of bX to obtain the corresponding value of Y.

Table 8-2

Subject	Push-ups (X)	Pull-ups (Y)
A	1	14
B	3	13
C	5	12
D	7	11
E	9	10
F	11	9
G	13	8
H	15	7

For the data in Table 8-2, $a=14.5$ and $b=-.5$. Thus, to find the value of Y when $X=5$,

$$Y=a+bX$$
$$Y=14.5+(-.5)(5)$$
$$Y=14.5-2.5$$
$$Y=12$$

which is precisely the value of Y in our original data. Since both these cases represent perfect correlations, all the points for X and Y fall on a single straight line. If we were to graph the data in Table 8-1, we would see that each time there is an increase of 2 units on the X axis, there is a corresponding increase of 3 units on the Y axis. We can state that b indicates the rate at which Y changes with change in X, and this can be determined directly from our graph in Fig. 8-1. Let us choose any two consecutive points on the line with the coordinates (X_1, Y_1) and (X_2, Y_2); then:

$$b=\frac{Y_2-Y_1}{X_2-X_1}$$

If we choose the coordinates (8, 12) and (10, 15), we have the following:

$$b=\frac{15-12}{10-8}$$

$$b=1.5$$

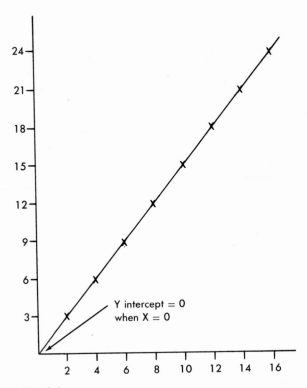

Fig. 8-1

The value of b is geometrically termed the slope of a straight line. Knowing b we can readily determine a by setting X equal to zero. The value of a is thus the value of Y when X is zero and can be graphically determined by extension of the regression line and is actually the Y intercept of the line (see Figs. 8-1 and 8-2). Notice that in the data representing a positive correlation the slope of the regression line is positive and that in the data representing a negative correlation the slope of the regression line is negative. In both cases just discussed, the correlations are perfect, and we can perfectly predict Y, given X, with our formula. In actual practice such correlations are rarely, if ever, found. In many cases the trend is linear, but all points will not fall precisely on the regression line.

The line of best fit, which best relates Y to X, is known as the regression line of Y on X. The equation used to represent this line is called a regression equation, and the value of b in this equation is called the regression coefficient. If we are not dealing with a perfect correlation between X and Y, our formula is

$$\widetilde{Y} = a + bX$$

where $\widetilde{Y}$ (Y tilde or predicted Y) is a value of Y given by the regression equation. This is not always equal to the observed value of Y corresponding

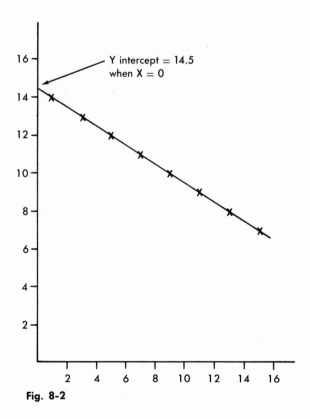

Fig. 8-2

to a given value of X. If $\tilde{Y}$ is the predicted value of Y, an error of prediction is the following:

$$Y - \tilde{Y} = Y - (a + bX)$$

We shall use the least squares method to determine the line of best fit. This means that we wish a and b to be those values that will make the sum of squares for errors of prediction less than for any other values. In other words

$$\Sigma(Y - \tilde{Y})^2 = \Sigma[Y - (a + bX)]^2$$

must be minimal. We will not develop this point but will simply present the final derived equations:

$$b = \frac{\Sigma XY - \dfrac{(\Sigma X)(\Sigma Y)}{N}}{\Sigma X^2 - \dfrac{(\Sigma X)^2}{N}}$$

$$a = \bar{Y} - b\bar{X}$$

If we now expand the data in Table 8-2, we have the values $\Sigma X = 64$, $\Sigma Y = 84$, $\Sigma X^2 = 680$, $\Sigma XY = 588$, $\bar{X} = 8$, $\bar{Y} = 10.5$, and $N = 8$. The student is advised to verify these values by his own computations. To obtain the value of b:

$$b = \frac{588 - \dfrac{(64)(84)}{8}}{680 - \dfrac{(64)^2}{8}}$$

$$b = \frac{-84}{168}$$

$$b = -.5$$

To obtain the value of a:

$$a = 10.5 - (-.5)(8)$$
$$a = 10.5 + 4 \cdot$$
$$a = 14.5$$

For the data in Table 8-2 our regression equation is

$$\tilde{Y} = 14.5 + (-.5)X$$

which we can use to predict the value of Y given a value of X. For example, for $X = 6$:

$$\tilde{Y} = 14.5 + (-.5)(6)$$
$$\tilde{Y} = 14.5 - 3$$
$$\tilde{Y} = 11.5$$

The regression equation may also be determined by using the values of x and y, which are especially helpful when the raw scores are large. (Note that in using deviations from the means of two distributions, it will be

$$r = \frac{\Sigma xy}{\sqrt{(\Sigma x^2)(\Sigma y^2)}}$$

simpler to use the notation x=deviations from the mean of the X distribution and y=deviations from the mean of the Y distribution than the term d as used in Chapter 4.) If we again look at the formula for the regression coefficient

$$b = \frac{\Sigma XY - \dfrac{(\Sigma X)(\Sigma Y)}{N}}{\Sigma X^2 - \dfrac{(\Sigma X)^2}{N}}$$

we can see that the denominator is the sum of the squared deviations of X from $\bar{X}$. We may simply call this value Σx^2. The numerator is the sum of the products of the deviations of X and Y from $\bar{X}$ and $\bar{Y}$, respectively. We may simply call this value Σxy. Therefore:

$$b = \frac{\Sigma xy}{\Sigma x^2}$$

short formula used

To illustrate, let us determine the value of b for the data in Table 8-2 by this formula. The full data are shown in Table 8-3.

Table 8-3

X	Y	x	y	xy	x²
1	14	−7	3.5	−24.5	49
3	13	−5	2.5	−12.5	25
5	12	−3	1.5	−4.5	9
7	11	−1	.5	−.5	1
9	10	1	−.5	−.5	1
11	9	3	−1.5	−4.5	9
13	8	5	−2.5	−12.5	25
15	7	7	−3.5	−24.5	49
$\bar{X}=8$	$\bar{Y}=10.5$			$\Sigma=-84$	$\Sigma=168$

Substituting these values into our formula we get

$$b = \frac{-84}{168}$$

$$b = -.5$$

which is the same value obtained by use of the first formula for b.

STANDARD ERROR OF ESTIMATE

The standard error of estimate is a measure of the variability of the Y values about the regression line of Y on X. The formula for standard error of estimate is

$$S_{Y \cdot X} = \sqrt{\frac{\Sigma(Y-\tilde{Y})^2}{N-2}}$$

where

$$\Sigma(Y-\tilde{Y})^2 = \Sigma Y^2 - \frac{(\Sigma XY)^2}{\Sigma X^2}$$

✓ small letters

$$\Sigma(Y-\tilde{Y})^2 = \Sigma y^2 - \frac{(\Sigma xy)^2}{\Sigma x^2}$$

small letter

For the data in Table 8-3 the value for ΣY^2 is 42. The student is advised to verify this for himself. Using these values we have

$$\Sigma(Y-\tilde{Y})^2 = 42 - \frac{(-84)^2}{168}$$

$$\Sigma(Y-\tilde{Y})^2 = 42 - 42$$

$$\Sigma(Y-\tilde{Y})^2 = 0$$

and

$$S_{Y \cdot X} = \sqrt{\frac{0}{6}}$$

$$S_{Y \cdot X} = 0$$

Since the data we are using for our example represent a perfect correlation, we would expect $S_{Y \cdot X} = 0$ because this means the Y values do not vary at all about the regression line of Y on X.

We may also determine the standard error of estimate by

$$S_{Y \cdot X} = S_Y \sqrt{1 - r^2}$$

when we know the standard deviation of the Y variable, and N is a large number ($> 1,000$). If N is less than 1,000, the formula just stated gives us a biased value for standard error of estimate that will generally underestimate the true value of $S_{Y \cdot X}$. To correct for this bias, we will use the formula:

$$S_{Y \cdot X} = \sqrt{\frac{N-1}{N-2}} \; S_Y \sqrt{1 - r^2}$$

It can be seen that the value of $N-1/N-2$ approaches unity as N becomes larger. Therefore the first term drops out when $N > 1,000$ and we have the formula introduced above.

We may interpret standard error of estimate in a way that is analogous to standard scores. Let us assume we have variables X and Y with the following values for the regression equation:

$$b = .5 \qquad a = 3 \qquad S_{Y \cdot X} = 2$$

The regression equation for Y on X is therefore:

$$\tilde{Y} = 3 + .5X$$

If we wish to predict a value of Y that will correspond to a given value of $X = 8$ we have the following:

$$\tilde{Y} = 3 + .5(8)$$
$$\tilde{Y} = 7$$

This is our best predicted value of Y for $X = 8$. Since $S_{Y \cdot X} = 2$, we may further state that approximately 68% of the distribution of values for Y when $X = 8$ will lie between $\tilde{Y} \pm S_{Y \cdot X}$ or between the values of 5 and 9. Stated in another way, we are 68% confident that the Y score corresponding to $X = 8$ is between the values of 5 and 9.

Problems

1. Determine the regression equation for the following data by means of both formulas.

X	Y	X	Y
13	8	15	4
12	10	7	20
8	18	9	16
10	14	6	22
11	12	14	6

2. For the data in problem 1, determine the value of the Y intercept of the regression line by means of a graph.
3. What value of the regression equation found in problem 1 is the Y intercept equal to?
4. For the data in problem 1, what value would you predict for Y when $X = 20$?
5. What is the standard error of estimate for the data in problem 1? Is this reasonable? Why?
6. Given the following X (height) and Y (vertical jump score) data, find the regression equation by means of both formulas.

X	Y	X	Y
68	20	70	24
70	23	67	20
68	25	71	21
66	15	74	26
75	21	63	18
70	22	71	22
69	19	72	20
65	19		

7. What would be the predicted value of Y for the data in problem 6 when $X = 76, 60, 75, 62, 73$?
8. What would be the predicted value of Y for the data in problem 6 when $X = 68, 70, 72, 74$?
9. Are the predicted values of Y in problem 9 the same as the observed values of Y? Is this reasonable? Why?
10. What is the standard error of estimate for the data in problem 6?
11. Between what values would you be approximately 68% confident of finding Y when $X = 60, 64, 62, 70$?

Chapter **9**

Chi square

The chi square (χ^2) test is used in cases where our concern is primarily with how many subjects, measurements, objects, and so on fall into each of a number of categories. These categories might be exemplified by:

1. Number of students who pass or fail a test
2. An animal choosing one of three doors in a maze
3. Schools using brand A, B, C, or D basketballs

In problems such as these, where we are dealing with the *observed* number of cases in various categories, we may test any null hypothesis from which we can predict an *expected* number of cases. In the general cases of k categories we would expect N/k observations in each category. For instance, let us assume a case in which we sample 500 coaches as to whether they prefer the National or American Football League for exciting play. If the null hypothesis were true, we would expect to find 250 who choose the NFL and 250 who choose the AFL. Of course, we would not expect to find exactly these numbers. Our real question is, how far from these expected frequencies may our responses be and still allow us to consider the null hypothesis as acceptable? Chi square tells us whether our *observed frequencies differ significantly from our expected frequencies*. Essentially, our interest is in the magnitude of differences between observed and expected frequencies. For our computational form, we find the difference between each observed and expected frequency, square these differences, divide this value by the expected frequency, and sum to find the chi square. Mathematically we state this as

$$\chi^2 = \sum_{i=1}^{k} \frac{(F_o - F_E)^2}{F_E}$$

where χ^2 = chi square, F_o = observed frequency in each category, and F_E = expected frequency in each category.

In our present example let us assume that $\alpha = .05$ or that we are willing to accept a 5% risk of rejecting a true null hypothesis. If we find 275 coaches who prefer the NFL and 225 coaches who prefer the AFL, our computations are as follows:

(1)

$$\chi^2 = \frac{(275-250)^2}{250} + \frac{(225-250)^2}{250}$$

$$\chi^2 = \frac{625}{250} + \frac{625}{250}$$

$$\chi^2 = 2.5 + 2.5$$

$$\chi^2 = 5.0$$

To determine if this value of χ^2 indicates whether the null hypothesis is tenable, we must compare it to tabled χ^2 values. To do this we must know the number of degrees of freedom with which to enter the table. We use the term degrees of freedom to denote pieces of information independent of each other or which cannot be deduced from each other. In the present example, since we have 500 subjects in our study, if we know the number of coaches favoring the NFL, we could deduce the number favoring the AFL. Therefore we may say that the first of our two frequencies is free to vary but that the second is not. In other words, if we knew one frequency, we could deduce the other. In this case we have 1 degree of freedom. In general, the number of degrees of freedom in this type of problem $= k-1$, where k is the number of possible categories. Entering Table C-7, Appendix C we see that the tabled value of χ^2 with 1 degree of freedom and with $\alpha = .05$ is 3.84146. Since our derived value of χ^2 exceeds the tabled value, we may reject the null hypothesis with 95% certainty that differences between observed and expected frequencies of the magnitude found in this example did not occur by chance. Another way of saying this is that we are 95% certain that a real factor of choice is in operation and that the results obtained are not due merely to chance. The same procedure is followed in cases where more than two categories are used.

Example: A ticket manager for athletic events wishes to know if patrons have a preference for sitting in any particular section of a football stadium. He questions 100 people and finds their preferences are North, 30; South, 20; East, 10; West, 40. Are these responses within the limits you would expect due to only chance factors being in operation?

	North	South	East	West
F_O	30	20	10	40
F_E	25	25	25	25

(2)

$$\chi^2 = \frac{(30-25)^2}{25} + \frac{(20-25)^2}{25} + \frac{(10-25)^2}{25} + \frac{(40-25)^2}{25}$$

$$\chi^2 = \frac{25}{25} + \frac{25}{25} + \frac{225}{25} + \frac{225}{25}$$

$$\chi^2 = 1+1+9+9$$

$$\chi^2 = 20$$

Entering our table with degrees of freedom $= k - 1 = 3$ and $\alpha = .05$, we find $\chi^2 = 7.815$. Since $20 > 7.815$, we reject the null hypothesis.

CONTINGENCY TABLES

In the same concept of categorical classification, the individual's interest may often concern two variables rather than one as in the preceding discussion. In this case our interest is in whether the two variables are dependent or independent. As an example let us consider the variable of sex as related to agreeing or disagreeing with a proposal that physical education should be required of all students in college. To determine if any relationship exists, we sample 120 men and 80 women. The results are shown in Table 9-1, which is termed a contingency table.

Table 9-1

	Agree	Disagree	Totals
Male	75	45	120
Female	35	45	80
Totals	110	90	200

We can see that 75 men and 35 women agree with the proposal, and 45 men and 45 women disagree. The marginal totals for columns are 110 and 90, and the marginal totals for rows are 120 and 80. Again we are interested in determining if the observed frequencies in each cell differ significantly from the expected frequencies. Our computations will be essentially the same as in the case of one variable. However, we must first determine the expected frequency for each cell. To do this we will make use of the marginal totals. Notice that 110 of the 200 subjects in our sample favor the proposal. To determine the expected frequency for the cells in column 1 we multiply 110/200 by the total number of males to give us F_E for cell 1. The same is done for cell 3 by multiplying 110/200 by the total number of females. For the cells in column 2 we multiply 90/200 by the total number of males to find F_E for cell 2 and then multiply 90/200 by the total number of females to find F_E for cell 4. The complete contingency table with expected frequencies in parentheses is shown in Table 9-2.

Table 9-2

	Agree	Disagree	Totals
Male	75 (66)	45 (54)	120
Female	35 (44)	45 (36)	80
Totals	110	90	200

To compute χ^2 we again square the differences between observed and expected frequencies, divide each of these values by its expected value, and sum. Thus our computational formula is

$$\chi^2 = \sum_{i=1}^{r} \sum_{i=1}^{k} \frac{(F_o - F_E)^2}{F_E}$$

where F_o = observed frequency in each cell and F_E = expected frequency in each cell. For our data the computations are as follows:

(3)
$$\chi^2 = \frac{(75-66)^2}{66} + \frac{(45-54)^2}{54} + \frac{(35-44)^2}{44} + \frac{(45-36)^2}{36}$$

$$\chi^2 = \frac{81}{66} + \frac{81}{54} + \frac{81}{44} + \frac{81}{36}$$

$$\chi^2 = 1.22 + 1.50 + 1.84 + 2.25$$

$$\chi^2 = 6.81$$

We now enter the χ^2 table with $(k-1)(r-1) = (1)(1) = 1$ degree of freedom. When $\alpha = .05$, our table value = 3.841. Since $6.81 > 3.841$, we must reject the null hypothesis. Our conclusion is that sex and agreement or disagreement with the proposal are not independent. The reader is urged to note that, given the restriction of the marginal totals, knowing the value of any of the four cells leads to deducing the value of the other three cells. Therefore we have only 1 degree of freedom as previously stated. The same procedure is followed in cases where one or both variables contain more than two categories.

Example: To determine if educational level and leisure time activities are related, we surveyed 300 subjects. We categorized educational level as those with college degrees and those without college degrees. Leisure time activities are categorized as vigorous activities, quiet activities, and no activity. The observed and expected frequencies are presented in Table 9-3.

Table 9-3

	Vigorous	Quiet	None	Totals
With	80 (45)	10 (27)	10 (28)	100
Without	55 (90)	70 (53)	75 (57)	200
Totals	135	80	85	300

(4)
$$\chi^2 = \frac{(80-45)^2}{45} + \frac{(10-27)^2}{27} + \frac{(10-28)^2}{28} + \frac{(55-90)^2}{90} + \frac{(70-53)^2}{53} + \frac{(75-57)^2}{57}$$

$$\chi^2 = \frac{1,225}{45} + \frac{289}{27} + \frac{324}{28} + \frac{1,225}{90} + \frac{289}{53} + \frac{324}{57}$$

$$\chi^2 = 27.22 + 10.70 + 11.57 + 13.61 + 5.45 + 5.68$$

$$\chi^2 = 74.23$$

The tabled value of x^2 with $(2)(1) = 2$ degrees of freedom and with $\alpha = .05$ is 5.991. Since $74.23 > 5.991$, we may reject the null hypothesis and assume that educational level and leisure time activity are related.

CORRECTION FOR CONTINUITY

It can be shown that in cases where there is only 1 degree of freedom (i.e., in the case where there are only two categories or where there is a 2 by 2 contingency table), the usual method of computing chi square gives too large a value. The net effect is, of course, to cause rejection of the null hypothesis when this is not actually justified. To compensate for this, correction for continuity, or Yates' correction, is employed. The correction for continuity is accomplished simply by subtracting .5 from the absolute value of the difference between expected and observed frequencies, prior to squaring the difference. This will lower the generated value of chi square. As an example of how the correction for continuity works, let us recompute examples 1 and 3 in this chapter.

Example 1

$$\chi^2 = \frac{(275-250-.5)^2}{250} + \frac{(225-250-.5)^2}{250}$$

$$\chi^2 = \frac{(25-.5)^2}{250} + \frac{(25-.5)^2}{250}$$

$$\chi^2 = \frac{24.5^2}{250} + \frac{24.5^2}{250}$$

$$\chi^2 = \frac{600.25}{250} + \frac{600.25}{250}$$

$$\chi^2 = 2.401 + 2.401$$

$$\chi^2 = 4.802$$

Example 3

$$\chi^2 = \frac{(75-66-.5)^2}{66} + \frac{(45-54-.5)^2}{54} + \frac{(35-44-.5)^2}{44} + \frac{(45-36-.5)^2}{36}$$

$$\chi^2 = \frac{8.5^2}{66} + \frac{8.5^2}{54} + \frac{8.5^2}{44} + \frac{8.5^2}{36}$$

$$\chi^2 = \frac{72.25}{66} + \frac{72.25}{54} + \frac{72.25}{44} + \frac{72.25}{36}$$

$$\chi^2 = 1.09 + 1.33 + 1.64 + 2.00$$

$$\chi^2 = 6.06$$

Note that in both cases the new value of chi square, obtained using the correction for continuity, is lower than the original value obtained without this correction.

Problems

1. You have given a true-false test to a student. The test contains eighty items and the student has answered forty-six items correctly. Do you think the student studied at all for the test?
2. You have rolled a single die ninty times and have recorded the following results:

Number 1, 12 rolls	Number 4, 18 rolls
Number 2, 18 rolls	Number 5, 15 rolls
Number 3, 10 rolls	Number 6, 17 rolls

   Is this within the limits you would expect due to chance?
3. A player tosses darts at a 5-circle target. The first forty tosses that hit one of the circles are counted. The colors hit are as follows:

Red, 10 hits	White, 7 hits	Green, 9 hits
Yellow, 6 hits	Blue, 8 hits	

   If the player is trying to hit the red circle and all circles are of equal size, do you think he is exhibiting any real degree of skill?

4. You have administered a teacher preference sheet to 150 major students in your departments. The number of first preference choices received by each of the five teachers in the department are as follows:

Teacher 1, 18 choices   Teacher 4, 48 choices

Teacher 2, 36 choices   Teacher 5, 27 choices

Teacher 3, 21 choices

How do you interpret these results?

5. College graduates and nongraduates are asked if they play bridge. The results are as follows:

	Graduate	Nongraduate
Play	60	40
Don't play	40	160

Is there sufficient reason to believe that there is a relation between whether an individual graduates from college and whether he plays bridge?

6. Obese and nonobese males are observed as to their activity patterns. The following results are noted:

	Vigorous	Moderate	Slight
Obese	20	30	40
Nonobese	50	40	30

Do you believe on the basis of these results that activity pattern and obesity are related?

7. Pubescent and prepubescent boys are questioned as to interest in sports. The responses are as follows:

	Interested	Not interested
Pubescent	65	35
Prepubescent	55	45

Are these variables related?

8. Male and female college students are asked to respond to a statement that physical education should be required. The responses are as follows:

	Agree	Disagree	No reaction
Male	35	20	25
Female	20	30	20

Are these variables related?

9. Basketball players, cross-country runners, and nonathletes are tested to determine if their pulse rates are above or below the median for their age. The results are as follows:

	Above	Below
Basketball	22	38
Cross-country	10	30
Nonathlete	80	40

Are these variables related?

10. Two hundred baseball coaches are asked to pick the best catcher from among four candidates chosen by a committee. The votes are as follows:

Player A, 63 votes   Player C, 41 votes

Player B, 44 votes   Player D, 52 votes

Is any player significantly more preferred than the other?

Chapter **10**

Other measures of association

In Chapter 7 on linear correlation we discussed the computation and interpretation of r, the coefficient of correlation. In all the cases previously discussed, both the X and Y data were measured on an interval scale. However, there are many cases in which either or both of our variables may be on a nominal scale, that is, when data are categorized into one of a number of possible classes. Another case may arise in which data are not subject to specific measurement, as on an interval scale, but are simply presented in rank order. The measures of association presented in this chapter are designed to enable us to handle data of this nature.

PHI COEFFICIENT

The phi coefficient (r_ϕ) is an appropriate statistic to use when both the X and Y data are measured on a nominal scale. In this case both variables can be categorized in one of two categories. The phi coefficient normally assumes that both X and Y represent true dichotomies. If X and Y represent artificial dichotomies, the phi coefficient is not appropriate. In such a case the *tetrachoric coefficient* is used. The tetrachoric coefficient will not be discussed in this text.

To begin our discussion of the phi coefficient let us consider the data in Table 10-1, where the Y variable is sex and the X variable is the response to the question, "Do you enjoy physical education?"

Table 10-1

	X_0	X_1
Y_0	20	20
Y_1	35	25

Let $Y_0 =$ girls, $Y_1 =$ boys, $X_0 =$ a yes response, and $X_1 =$ a no response. In

Table 10-2

	X_0	X_1
Y_0	a	b
Y_1	c	d

the case of the phi coefficient, or fourfold point coefficient as it is some-times called, the general model is shown in Table 10-2, and:

$$r_\phi = \frac{bc - ad}{\sqrt{(a+c)(b+d)(a+b)(c+d)}}$$

In our example:

$$r_\phi = \frac{(20)(35) - (20)(25)}{\sqrt{(20+35)(20+25)(20+20)(35+25)}}$$

$$r_\phi = \frac{700 - 500}{\sqrt{(55)(45)(40)(60)}}$$

$$r_\phi = \frac{200}{2,437}$$

$$r_\phi = .082 \qquad \text{Correlation Value}$$

To determine if this value represents a significant relationship between X and Y we will again make use of the chi square statistic. In this case

$$\chi^2 = Nr_\phi^2$$

with 1 degree of freedom. For the data in Table 10-1:

$$\chi^2 = 100(.082)^2$$
$$\chi^2 = 100(.006724)$$
$$\chi^2 = .6724$$

If we now compare this value of chi square with the tabled value, as-suming $\alpha = .05$, we find our value is not significant and thus we accept the null hypothesis that these variables are independent.

An additional coefficient, the *contingency coefficient,* is used in cases where the X and Y variables contain more than two categories. This coefficient is seldom used and will not be discussed here.

POINT BISERIAL COEFFICIENT

The point biserial coefficient is an appropriate statistic to use when one variable is measured on an interval scale and the other variable is mea-sured on a nominal scale. The point biserial coefficient assumes that the variable on a nominal scale is a true dichotomy. If this variable is an arbitrary dichotomy, the point biserial coefficient is not appropriate. In such a case the *biserial coefficient* is used. The biserial coefficient will not be discussed in this text.

We normally call the dichotomized variable the X variable and the interval variable the Y variable. Let us consider the data in Table 10-3.

Table 10-3

X_0		X_1	
Y_0	Y_0^2	Y_1	Y_1^2
8	64	4	16
6	36	3	9
5	25	2	4
7	49	6	36
4	16	4	16
8	64	3	9
3	9	6	36
5	25	3	9
2	4		
9	81		
3	9		
4	16		
64	398	31	135

In this case the X variable is sex and the Y variable is the number of foul shots made in ten attempts. Let X_0 = boys and X_1 = girls.

Solving for the point biserial coefficient involves a number of new terms that will be more fully discussed in Chapter 12. However, it will be helpful to remember that in the following discussion the term "sums of squares" refers to squared deviations from the mean of a distribution.

The formula for point biserial coefficient is

$$r_{pb} = \sqrt{\frac{\Sigma y_b^2}{\Sigma y_t^2}}$$

where Σy_b^2 = sum of squares between groups = $\dfrac{(\Sigma Y_0)^2}{N_0} + \dfrac{(\Sigma Y_1)^2}{N_1} - \dfrac{(\Sigma Y)^2}{N}$

and Σy_t^2 = total sum of squares = $\Sigma Y^2 - \dfrac{(\Sigma Y)^2}{N}$.

For the data in Table 10-3:

$$\Sigma y_b^2 = \frac{(64)^2}{12} + \frac{(31)^2}{8} - \frac{(95)^2}{20}$$

$$\Sigma y_b^2 = \frac{4{,}096}{12} + \frac{961}{8} - \frac{9{,}025}{20}$$

$$\Sigma y_b^2 = 341.33 + 120.12 - 451.25$$

$$\Sigma y_b^2 = 10.20$$

and

$$\Sigma y_t^2 = 533 - \frac{(95)^2}{20}$$

$$\Sigma y_t^2 = 533 - \frac{9{,}025}{20}$$

$$\Sigma y_t^2 = 533 - 451.25$$

$$\Sigma y_t^2 = 81.75$$

Now we substitute in our formula for point biserial coefficient as follows:

$$r_{pb} = \sqrt{\frac{10.20}{81.75}}$$

$$r_{pb} = \sqrt{.124}$$

$$r_{pb} = \quad .34$$

We must now test the null hypothesis that these two variables are independent. To do this we must find the within sum of squares as follows:

$$\Sigma y_w^2 = \Sigma y_t^2 - \Sigma y_b^2$$

In this case:

$$\Sigma y_w^2 = 81.75 - 10.20$$

$$\Sigma y_w^2 = 71.55$$

The next step is to find the mean square between groups and the mean square within groups. These are found by dividing the appropriate sum of squares by its degrees of freedom. The between sum of squares has $k-1=1$ degree of freedom. The within sum of squares has $N-2=18$ degrees of freedom. Therefore:

$$MSB = \frac{10.20}{1}$$

$$MSB = 10.20$$

and

$$MSW = \frac{71.55}{18}$$

$$MSW = \quad 3.97$$

The final step is to form a ratio, known as an F ratio, between the mean square between groups and the mean square within groups. If this value of F exceeds the table value (Table C-9, Appendix C) at the appropriate number of degrees of freedom $(k-1, N-2)$, we reject the null hypothesis. For our data:

$$F = \frac{MSB}{MSW}$$

$$F = \frac{10.20}{3.97}$$

$$F = \quad 2.57$$

In this case the obtained value, 2.57, does not exceed the tabled value, 4.41, with $\alpha = .05$. Therefore we conclude that these variables are independent.

An additional statistic, the *correlation ratio*, is used in cases where the X variable contains more than two categories. This is another seldom used statistic and will not be discussed further.

RANK-ORDER COEFFICIENT

The rank-order coefficient (R), or Spearman Rho as it is also called, is used in cases where both the X and Y data are presented in rank order. Let us consider the data in Table 10-4.

Table 10-4

Gymnast	X	Y	R_x	R_y	$R_x - R_y$	$(R_x - R_y)^2$
A	8.7	8.5	3	3.5	−0.5	0.25
B	8.0	7.5	6	8.5	−2.5	6.25
C	9.1	9.1	2	1	1	1
D	7.5	8.0	8	6	2	4
E	5.8	5.0	10	10	0	0
F	9.4	9.0	1	2	−1	1
G	7.6	8.2	7	5	2	4
H	8.3	7.5	5	8.5	−3.5	12.25
I	8.5	8.5	4	3.5	0.5	0.25
J	6.8	7.6	9	7	2	4
						33

In this case X and Y represent the scores given to ten gymnasts by two different judges. R_x and R_y represent the rank order of each gymnast according to the scores given by judges X and Y. Notice that judge Y gave gymnasts A and I the same score (8.5) and also gave gymnasts B and H the same score (7.5). In such a case the rank order for those gymnasts is the average of the ranks they are tied for. The formula for rank-order coefficient is as follows:

$$R = 1 - \frac{6\Sigma(R_x - R_y)^2}{N(N^2 - 1)}$$

For the data in Table 10-4:

$$R = 1 - \frac{6(33)}{10(100 - 1)}$$

$$R = 1 - \frac{198}{990}$$

$$R = 1 - .20$$

$$R = .80$$

To test the null hypothesis, when N is equal to or greater than 10, we use the formula

$$t = \frac{R}{\sqrt{1 - R^2}}\left(\sqrt{N - 2}\right)$$

with $N - 2$ degrees of freedom. For our data:

$$t = \frac{.80}{\sqrt{1 - (.80)^2}} \sqrt{10 - 2}$$

$$t = \frac{.80}{\sqrt{1 - .64}} \sqrt{8}$$

$$t = \frac{.80}{\sqrt{.36}} \sqrt{8}$$

$$t = \frac{.80}{.60} \ (2.82)$$

$$t = 3.76$$

This t value may now be compared to the tabled value of t with $N-2$ degrees of freedom to test whether these variables are independent. (See Table C-8 in Appendix C.) When $\alpha = .05$ the table value of t with 8 degrees of freedom is 2.31, which is less than our obtained value. Therefore we reject the null hypothesis that there is no significant relationship between X and Y.

Problems

1. For what type of X and Y variables is the phi coefficient an appropriate measure of association?
2. When is the tetrachoric coefficient used instead of the phi coefficient?
3. When is the contingency coefficient used instead of the phi coefficient?
4. Determine the phi coefficient for the following X and Y data where X_0 = athlete, X_1 = nonathlete, Y_0 = those able to swim, and Y_1 = those unable to swim.

	X_0	X_1
Y_0	25	25
Y_1	5	25

5. Are the X and Y data presented in problem 4 significantly related?
6. Determine the phi coefficient for the following X and Y data where X_0 = males, X_1 = females, Y_0 = those who major in physical education, and Y_1 = those who do not major in physical education.

	X_0	X_1
Y_0	30	20
Y_1	70	80

7. Are the X and Y data presented in problem 6 independent or dependent?
8. For what type of X and Y variables is the point biserial coefficient an appropriate measure of association?
9. When is the biserial coefficient used instead of the point biserial coefficient?
10. When is the correlation ratio used instead of the point biserial coefficient?
11. Determine the point biserial coefficient for the following X and Y data where X_0 = those who have taken a badminton course, X_1 = those who have not taken a badminton course, and Y = scores on a badminton serving test.

X_0	X_1
Y_0	Y_1
24	10
30	13
18	20
22	12
20	15
16	23
15	14
	9
	11

12. Are the X and Y variables in problem 11 independent?
13. For what type of X and Y variables is the rank-order coefficient an appropriate measure of association?

14. Determine the rank-order coefficient for the following X and Y data that represent the scores obtained by fifteen men on two different tests of physical fitness.

X	Y	X	Y
81 8	31 8.5	73 14	24 14
83 5.5	33 6	79 10	31 8.5
92 2	40 1	85 3	37 3
80 9	32 7	65 15	22 15
94 1	38 2	77 11.5	28 12.5
83 5.5	36 4.5	82 7	30 10.5
77 11.5	30 10.5	76 13	28 12.5
84 4	36 4.5		

15. Does the rank-order coefficient obtained in answer to problem 14 indicate a significant degree of association between X and Y?

Chapter 11

t **tests**

W. S. Gosset, in 1931, developed a *t* statistic to test hypotheses about the means of populations having unknown variances. Since he wrote this article under the pseudonym of "Student," the test has come to be known as Student's *t* test. This statistic can be used to test hypotheses about one mean, two means from independent samples, or two means from related samples.

DISTRIBUTION OF *t*

The distribution of *t* is actually many distributions, one for each sample size. All these distributions look quite similar to the normal curve (Fig. 3-1), and for sample sizes greater than 50 a normal-curve *z* distribution is practically identical to the *t* distribution. As sample sizes get smaller, the shoulders of the bell curve for *t* are broadened, and the tails are lengthened. The *t* values are given in Table C-8, Appendix C. The student should note that two values are needed to enter the table—the degrees of freedom in the left-hand column, and alpha across the top. The degrees of freedom value is simply $n-1$ where n is the size of the sample. The "degrees of freedom" is a measure of the accuracy with which one can estimate the variance of a population from a given sample. As the size of the sample increases, the probable accuracy of the variance estimate also increases. Alpha is the probability of rejecting a test hypothesis (usually the null hypothesis) when that hypothesis is true and also represents the critical area of rejection under the curve for the distribution of *t* with the given number of degrees of freedom.

If, for example, only large values of *t* will cause the rejection of the test hypothesis at the .05 level, then the critical area of rejection is the 5% of the area under the extreme right of the curve of *t* (Fig. 11-1, *A*). On the other hand, if only small values of *t* will cause rejection of the test hypothesis at the .05 level, the 5% of the area under the curve at the far left (Fig. 11-1, *B*) represents the critical area of rejection. Finally, if the test hypothesis will be rejected by either large or small values of *t*, the critical area of rejection is represented by the extreme right 2.5% of the area under the *t* curve and by the extreme left 2.5% (Fig. 11-1, *C*). A test whose critical

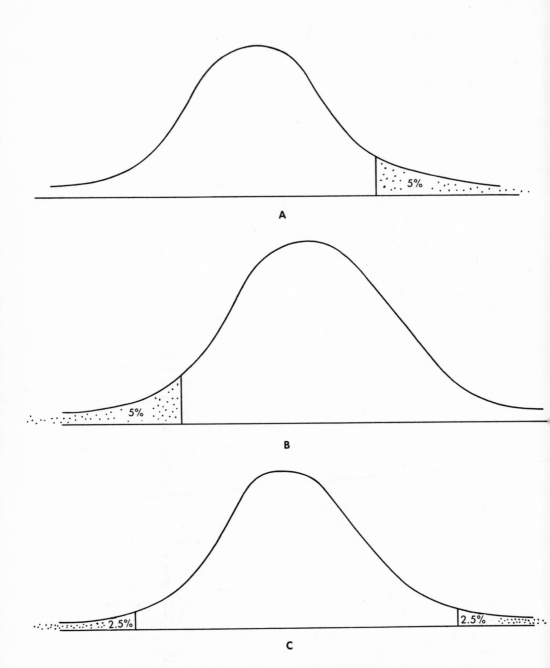

Fig. 11-1. The critical area of rejection under the *t* distribution. **A,** Upper 5% one-tailed critical area of rejection. **B,** Lower 5% one-tailed critical area of rejection. **C,** 5% two-tailed critical area of rejection.

area of rejection lies only at the right or only at the left of the curve is called a one-tailed test, and one that rejects for both high and low values is known as a two-tailed test. If a two-tailed test is desired, alpha is located in the second row across the top heading of Table C-8, Appendix C, and the one-tailed alpha values are found in the first row. The tabled t value should be compared with the absolute values of the t computed from the sample data, since only the positive values are tabled.

t TESTS INVOLVING ONE MEAN

Suppose that Harvey Mallace noticed that the ninth-grade boys in his high school physical education classes seemed to have much greater grip strengths this year as compared with those of the last ten years. Since he had available the mean grip-strength scores (based on about 400 students each year) of ninth graders in his school for the last ten years, Harvey thought that a pooled mean value (there was little variance from year to year) would be an accurate representation of a population mean for ninth graders at his school. Unfortunately the individual data were discarded, and no standard deviations had been computed. The pooled mean was 47 pounds for grip strength. This year, however, the average grip strength of the fifty students in his class was 54 pounds with a standard deviation of 9 pounds.

Harvey wondered if the increase of 7 pounds was just a chance occurrence or if ninth graders this year were actually stronger, perhaps because of an increased emphasis on strength training in the lower grades. Because Harvey wanted to avoid saying that the present ninth graders were stronger if there were no real differences, his test hypothesis and its alternative were the following:

$$H_o: \ \mu \text{ present} \leq \mu \text{ past} = 47$$
$$H_A: \ \mu \text{ present} > 47$$

This obviously required a test to compare a sample mean with a fixed value. Not knowing the population variance of grip-strength measures for the past ten years' students, Harvey decided to use the t distribution.

Assumptions of the t test involving one̸sample̸mean

When one sample mean is being compared to a given value, the only assumptions necessary for a t test are (1) the observations are measured on at least an interval scale, (2) the sample is a random sample of the population under consideration, and (3) the population has a normal distribution. If n is fairly large ($n > 30$), deviations from normality are not usually important, but may serve to increase alpha slightly. When these assumptions are satisfied, the t statistic can be used to help choose between the following hypotheses involving one mean:

(a) _Two tails_
$H_o: \ \mu = k$
$H_A: \ \mu \neq k$

(b) $H_o: \ \mu \geq k$
$H_A: \ \mu < k$

(c) $H_o: \ \mu \leq k$
$H_A: \ \mu > k$

where $k =$ the given value of some population mean with which μ is being compared. Notice that hypothesis (a) requires a two-tailed test, and hypotheses (b) and (c) require one-tailed tests.

The statistic to use for making choices between these hypotheses when the variance of the population sampled is unknown is

$$t_{n-1} = \frac{\bar{X}-k}{\frac{S}{\sqrt{n}}} = \frac{\sqrt{n}\,(\bar{X}-k)}{S}$$

where α is the level of significance desired, S is the sample standard deviation, and n is the number of observations in the sample. Note the similarity between z and t, with the principal difference being the substitution of S, the sample estimate of the population standard deviation, for σ which is now unknown. The $n-1$ subscript for t is the degrees of freedom value used to enter the table of the t distribution.

Example of a t test involving one mean

Let us return to the Mallace case for an illustration of the use of the t test involving one mean. The data collected were as follows:

$\bar{X}=$ 54 pounds = mean grip strength for this year's sample of $n=$ fifty students
$k=$ 47 pounds = ten-year population mean grip strength for ninth graders at Westwood High
$S=$ 9 pounds = sample standard deviation

To test H_0, this year's mean grip strength equaling 47, Harvey computed

$$t_{50-1} = \frac{\sqrt{50}\,(54-47)}{9} = 5.5$$

with $\alpha=.05$. Since only high positive t values could fall in the critical rejection region, Harvey wanted to conduct a one-tailed test. Therefore he entered the table of the t distribution with 49 degrees of freedom in the left hand column and with $\alpha=.05$ in the top row of the table headings. The t value for $t_{.05,49}$ is approximately 1.68. Harvey could now conclude that the present year's freshmen were indeed stronger as measured by grip-strength dynamometers because 5.5 falls far to the right of the critical value

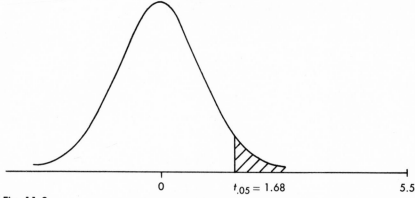

Fig. 11-2

for *t*, 1.68 (Fig. 11-2). There is a .05 probability of incorrectly rejecting H_o whenever one runs such a test.

Summary of procedures for using *t* to test the divergence of one sample mean from some value

1. Try to ascertain the validity of the test assumptions. In most physical education research the normality assumption is acceptable, especially when $n > 30$.

2. Establish the null and alternative hypotheses and determine whether a one- or two-tailed test is appropriate.

3. Set α before collecting the data.

4. Calculate the sample mean and standard deviation.

5. Compute *t* for the sample data.

6. Compare the absolute value of the computed *t* and the *t* found in the table, using the appropriate degrees of freedom and α.

7. If the absolute value of the computed *t* is larger than the tabled value, reject the test hypothesis and accept the alternative hypothesis at a level of confidence equal to alpha.

8. If the computed *t* is smaller than the tabled value, retain the test hypothesis, since insufficient evidence has been found to reject it. There will be some large probability, β, that the choice to retain the test hypothesis is incorrect.

t TESTS INVOLVING TWO MEANS FROM INDEPENDENT SAMPLES

Although *t* tests involving one mean are sometimes used in physical education testing programs, a far more common use of *t* is in research where two sample means are compared, typically to see if one type of exercise program produced different results from another type. Sometimes the means are from two independent samples, for example, resting heart rates in Mr. Gradner's class, which did interval training, and from Mr. Emstrog's class, which used only isometric exercises. (Comment on sampling procedures for such a comparison. Is there a possibility of self-selection here; that is, are the students in their respective classes possibly because they knew about the training techniques used by each instructor?) At other times the means are from dependent or related samples, for example, pre-training and posttraining body weights of a single group of obese students. With dependent samples the data from one sample are correlated with the data from the other; for example, a heavy subject will still be quite heavy even after a training program. In this section only independent data will be considered.

The usual hypotheses concerning two population means using data from two independent samples are as follows:

(a) $H_o : \mu_1 = \mu_2$ (b) $H_o : \mu_1 \geq \mu_2$ (c) $H_o : \mu_1 \leq \mu_2$
      $H_A : \mu_1 \neq \mu_2$ $H_A : \mu_1 < \mu_2$ $H_A : \mu_1 > \mu_2$

Once again a two-tailed test is appropriate for testing hypothesis a, whereas one-tailed tests are the choice for hypotheses b and c.

The appropriate test for hypotheses a, b, and c is

$$t_{\alpha,\, n_1+n_2-2} = \frac{\bar{X}_1 - \bar{X}_2}{\sqrt{\dfrac{(n_1-1)s_1^2 + (n_2-1)s_2^2}{n_1+n_2-2} \times \dfrac{n_1+n_2}{n_1 n_2}}}$$

where α = level of significance desired, n_1 = size of sample 1, n_2 = size of sample 2, $\bar{X}_1$ = mean of sample 1, $\bar{X}_2$ = mean of sample 2, s_1^2 = variance of sample 1, and s_2^2 = variance of sample 2. The denominator of this statistic is a pooled estimate of the standard error of the difference between means.

Assumptions for a *t* test involving two means from independent samples

For a *t* test of the hypotheses a, b, or c to be meaningful, the following assumptions must be approximately true:
1. The data must be measured on at least an interval scale.
2. The data must be from two random samples drawn from the populations of interest.
3. The populations from which the samples are drawn must be normal.
4. The populations must have the same variance.

Mild departures from assumptions 3 and 4 do not seem to seriously affect the conclusions derived from the *t* test as long as the sample sizes are equal and fairly large. The probability of committing a type I error may be slightly increased with such departures from the assumptions. In most physical education research, assumptions 3 and 4 are usually accurate.

Example of a *t* test involving two means from independent samples

Dr. Gillespie believed that growth hormone from the pituitary (hypophysis) was partly responsible for causing an increase in muscle glycogen stores 48 hours after rats were exercised to exhaustion. To investigate this matter she hypophysectomized sixteen animals and treated them with all the pituitary hormones except growth hormone. She then compared the 48-hour postexercise glycogen values of this group of rats with another group of sixteen exercised normals. Her null hypothesis and alternative hypothesis were the following:

$$H_0:\ \mu_{\text{Hypophysectomized}} \geqq \mu_{\text{Normal}}$$
$$H_A:\ \mu_H < \mu_N$$

She decided on a one-tailed *t* test to choose between the two hypotheses and set $\alpha = .01$ before the experiment was begun. The results were $\bar{X}_H = 0.6\%$, $S_H = 0.07\%$, $\bar{X}_N = 2.1\%$, $S_N = 0.10\%$. The *t* value was computed as follows:

$$t_{01,\ 16+16-2} = \frac{0.6 - 2.1}{\sqrt{\dfrac{15(.0049) + 15(.01)}{16+16-2} \times \dfrac{16+16}{16\,(16)}}} = -3.50$$

Entering the *t* table with 30 degrees of freedom in the left-hand column and $\alpha = .01$ in the top row of the table headings, Dr. Gillespie found the tabled *t* value to be 2.457, which was much less than 1.668, the absolute value of the *t* she computed from her sample data. Dr. Gillespie concluded that a lack of growth hormone significantly reduced the ability of muscle to increase its glycogen stores as a response to exercise.

The procedures for testing the difference between means from two independent samples can be summarized in the same way as the procedures for testing one mean, except that two sample means and standard deviations must be computed, and the *t* formulas are different.

t TESTS INVOLVING TWO MEANS FROM DEPENDENT OR RELATED SAMPLES

Much physical education research involves before and after or preexperiments and postexperiments. The example of changes in body weights with training has already been given. Other variables often tested before and after intervening exercise programs are strength, speed, skill, heart rate, and oxygen consumption. As a rule the data collected for a subject after an exercise program will be highly correlated to his score before the program. Thus the data do not occur as two random samples, but rather as one random sample of paired values (Table 11-1). These data should be analyzed with the *t* test developed in this section, since such data violate the randomness assumption of the *t* for independent measures.

Table 11-1. Pretest-posttest experimental design

Subject	Pretest	Posttest	Difference (pretest-posttest)
1	X_{11}	X_{12}	$d_1 = X_{11} - X_{12}$
2	X_{21}	X_{22}	$d_2 = X_{21} - X_{22}$
⋮	⋮	⋮	⋮
n	X_{n1}	X_{n2}	$d_n = X_{n1} - X_{n2}$

Assumptions of the *t* test involving two means from dependent or related samples

The only change in assumptions for this new form of *t* as compared with those of the *t* for independent samples is that the paired differences, $X_i - X_j$, are a random sample from a normal population and that the equal variances assumption becomes unnecessary, since we are now dealing with one population, the population of paired differences.

Sometimes an investigator may choose to gather data as correlated pairs in order to remove extraneous variability from the data. Thus, if leg strength strongly influences scores in the long jump, to compare the effectiveness of two different training methods on long-jump performance, one might match pairs of novice jumpers on leg strength and then randomly assign each member of the pairs to one of the training methods. By analyzing only the differences between the pairs, the effects of leg strength could hopefully be eliminated, and any large difference should then be caused by the effects of the training methods. In designing such an experiment, it is wise to have very small differences on the matching variable within a pair, but wide differences between pairs. In the case of leg strength, it would be best to have each member of a pair differ only by 3 pounds or less, but have differences between pairs of 10 pounds or more.

If the matching variable is an important factor in determining the test score, then matching will decrease the variability of the data and thus decrease the probability of committing a type II error. If the matching variable is unimportant, then the matching procedure will be wasteful of data, since the number of degrees of freedom for the t test for dependent or matched data is only half as great as for the t test for independent data.

The appropriate t test for dependent or matched pairs of data is

$$t_{\alpha,\,n-1} = \frac{\bar{d} - \mu_d}{\frac{S_d}{\sqrt{n}}} = \frac{\sqrt{n}\,(\bar{d} - \mu_d)}{S_d}$$

where α = level of significance desired, n = number of matched or dependent pairs, $\bar{d}$ = mean difference within pairs, μ_d = population mean difference within pairs under H_o, and S_d = standard deviation of differences within pairs. Usually H_o will hold that $\mu_d = 0$ or that the average difference within pairs is zero. These symbols can be better understood by an illustration.

Example of a t test involving two means from dependent or related samples

Suppose in the leg-strength and long-jump experiment eight matched pairs of jumpers were selected. After the training period each jumper would be tested on performance in the long jump. Assume the scores in feet were as follows:

Type of training	Pair							
	1	2	3	4	5	6	7	8
Method 1	20	19	18	23	24	17	21	21
Method 2	19	18	22	19	18	14	19	18
$d_i(1-2)$	1	1	-4	4	6	3	2	3

$$n = 8$$
$$\Sigma d_i = 16$$
$$\bar{d} = 16/8 = 2$$
$$S_d{}^2 = \frac{\Sigma d_i{}^2 - \frac{(\Sigma d_i)^2}{n}}{n-1} = \frac{92 - \frac{256}{8}}{7} = 8.57$$
$$S_d = \sqrt{S_d{}^2} = \sqrt{8.57} = 2.93$$
$$\alpha = .05$$
$$t_{.05,\,8-1} = \frac{\sqrt{8}\,(2-0)}{2.93} = 1.93$$

The tabled t for 7 degrees of freedom with $\alpha = .05$ for a two-tailed test is 2.365. With this experiment the investigator would have to retain the null hypothesis that there is no difference in long-jumping ability caused by the different training methods. Although seven of eight jumpers trained by method 1 were better jumpers than their partners of method 2, these results were quite likely just by chance. The reader should use the same data as though they were from two independent samples and compute a *t* according to the formula presented in the previous section for independent samples. Note that the newly computed *t* still does not exceed the tabled critical value. With data such as these that point to a meaningful difference in training methods (an average performance increase of more than 2 feet in seven of eight athletes), although no statistical significance is indicated, the investigator should proceed to replicate his experiment with more subjects so that a better estimate of the standard error of the difference is obtained. It is quite likely that a significant difference would have been detected had there been fifteen instead of eight matched pairs. Also, the experimenter should attempt to obtain a greater range of abilities between the pairs, for example, more pairs who jump only 13 to 15 feet.

Problems

1. Analyze these data from an experiment to test the effects of 1 hour of daily practice on free-throw shooting performance.

Percentage of shots made

Subject	Pretest	Posttest
1	40	51
2	29	39
3	53	59
4	62	63
5	50	56
6	33	39
7	28	35
8	47	53
9	78	60
10	69	73

dependent sample
1 tail

2. Analyze the results of this experiment to determine the effect of training on body composition of two groups of subjects matched on pretraining percent body fat.

Effect of training on body fat (percent) *dependent σ* *Solve* *one tail*

					Matched pairs							
Group	1	2	3	4	5	6	7	8	9	10	11	12
Untrained	20	18	16	15	15	14	14	14	13	13	13	12
Trained	14	13	12	12	13	12	11	14	12	12	11	10

Comment on the efficiency of this design as opposed to the pretest-posttest type of design. Are there any reasons why the matched groups design might be better than a pretest-posttest design?

3. The following X_1 and X_2 data represent 100-yard-dash times for two groups receiving different starting method instructions. Are the means significantly different?

Independent *2 tail*

X_1	X_2	X_1	X_2
10.3	11.2	11.7	11.1
12.2	10.3	12.4	12.0
10.7	10.5	10.2	11.1
12.1	11.0	11.4	10.4
10.0	9.8	11.2	10.6

4. Given the following means, N's, and standard deviations, determine if the means are significantly different. (Use $\alpha = .05$.)

$\bar{X}_1 = 125$ $\bar{X}_2 = 115$
$S = 10$ $S = 9$
$N_1 = 13$ $N_2 = 9$

5. Given the following means, N's, and standard deviations, determine if the means are significantly different. (Use $\alpha = .05$.)

$\bar{X}_1 = 21$ $\bar{X}_2 = 28$
$S = 1$ $S = 3$
$N_1 = 50$ $N_2 = 50$

6. Given the following means, N's, and standard deviations, determine if the means are significantly different. (Use $\alpha = .01$.)

$\bar{X}_1 = 94$ $\bar{X}_2 = 85$
$S = 2$ $S = 2$
$N_1 = 25$ $N_2 = 30$

7. Given the following means, N's, and standard deviations, determine if the means are significantly different. (Use $\alpha = .01$.)

$\bar{X}_1 = 230$ $\bar{X}_2 = 208$
$S = 3$ $S = 8$
$N_1 = 45$ $N_2 = 25$

Chapter 12

One-way analysis of variance

ANALYSIS OF VARIANCE

The t test and its derivatives as described in Chapter 11 are methods for testing hypotheses about two population means. Often these hypotheses take the following form:

$$H_o: \quad \mu_1 = \mu_2$$
$$H_A: \quad \mu_1 \neq \mu_2$$

Many types of physical education problems require tests of hypotheses about more than two means:

$$H_o: \quad \mu_1 = \mu_2 = \cdots = \mu_r$$
$$H_A: \quad \text{at least two means are not equal}$$

An example of such a problem is the typical weight-training experiment where three or more progressive resistance routines are tested for their relative value in strength training. If these routines were 1, 3, and 10 RM,* for instance, then the hypotheses of interest would probably be

$$H_o: \quad \mu_{1\,RM} = \mu_{3\,RM} = \mu_{10\,RM}$$
$$H_A: \quad \text{at least two of the means for strength gain are not equal.}$$

The analysis of variance can be considered as an extension of the t test for more than two groups. The test is named analysis of variance because a statistic is derived by partitioning sums of squares into different components so that an estimation of variance or variability due to different sources (e.g., training methods and random or uncontrolled error) can be estimated. There are many different mathematical models of the analysis of variance, but we shall describe only four—the one-way, fixed effects, completely randomized model; the one-way, fixed effects, randomized blocks model; the one-way, fixed effects model with repeated observations on the same subjects; and the two-way, fixed effects, completely randomized model. These are the models most frequently encountered in physical education research.

*An RM (repetition maximum) is the maximum load with which a given movement (e.g., military press) can be correctly executed for the given number of repetitions.

103

ONE-WAY, FIXED EFFECTS, COMPLETELY RANDOMIZED MODEL
Purpose

The one-way, fixed effects, completely randomized model, also known as the one-way analysis of variance, is the most often used type of analysis of variance in physical education. Its purpose is to compare r ($r \geq 2$) population means by selecting r independent random samples from those populations and testing the equality of the sample means. Let us assume, for example, that we want to compare the effects of 1, 3, and 10 RM elbow flexion exercises on strength gain as measured by cable tensiometer techniques in a weight-lifting class of forty-five students. One way to do this would be to randomly assign fifteen students to each of the three routines and compare strength measurements after a given period of training, say 9 weeks. Although there are better ways to compare the training effects (see randomized blocks and analysis of covariance), the data as described could readily be analyzed with the one-way analysis of variance. This analysis will tell with a given degree of confidence whether the mean strengths of the three groups could have come from the same population. Another way of stating the purpose of the analysis for these data is that the test will tell us with some confidence whether the effects of the three training methods on strength are different from each other.

Layout of the data

The data for the one-way, fixed effects, completely randomized analysis of variance can be organized in the manner of Table 12-1. In this table, X_{11} represents the first observation from a random sample of size n_1 drawn from a population that has received treatment 1, whereas X_{32} represents the second observation from a random sample of size n_3 drawn from a population that has received treatment 3. In our weight-training example, treatment 1 might be the 1 RM regimen, and treatments 2 and 3 the 3 and 10 RM regimens, with the X values being the strength measurements.

Table 12-1. Layout of data for the one-way analysis of variance

	Treatments					
	1	*2*	*3*	$\cdots$	*r*	
Observations	X_{11}	X_{21}	X_{31}		X_{r1}	
	X_{12}	X_{22}	X_{32}		X_{r2}	
	$\vdots$	$\vdots$	$\vdots$		$\vdots$	
	$\bar{X}_{1n_1}$	$\bar{X}_{2n_2}$	$\bar{X}_{3n_3}$		$\bar{X}_{rn_r}$	
Totals	T_1	T_2	T_3		T_r	Grand total
Means	$\bar{X}_1$	$\bar{X}_2$	$\bar{X}_3$		$\bar{X}_r$	
$\sum\limits_{i=1}^{r} X_i^2$	$\sum X_1^2$	$\sum X_2^2$	$\sum X_3^2$		$\sum X_r^2$	Grand $\sum X^2$
$\dfrac{\text{Total}^2}{n_i}$	$\dfrac{T_1^2}{n_1}$	$\dfrac{T_2^2}{n_2}$	$\dfrac{T_3^2}{n_3}$		$\dfrac{T_r^2}{n_r}$	$\sum\limits_{i=1}^{r} \dfrac{T_i^2}{n_i}$

Assumptions of the test

The assumptions of the one-way analysis of variance are the following:
1. The data are measured on an interval (or ratio) scale.
2. The columns of data are independent, random samples from the treatment populations.
3. The treatment populations are normal.
4. The treatment populations have the same variance.

Assumptions 1 and 2 are very important and must be met if one is to have any confidence about his results. The third assumption is not too important if the sample sizes are fairly large ($n > 10$), and the fourth is not important if sample sizes are equal and fairly large. It is always wise when using analysis of variance techniques to study samples of equal size, not only to avoid the problem of unequal population variances, but also for purposes of efficient comparisons between means, that is, Tukey tests.

Analytical procedure

These steps should be followed for the one-way analysis of variance:

Step 1. Determine whether the assumptions of the test are tenable for the data at hand. If they are not, consult Chapter 18 for an appropriate test.

Step 2. State the hypothesis and the alternative. They usually will take the following form:

H_o: $\mu_1 = \mu_2 = \cdots = \mu_r$
H_A: at least two treatment means are different.

Step 3. Choose the level of significance (probability of committing a type I error) you will accept. Usually this level is .05 or .01, but you may decide on another. This step should always be taken before the data analysis is begun.

Step 4. Arrange the data as in Table 12-1.

Step 5. Compute the column totals, means, sums of squares, total$^2/n_i$, the grand (overall) total, grand sum of squares, and $\sum\limits_{i=1}^{r} \dfrac{T_i^2}{n_i}$ in the usual fashion.

Step 6. Compute the total sum of squares (SS_T):

$$SS_T = \text{Grand } \Sigma x^2 - \frac{(\text{Grand total})^2}{\text{Total } N}$$

Step 7. Compute the treatment sum of squares (SS_{Tr}):

$$SS_{Tr} = \sum_{i=1}^{r} \frac{T_i^2}{n_i} - \frac{(\text{Grand total})^2}{\text{Total } N}$$

Step 8. Compute the error sum of squares (SS_E):

$$SS_E = SS_T - SS_{Tr}$$

Step 9. Compute the treatment mean square (MS_{Tr}):

$$MS_{Tr} = \frac{SS_{Tr}}{r-1}$$

This value is an estimate of the overall population variance plus an amount caused by differences between treatment effects.

Step 10. Compute the error mean square (MS_E):

$$MS_E = \frac{SS_E}{N-r}$$

This value is an estimate of the overall population variance.

Step 11. Compute the F ratio:

$$F = \frac{MS_{Tr}}{MS_E}$$

Since MS_E estimates the population variance, σ^2, and MS_{Tr} estimates σ^2 plus an amount caused by treatment effects, then the ratio of these two, $F = (\text{est. } \sigma^2 + \text{treatment effects})/\text{est. } \sigma^2$, should approach 1 if only insignificant differences between treatment effects exist, and should become progressively greater than 1 as the differences between treatment effects are greater.

Step 12. Summarize the results in an analysis of variance table as in Table 12.2.

Table 12-2. Summary of results for one-way analysis of variance

Source of variation	SS	Degrees of freedom	MS	F
Treatments	SS_{Tr}	$r-1$	MS_{Tr}	$\dfrac{MS_{Tr}}{MS_E}$
Error	SS_E	$N-r$	MS_E	
Total	SS_T			

Step 13. Consult a table of the F distribution (Table C-9, Appendix C) to compare the obtained F value with that found in the table at the predetermined alpha level and with the appropriate degrees of freedom, $r-1$ and $N-r$. If the experimentally obtained F value is greater than the tabled value, reject the null hypothesis, H_o: $\mu_1 = \mu_2 = \cdots = \mu_r$, and conclude that at least two of the treatment means are different, knowing that there is a probability, alpha, that this conclusion is incorrect. If the obtained F value is less than the tabled value, the appropriate conclusion is that insufficient evidence was obtained to warrant rejection of the null hypothesis. It is *not* appropriate to conclude that there are no differences between treatment means, unless the probability of committing a type II error was less than some small value, say 20%. In most cases this probability will be much greater than 20%, often as high as 85%. If an estimate of the probability of committing a type II error is desired, one should consult an appropriate reference.*

---

*See Guenther, W. C.: Analysis of variance, Englewood Cliffs, N. J., 1964, Prentice-Hall, Inc., p. 47.

Step 14. If the obtained F ratio is greater than the tabled value, use the Tukey or Scheffé procedures (discussed later in this chapter) to discover which means are significantly different from each other. The F test only indicates that at least two means are different, but once a significant F ratio is obtained, the Tukey (for samples of equal size) or Scheffé (samples of unequal size) procedures can be used to compare all pairs of means to determine which are different.

Performing multiple t tests of differences between various means is not the best way to compare means after the F test because more than one t test must be performed. Since the probability of incorrectly rejecting a null hypothesis, H_o: $\mu_A = \mu_B$, is α for one t test, the probability of incorrectly rejecting one or more null hypotheses when several tests are performed is considerably greater, with a maximum probability equal to the sum of all the α levels. Both the Tukey and Scheffé methods have a known overall α associated with all possible comparisons. With multiple t tests one has no way of accurately determining an overall α level.

Example of one-way analysis of variance

Returning to our example of studying the effects of three different weight-training techniques on elbow flexion strength, we can follow the above analytical procedure step by step.

Table 12-3. Cable tensiometer measures of elbow flexion strength (pounds)

	1 RM	3 RM	10 RM	
		Treatments		
Observations	45	68	28	
	40	47	34	
	58	63	42	
	33	40	43	
	70	38	29	
	67	38	37	
	50	59	45	
	41	45	29	
	48	48	33	
	62	40	53	
	50	39	53	
	47	50	26	
	43	47	50	
	69	70	40	
	48	64	39	
Totals	771	756	581	2,108
Means	51.4	50.4	38.7	
$\sum_{i=1}^{3} X_i^2$	~~37,575~~ 41,419	39,926	23,633	~~101,134~~ 104,978
$\frac{\text{Total}^2}{n_i}$	39,629	38,102	22,504	100,235

Step 1. The analysis of variance assumptions seem reasonable as our three samples were randomly drawn, the strength measures are on an interval scale, most biological populations are normal, and our large and equal sample sizes make the assumption of equal variances unimportant.

Step 2. The null hypothesis is to be tested against the alternative that at least two of the treatment means are different.

$$H_o: \quad \mu_{1RM} = \mu_{3RM} = \mu_{10RM}$$
$$H_A: \quad \text{At least two of the means are different.}$$

Step 3. An alpha level of .05 is chosen.

Step 4. The data are arranged in Table 12-3.

Step 5. The column and grand totals, means, sums of squares, and variances are computed and entered in Table 12-3.

Step 6. The total sum of squares is computed:

$$SS_T = \text{Grand } \Sigma X^2 - \frac{(\text{Grand total})^2}{\text{Total } N}$$

$$SS_T = 101,\text{\st{1}} \underset{\text{(hw)}}{1079} - \frac{(2,108)^2}{45}$$

$$SS_T = \text{\st{2,386}} \quad 6,230 \text{ (hw)}$$

Step 7. The treatment sum of squares is computed:

$$SS_{Tr} = \sum_{i=1}^{3} \frac{T_i^2}{n_i} - \frac{(\text{Grand total})^2}{\text{Total } N}$$

$$SS_{Tr} = 100,235 - \frac{(2,108)^2}{45}$$

$$SS_{Tr} = 1,487$$

Step 8. The error sum of squares is computed by subtraction:

$$SS_E = SS_T - SS_{Tr}$$

$$SS_E = \text{\st{6,230}} 6,230 \text{ (hw)} - 1,487$$

$$SS_E = \text{\st{899}} 4743 \text{ (hw)}$$

Step 9. The treatment mean square is computed:

(hw: r = #) experimental groups)

$$MS_{Tr} = \frac{SS_{Tr}}{r-1}$$

$$MS_{Tr} = \frac{1,487}{2}$$

$$MS_{Tr} = 743.5$$

Step 10. The error mean square is computed:

$$MS_E = \frac{SS_E}{N-r}$$

$$MS_E = \frac{\text{\st{899}} 4743 \text{ (hw)}}{45-3}$$

$$MS_E = \text{\st{214}} 112.92 \text{ (hw)}$$

Step 11. The F ratio is computed:

$$F = \frac{MS_{Tr}}{MS_E}$$

$$F = \frac{743.5}{2\text{++}} \quad 112.92$$

$$F = \text{3.74} \quad 6.58$$

Step 12. The results are summarized in Table 12-4.

Table 12-4. Summary of analysis of variance of strength measures

Source of variation	SS	Degrees of freedom	MS	F
Treatments (Due to training regimens)	1,487	2	743.5	
Error (Due to chance, instrumental error, and unknown factors)	~~899~~ 4743 ~~6230~~	42	~~21.4~~ 112.92	~~34.74~~ 6.58
Total	~~2,386~~ ~~2386~~			

Step 13. Entering Table C-9, Appendix C, of the F distribution, for $\alpha = .05$ with degrees of freedom for $MS_{Tr} = 2$ and degrees of freedom for $MS_E = 42$, a value of approximately 3.23 is found. Since this value is less than our experimentally obtained value, we reject the null hypothesis and conclude that at least two of the means for the three training methods are different, and that the sample differences are not due to chance, but most likely to the different training methods. We realize that there is about a 5% chance that data such as these will reject the null hypothesis incorrectly.

Step 14. Since we obtained a significant F ratio, we now wish to see if all three means are significantly different from each other or if only two are different. With equal sample sizes, the Tukey method is the most efficient for making comparisons between pairs of means.

TUKEY METHOD FOR COMPARING ALL PAIRS OF MEANS

The F test of the analysis of variance does not tell which means are significantly different from each other. We will present two methods for doing so—the Tukey and Scheffé methods.

The Tukey procedure compares the differences between pairs of sample means with a computed T value. If a difference is greater than the T value, then the two means are said to be significantly different from each other.

Tukey analytical procedure

Step 1. Set up a table of differences between sample means as in Table 12-5.

Table 12-5. Differences between sample means

Comparison means	Comparison mean − Smallest mean	Comparison mean − Second smallest mean	⋯	Comparison mean − Second largest mean
Largest mean	Largest − smallest	Largest − second smallest		Largest − second largest
Second largest mean	Second largest − smallest	Second largest − second smallest		_____
⋮	⋮	⋮		_____
		Third smallest − second smallest		_____
	Second smallest − smallest	_____		_____
Smallest mean	_____	_____		_____

Step 2.   Compare the differences with the T value

$$T = (q_{\alpha;\ r,\ N-r}) \sqrt{MS_E/n}$$

where q = a value found in Table C-6, Appendix C, α = the chosen level of significance, r = the number of treatments or groups, N = the total number of observations, n = the number of observations in each sample, and MS_E = the error mean square computed for the analysis of variance.

When a difference between sample means is greater than the computed T value, the appropriate conclusion is that the two means could not have come from the same population or that the treatment effects caused significant differences between the means. The probability that one or more of the conclusions drawn with this technique will be incorrect is alpha.

Example of the Tukey method for comparing all pairs of means

Using the data of the weight-training example from Table 12-3 and Table 12-4, we can illustrate the Tukey method as follows:

Step 1.   The table of differences between sample means is set up in Table 12-6.

Table 12-6. Differences between sample means

Comparison means	Comparison mean − Smallest mean	Comparison mean − Second smallest mean
51.4	51.4 − 38.7 = 12.7	51.4 − 50.4 = 1.0
50.4	50.4 − 38.7 = 11.7	—————
38.7	—————	

Step 2.   The T value is computed and compared with the differences between sample means:

$$T = (q_{\alpha;\ r,\ N-r}) \left(\sqrt{MS_E/n} \right)$$

$$T = (q_{.05;\ 3,\ 42}) \sqrt{}5$$

$$T = (3.44)()\ 2.74$$

$$T = \ 9.438$$

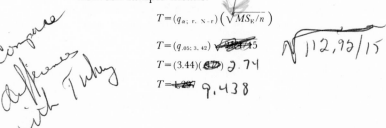

Since the difference between the 3 and 1 RM means is less than the T value, there is not enough evidence to conclude that the difference was due to the training regimens and not to error or chance. However, both the 1 and 3 RM means are significantly greater than the 10 RM mean. There is a probability, alpha (.05), that one or more of these conclusions is incorrect. The practical conclusion is that elbow-flexor strength is increased more by a training regimen of few (one to three) repetitions than by a regimen including ten repetitions.

SCHEFFÉ METHOD FOR COMPARING ALL PAIRS OF MEANS

If an analysis involves unequal sample sizes, the Tukey procedure is no longer applicable, but the Scheffé procedure can be used in such cases. The Scheffé test requires comparisons of differences between sample means with an S value. If a difference is greater than the S value, the two means are said to be significantly different from each other.

Scheffé analytical procedure

Step 1.   Set up a table of differences between sample means as in Table 12-5.

Step 2.   Compare the differences from the table with the S value:

$$S = \left[\sqrt{(r-1)(F_{\alpha;\ r-1,\ N-r})} \right] \left[\sqrt{MS_E \left(\frac{1}{n_i} + \frac{1}{n_j} \right)} \right]$$

where r = the number of experimental treatments, F = a tabled value (Table C-9), (usually the same value used for comparison with the obtained F ratio in the analysis of variance), α = the probability of making one or more false conclusions about the means, (it is usually the same α as that used for the F test of the analysis of variance), N = the total number of experimental observations, MS_E = the error mean square term (denominator) of the analysis of variance F test, and n_i and n_j = the sizes of the two samples from which the two compared means were computed. If sample sizes were equal, the term $(1/n_i) + (1/n_j)$ would become $(2/n)$.

Although all differences between sample means could be compared with a single T value in the Tukey procedure, several S values may need to be computed if samples are of several different sizes.

If the computed S value for the difference in question is smaller than the difference between sample means, the appropriate conclusion is that the two means are significantly different.

Example of the Scheffé method for comparing all pairs of means

We will use the data of the weight-training example to illustrate the use of the Scheffé method.

Step 1.   Assume the table of differences between sample means is the same as Table 12-6. In this case, however, assume the means were computed from sample sizes of 10, 9, and 8 rather than

15, 15, and 15 for the 1, 3, and 10 RM regimens, respectively. The total N of the experiment is now 27, rather than 45.

Step 2.   The S values for all possible pairs of means would be computed as follows:

1 RM vs. 10 RM $S = \left[\sqrt{(3-1)(F_{.05;\ 3-1,\ 27-3})} \right] \left[\sqrt{\frac{12.92}{27} \left(\frac{1}{10} + \frac{1}{8} \right)} \right]$

$S = \left[\sqrt{2(3.40)} \right] \left[\sqrt{\frac{12.92}{21} \left(\frac{9}{40} \right)} \right]$ *13.16*

$S = 3.72$

3 RM vs. 10 RM $S = \left[\sqrt{2(3.4)} \right] \left[\sqrt{\frac{12.92}{21} \left(\frac{1}{9} + \frac{1}{8} \right)} \right]$ *13.48*

$S = [(2.61)] \left[\sqrt{\frac{12.92}{21} (17/72)} \right]$

$S = 5.87$

1 RM vs. 3 RM $S = \left[\sqrt{2(3.4)} \right] \left[\sqrt{\frac{12.92}{21} \left(\frac{1}{10} + \frac{1}{9} \right)} \right]$ *12.74*

$S = [2.61] \left[\sqrt{\frac{12.92}{21} (19/90)} \right]$

$S = 5.56$

Since only the difference (1.0) between the means for the 1 and 3 RM treatments was less than the corresponding S value, one would conclude that this difference was not significant, whereas the other two were.

Problems

1. An experiment was performed to determine the effects of diets of cod-liver oil, peanut oil, or Fig Newtons on treadmill endurance time. The data were as follows:

Cod	Peanut	Fig
15	22	38
20	21	27
14	19	40
13	17	32
17	18	33
22	24	19
12	15	28
10	9	27
16	23	41
17	20	18

Analyze the data with a one-way analysis of variance and perform the Tukey test if necessary. Interpret your results.

2. Harry, Bob, Carl, and John were physical education instructors at Waddley High School. Their respective classes at the end of the year had the following fitness scores:

Harry	Bob	Carl	John
100	90	15	80
92	70	99	80
87	33	48	75
79	82	19	77
100	46		12
100			

Analyze their scores with the one-way analysis and use the Scheffé test if necessary.

Chapter **13**

Randomized blocks analysis of variance

ONE-WAY, FIXED EFFECTS, RANDOMIZED BLOCKS MODEL
Purpose

Recall that in the F test for the one-way, fixed effects, completely randomized model of the analysis of variance the error mean square (MS_E) was an estimate of the population variance that was divided into the treatment mean square (MS_{Tr})—an estimate of the population variance plus a factor due to the treatment effects. Now if the measurement variability of the experiment can be reduced or if a part of the variability known to be caused by some constant factor can be removed, then the denominator of the F test, $MS_{Tr}/MS_E =$ (est. $\sigma^2 +$ treatment effects)/est. σ^2, can be reduced, and the possibility of detecting significant treatment effects increased.

Measurement variability can be reduced in an experiment by using more reliable measurement techniques, by keeping testing equipment in constant repair and calibration, and by using experienced personnel. Sometimes a known factor causes variation in results, and the variance due to this factor can be removed from the estimate of the population variance (MS_E) by using a randomized blocks design in which experimental subjects are assigned randomly to groups or treatments only after they have been first placed in homogeneous groups or *blocks* based on the known factor.

In the weight-training experiment of Chapter 12, for instance, much of the variability of the strength measurements could be accounted for by body weight, heavier subjects generally having greater strength. To remove this source of variation we might have placed the forty-five subjects in fifteen "blocks" of three subjects each, the three heaviest subjects being placed in block 1, the next three heaviest in block 2, and so on, until the three lightest subjects were placed in block 15. Then the subjects within each block could have been randomly assigned to training regimens, one subject of each block being assigned to each of the three training methods. With the randomized blocks analysis, the variance in the strength measures due to body weight could then have been eliminated from the denominator of the F ratio so that effects due to training could be more readily detected.

Layout of the data

The data for the randomized blocks analysis of variance can be organized as in Table 13-1.

Table 13-1. Arrangement of data for a randomized blocks analysis of variance

Blocks$_j$ $j = 1, 2, \ldots, n$	Treatments$_i$ $i = 1, 2, \ldots, r$					Block totals	Block totals^2 r
	1	2	3	$\cdots$	r		
1	X_{11}	X_{21}	X_{31}	$\cdots$	X_{r1}	T_{B1}	$\dfrac{T_{B1}{}^2}{r}$
2	X_{12}	X_{22}	X_{32}	$\cdots$	X_{r2}	T_{B2}	$\dfrac{T_{B2}{}^2}{r}$
3	X_{13}	X_{23}	X_{33}	$\cdots$	X_{r3}	T_{B3}	$\dfrac{T_{B3}{}^2}{r}$
$\vdots$	$\vdots$	$\vdots$	$\vdots$		$\vdots$	$\vdots$	$\vdots$
n	X_{1n}	X_{2n}	X_{3n}	$\cdots$	X_{rn}	T_{BN}	$\dfrac{T_{BN}{}^2}{r}$
Treatment totals	T_1	T_2	T_3	$\cdots$	T_r	Grand total	$\displaystyle\sum_{j=1}^{n} \dfrac{\text{Block total}_j{}^2}{r}$
Treatment means	$\bar{X}_1$	$\bar{X}_2$	$\bar{X}_3$	$\cdots$	$\bar{X}_r$		
Treatment ΣX^2	ΣX_1^2	ΣX_2^2	ΣX_3^2	$\cdots$	ΣX_r^2	Grand ΣX^2	
Treatment totals^2 n	$\dfrac{T_1^2}{n}$	$\dfrac{T_2^2}{n}$	$\dfrac{T_3^2}{n}$	$\cdots$	$\dfrac{T_r^2}{n}$	$\displaystyle\sum_{i=1}^{r} \dfrac{\text{Tr. total}_i{}^2}{n}$	

In this table, X_{23} represents the observation for the subject of block 3 who was assigned to treatment 2. Note that with this model there must be an equal number of subjects in each treatment group. If in the course of an experiment one or more observations are lost, there are procedures for computing substitute values, but the efficiency of the F test is reduced progressively as more substitute data are entered. The procedure for filling in one missing observation is described elsewhere.*

Assumptions of the test

The assumptions for the randomized blocks analysis are as follows:
1. The data are measured on an interval or ratio scale.
2. Each of the m observations is a random sample of size 1 drawn from one of the m populations.
3. All m populations are normal.
4. All m populations have the same variance.
5. Treatment differences are constant between blocks, and blocking differences are constant between treatments. This is known as the additivity assumption.

---

*See Guenther, W. C.: Analysis of variance, Englewood Cliffs, N. J., 1964, Prentice-Hall, Inc., p. 77.

Comments about the one-way analysis assumptions 1 to 4 on p. 105 hold for the first four randomized blocks assumptions, but assumption 5 requires some explanation. Table 13-2 depicts data that illustrate this assumption.

Table 13-2. Illustration of constant treatment and blocking effects on the population means

Blocks	Treatments			
	1	2	3	4
1	10	5	13	9
2	30	25	33	29
3	15	10	18	14
4	7	2	10	6

Notice that the difference between block 1 and block 2 values is 20 for all four treatments and that the difference between treatment 3 and treatment 4 values is 4 for all four blocks. In the weight-training example, this assumption of additivity (assumption 5) means that a given training regimen must have the same effects on both heavy and light individuals and that the effect of placing subjects in blocks has the same effect on the results of all three training regimens. In other words, there are no interactions between the training methods and body weights.

Obviously, the sample values collected will never show perfect additivity. If there is a doubt about whether additivity can be assumed, a test for this assumption can be performed as described in Guenther.* Usually, the investigator has a fairly good idea of whether interactions exist. He would guess, for instance, that a training program consisting of a daily 10-mile run would affect the caloric expenditure of obese persons differently from that of lean ones. In that case one should not attempt to group or block subjects according to body weight but should rely either on the completely randomized analysis of variance or on the analysis of covariance (Chapter 15).

Analytical procedure

The following steps are appropriate for a randomized blocks analysis of variance:

Step 1.   Determine whether the assumptions of the test are tenable for the data at hand. If they are not, consult Chapter 18 for an appropriate test.

Step 2.   State the hypothesis and the alternative. Usually they will be of the following form:

$$H_0: \quad \mu_1 = \mu_2 = \cdots = \mu_r$$
$$H_A: \quad \text{At least two means are different.}$$

Step 3.   Choose the level of significance (α) before analyzing the data.

---

*Guenther, W. C.: Analysis of variance, Englewood Cliffs, N. J., 1964, Prentice-Hall, Inc., p. 76.

Step 4. Arrange the data as in Table 13-1. Procedures for filling in missing observations are presented in some texts.*

Step 5. Compute column and block totals, totals²/n or r, column means and sums of squares, and all grand totals.

Step 6. Compute the total sum of squares (SS_T) as before:

$$SS_T = \text{Grand } \Sigma X^2 - \frac{(\text{Grand total})^2}{\text{Total } N}$$

Step 7. Compute the sum of squares for treatments (SS_{Tr}):

$$SS_{Tr} = \sum_{i=1}^{r} \frac{\text{Tr. total}_i{}^2}{n} - \frac{(\text{Grand total})^2}{\text{Total } N}$$

This is the same formula as the treatment sum of squares in the completely randomized model except for the requirement of equal sample sizes.

Step 8. Compute the sum of squares for blocks (SS_B):

$$SS_B = \sum_{j=1}^{n} \frac{\text{Block total}_j{}^2}{r} - \frac{(\text{Grand total})^2}{\text{Total } N}$$

Step 9. Compute the sum of squares for error (SS_E) by subtraction:

$$SS_E = SS_T - SS_{Tr} - SS_B$$

Step 10. Compute the treatment mean square (MS_{Tr}):

$$MS_{Tr} = \frac{SS_{Tr}}{r-1}$$

This value is an estimate of the population variance plus an amount due to the effect of the treatments.

Step 11. Compute the error mean square (MS_E):

$$MS_E = \frac{SS_E}{(n-1)(r-1)}$$

This value is an estimate of the population variance.

Step 12. Compute the F ratio:

$$F = \frac{MS_{Tr}}{MS_E}$$

As was the case in the completely randomized analysis, the F ratio

$$F = \frac{\text{est. } \sigma^2 + \text{treatment effects}}{\text{est. } \sigma^2}$$

should approach 1 if there are no appreciable treatment effects and should increase as the treatment effects increase. Notice that the only changes in the F ratio from that which would

---

*Ostle, B.: Statistics in research, Ames, Iowa, 1956, Iowa State University Press; Guenther, W. C.: Analysis of variance, Englewood Cliffs, N. J., 1964, Prentice-Hall, Inc.

have been computed in the completely randomized model are a smaller error sum of squares brought about by subtracting the sum of squares due to blocking from the total sum of squares before computing the error sum of squares and a smaller denominator (degrees of freedom) for computing the error mean square. The analysis in effect reduces the estimate of population variance by eliminating the variance due to the blocking variable. This reduction in the denominator of the F test will make it more likely that significant treatment effects are detected by increasing the probability of rejecting false null hypotheses. This is equivalent to saying that when the blocking variable is an important contributor to the population variance, the randomized blocks design will reduce the probability of committing a type II error. If the blocking variable is not an important contributor to the population variance, the randomized blocks design will be less powerful than the completely randomized model because of the loss of degrees of freedom (denominator) for the error mean square.

To make this final point clear, consider the data in Table 13-3.

Table 13-3. Contrast between randomized blocks and completely randomized models for power of F test

$r = 3$, $n = 10$ $\alpha = .05$	Case 1		Case 2	
	Randomized blocks	Completely randomized	Randomized blocks	Completely randomized
Total SS	1,000	1,000	1,000	1,000
Treatment SS	100	100	200	200
Blocks SS	700	----	125	----
Error SS	200	900	675	800
Degrees of freedom for F test	2/18	2/27	2/18	2/27
Treatment MS	50	50	100	100
Error MS	11.1	33.3	37.5	29.6
F ratio	4.34	1.50	2.67	3.38
$F_{.05}$	3.55	3.34	3.55	3.34

In the data for case 1 of this table the blocking variable accounted for much of the total variance as indicated by the blocks sum of squares term of 700. Thus, even though the degrees of freedom for the F test denominator are less for the randomized blocks model than for the completely randomized model (18 vs. 27), the error mean square for the randomized blocks design is much less than for the other (11.1 vs. 33.3). In case 1, therefore, it was wise to use the randomized blocks model because the smaller F test denominator resulted in a larger F value than with the completely randomized model (4.34 vs. 1.50). In case 2, however, the blocking variable accounted for much less of the total variance, and the smaller error sum of squares was nullified by the smaller degrees of freedom value so that the error mean square of the randomized blocks model ended up larger than that for the other model (37.5 vs. 29.6). In case 2 it would have been unwise to use a randomized blocks design. The judgement on whether to conduct an experiment as a randomized blocks or as a completely randomized design should be made on the basis of previous experience or evidence from the scientific literature that shows whether the proposed blocking variable (e.g., body weight, strength, leg length) can be expected to account for a large share of the total experimental variance.

Step 13. Summarize the results in an analysis of variance table such as Table 13-4.

Table 13-4. Summary of results for randomized blocks analysis of variance

Source of variation	SS	Degrees of freedom	MS	F
Treatments	SS_{Tr}	$r-1$	MS_{Tr}	$\dfrac{MS_{Tr}}{MS_E}$
Blocks	SS_B	$n-1$		
Error	SS_E	$(r-1)(n-1)$	MS_E	
Total	SS_T			

Step 14. Consult a table of the F distribution (Table C-9, Appendix C) to compare the obtained F value with that found in the table at the predetermined alpha level and with the appropriate degrees of freedom, $r-1$ and $(r-1)(n-1)$. If the experimentally obtained F value is greater than the tabled value, reject the null hypothesis, H_o: $\mu_1 = \mu_2 \cdots = \mu_r$, and conclude that at least two of the treatment means are different, with the knowledge that there is a probability, alpha, that this conclusion is incorrect. If the tabled F value is greater than the obtained value, conclude that insufficient evidence was obtained to warrant rejection of the null hypothesis.

Step 15. If the obtained F ratio is greater than the tabled value, use the Tukey procedure to discover which means are significantly different from each other. The only difference in the Tukey procedure from that of the completely randomized design procedure is in the substitution of $(n-1)(r-1)$ degrees of freedom for $N-r$ degrees of freedom.

An example of the randomized blocks analysis of variance

Let us assume that Dr. Wallace wanted to study changes in liver glycogen concentration as the result of single and repeated bouts of exercise in guinea pigs. He read in the scientific literature that liver glycogen content varies markedly from one litter of animals to another but that it is quite similar among animals of the same litter. Most litters of guinea pigs have three animals at most. Therefore, to improve his chances of detecting any changes in glycogen as a result of exercise, Dr. Wallace decided to purchase nine different litters of three animals each and randomly assign each of the three animals per litter to a different experimental treatment: no exercise, one exercise bout, or ten exercise bouts over a 2-week period. The animals were sacrificed after 24 hours of rest.

Analytical procedure

Step 1. The assumptions of the randomized blocks analysis seemed reasonable.

Step 2. The hypotheses were as follows:

H_o: $\mu_1 = \mu_2 = \mu_3$ where 1, 2, 3 were the experimental treatments.
H_A: At least two means are different.

Step 3. Dr. Wallace decided upon an alpha level of .01.

Step 4. The data were displayed as in Table 13-5.

Table 13-5. Liver glycogen concentrations as percent tissue weight

Litters (blocks)	No exercise	Treatments 1 exercise bout	Treatments 10 exercise bouts	Block totals	Block totals² / 3
1	2.82	4.80	8.00	15.62	81.33
2	2.01	2.78	4.32	9.11	27.66
3	1.75	2.55	3.18	7.48	18.65
4	1.92	2.98	5.79	10.69	38.09
5	2.55	4.09	7.11	13.75	63.02
6	2.20	3.55	6.43	12.18	49.45
7	1.80	2.38	5.22	9.40	29.45
8	2.93	5.00	9.57	17.50	102.08
9	2.70	4.63	7.88	15.21	77.11
Treatment totals	20.68	32.76	57.50	110.94	486.84
Treatment means	2.30	3.64	6.39		
Treatment ΣX^2	49.20	127.58	399.12	575.90	
Treatment totals² / 9	47.52	119.25	367.36	534.13	

Step 5. The column and block totals and means, column sums of squares and variances, and the grand total, mean, sum of squares and variance were computed and entered in Table 13-5.

Step 6. The total sum of squares was computed:

$$SS_T = \text{Grand } \Sigma X^2 - \frac{(\text{Grand total})^2}{\text{Total } N}$$

$$SS_T = 575.90 - \frac{(110.94)^2}{27}$$

$$SS_T = 120.09$$

Step 7.   The treatment sum of squares was computed:

$$SS_{Tr} = \sum_{i=1}^{3} \frac{Tr.\ total_i{}^2}{9} - \frac{(Grand\ total)^2}{Total\ N}$$

$$SS_{Tr} = 543.13 - \frac{(110.94)^2}{27}$$

$$SS_{Tr} = 78.32$$

Step 8.   The sum of squares for blocks was computed:

$$SS_{B} = \sum_{j=1}^{9} \frac{Block\ total_j{}^2}{3} - \frac{(Grand\ total)^2}{Total\ N}$$

$$SS_{B} = 486.84 - \frac{(110.94)^2}{27}$$

$$SS_{B} = 31.03$$

Step 9.   The error sum of squares was computed:

$$SS_{E} = SS_{T} - SS_{Tr} - SS_{B}$$

$$SS_{E} = 120.09 - 78.32 - 31.03$$

$$SS_{E} = 10.74$$

Step 10.   The mean square for treatments was computed:

$$MS_{Tr} = \frac{SS_{Tr}}{r-1}$$

$$MS_{Tr} = \frac{78.32}{3-1}$$

$$MS_{Tr} = 39.16$$

Step 11.   The error mean square was computed:

$$MS_{E} = \frac{(SS_{E})}{(n-1)(r-1)}$$

$$MS_{E} = \frac{(10.74)}{(9-1)(3-1)}$$

$$MS_{E} = 0.67$$

Step 12.   The F ratio was computed:

$$F = \frac{MS_{Tr}}{MS_{E}}$$

$$F = \frac{39.16}{0.67}$$

$$F = 58.45$$

Step 13.   The results are summarized in Table 13-6.

Table 13-6. Summary of results of glycogen data analysis

Source of variation	SS	Degrees of freedom	MS	F
Treatments	78.32	2	39.16	
Blocks	31.03	8		58.45
Error	10.74	16	0.67	
Total	120.09			

Step 14. The F table (Table C-9, Appendix C) shows an F value of 6.23 for $\alpha = .01$, with $r - 1 = 2$ and $(r - 1)(n - 1) = 16$ degrees of freedom for the numerator and denominator, respectively. Since the obtained F ratio, 58.45, was larger than the tabled value, the appropriate conclusion is that at least two of the treatment means are significantly different. There is a probability of .01 that this conclusion is incorrect.

Step 15. Since a significant F ratio was determined, it is appropriate to compare all possible pairs of means with the Tukey procedure to determine which means are significantly different.

Tukey procedure example

Step 1. The differences between means are displayed in Table 13-7.

Table 13-7. Differences between sample means

Comparison means	Comparison mean $-$ Smallest mean	Comparison mean $-$ Second smallest mean
6.39	$6.39 - 2.30 = 4.09$	$6.39 - 3.64 = 2.75$
3.64	$3.64 - 2.30 = 1.34$	------
2.30	------	

Step 2. The T value is computed and compared with the differences between sample means. (See Chapter 12 for an explanation of the Tukey procedure.)

$$T = (q_{.01;\, 3,\, 16})\ \sqrt{0.67/9}$$

$$T = 4.79(.27)$$

$$T = 1.29$$

Since all differences between means are greater than the computed T value, the appropriate conclusion is that all treatments had significant effects. In other words, exercise only once increased the concentration of glycogen over that of sedentary animals, and chronic exercise increased the glycogen still further. There is a probability of .01 that one or more of those conclusions is incorrect.

Problems

1. Dr. Putton studied the heart rate changes caused by physical training of three different types. To remove the variability in response due to differences in pretraining heart rates

(those with higher initial heart rates could expect greater decreases with training), he grouped his thirty-two subjects into eight blocks of four subjects each on the basis of pretraining heart rates. One subject of each block was then randomly assigned to one of the three training regimens or to a sedentary control group. The changes in heart rate after 6 weeks were recorded. Analyze these data with a randomized blocks analysis of variance and the appropriate multiple comparison of means technique. Interpret the results of the experiment.

Blocks	Treatments			
	Untrained	Bicycling	Weight lifting	Running
1	+ 5	− 15	− 1	− 20
2	+ 2	− 13	− 2	− 18
3	− 3	− 9	0	− 14
4	+ 4	− 6	+ 5	− 11
5	− 6	− 5	− 2	− 10
6	− 2	+ 2	+ 5	− 9
7	+ 1	− 6	− 3	− 8
8	+ 5	− 4	+ 1	− 2

2. Jon Loi analyzed the results of a written fitness knowledge test taken by twenty-one students who had been matched on the basis of I.Q. into seven blocks of three students each. One student from each block had then been randomly assigned to one of three different teachers. Analyze the test scores and determine whether one teacher did a better teaching job for this particular test.

Blocks	Teachers		
	A	B	C
1	95	90	87
2	89	84	82
3	83	78	80
4	76	70	71
5	70	68	65
6	65	62	58
7	60	61	50

Chapter **14**

Two-way analysis
of variance

TWO-WAY, FIXED EFFECTS, COMPLETELY RANDOMIZED MODEL
Purpose

Many times a research hypothesis in physical education involves the relationship between two independent variables and a dependent variable. One might hypothesize, for instance, that the reason physical training lowers one's resting heart rate is that the exercise somehow increases the amount of stimulation the heart receives from the vagus nerves, which act to lower the heart rate. To investigate this hypothesis, the scientist might study normal exercised and sedentary rats and compare their heart rates with exercised and sedentary rats that have been vagotomized (vagus nerves to the heart have been severed). The most efficient way to make this study is by a two-way analysis of variance in which the effects of two independent variables, exercise state and vagus condition, and their interaction effects on the dependent variable, resting heart rate, are analyzed. This design is illustrated in Table 14-1.

Table 14-1. Effects of exercise state and vagus condition on resting heart rate

	Sedentary	Single exercise	Repeated exercise
Normal vagus	X X X X	X X X X	X X X X
Vagotomized	X X X X	X X X X	X X X X

If the vagotomized rats that have been repeatedly exercised showed heart rates lower than the sedentary vagotomized group, the investigator would have evidence that the bradycardia (heart rate reduction) of training was not simply due to increased vagal stimulation. The other groups of animals serve as controls in the experiment.

In the two-way analysis of variance the total sum of squares is partitioned into a sum of squares for effects due to independent variable A, a sum of squares for independent variable B, one for AB interaction effects, and finally, a sum of squares for effects due to error and other uncontrolled factors. The two-way analysis is more efficient than two one-way analyses (e.g., effects of exercise state and effects of vagus condition) because fewer subjects are needed to get equivalent information and because only with the two-way analysis can one detect interaction effects, that is, effects of particular combinations of variable A and variable B.

Layout of the data

The data for the two-way, completely randomized model of the analysis of variance can be summarized in a table such as Table 14-2.

Table 14-2. Layout of data for the two-way analysis of variance

Variable A \ Variable B	Level 1	Level 2	$\cdots$	Level b	Row totals	Row means	Row totals²
Level 1	X_{111} $\vdots$ X_{11n} Cell total Cell mean	X_{211} $\vdots$ X_{21n} Cell total Cell mean	$\cdots$	X_{b11} $\vdots$ X_{b1n} Cell total Cell mean	RT_1	$R\bar{X}_1$	RT_1^2
Level 2	X_{121} $\vdots$ X_{12n} Cell total Cell mean	X_{221} $\vdots$ X_{22n} Cell total Cell mean	$\cdots$	X_{b21} $\vdots$ X_{b2n} Cell total Cell mean	RT_2	$R\bar{X}_2$	RT_2^2
$\vdots$	$\vdots$	$\vdots$		$\vdots$	$\vdots$	$\vdots$	$\vdots$
Level a	X_{1a1} $\vdots$ X_{1an} Cell total Cell mean	X_{2a1} $\vdots$ X_{2an} Cell total Cell mean	$\cdots$	X_{ba1} $\vdots$ X_{ban} Cell total Cell mean	RT_a	$R\bar{X}_a$	RT_a^2
Column totals	CT_1	CT_2	$\cdots$	CT_b	Grand total	-----	$\sum_{j=1}^{a} RT_j^2$
Column means	$C\bar{X}_1$	$C\bar{X}_2$	$\cdots$	$C\bar{X}_b$	-----		
ΣX^2, columns	ΣX_1^2	ΣX_2^2	$\cdots$	ΣX_b^2	Grand ΣX^2		
Column totals²	CT_1^2	CT_2^2	$\cdots$	CT_b^2	$\sum_{i=1}^{b} CT_i^2$		

The notation for the two-way layout becomes slightly altered from that of the one-way and randomized blocks designs. In this layout there are n

observations for each cell, with a cell being made up of all the observations for the ith level of variable B, and the jth level of variable A, where $i = 1, 2, \ldots, b$ and $j = 1, 2, \ldots, a$. The totals and means for the columns (variable B) are presented at the bottom of the table, and those for the rows (variable A) at the right. We will consider only the case where there is more than one observation per cell and where there is an equal number of observations for each cell. Consult other statistics texts for the case of unequal n or where $n = 1$.[*]

Assumptions of the test

The assumptions of the two-way analysis of variance are the following:
1. The data are measured on an interval or ratio scale.
2. The ab cells represent ab random samples of size n drawn from ab populations. This means that subjects must be randomly assigned to cells or treatment combinations.
3. Each of the ab populations is normal.
4. Each of the ab populations has the same variance.

As before, assumptions 3 and 4 are not vital if the sample sizes are equal and fairly large ($n > 10$).

Analytical procedure

Data can be analyzed with the two-way analysis of variance by the following steps:

Step 1.   Determine whether the assumptions of the test are tenable.

Step 2.   State the hypotheses and alternatives. With the two-way analysis there are usually three main hypotheses:

(a) H_o: $\mu_{1A} = \mu_{2A} = \cdots = \mu_{aA}$

   H_A: At least two levels of variable A have different means (have significantly different effects).

(b) H_o: $\mu_{1B} = \mu_{2B} = \cdots = \mu_{bB}$

   H_A: At least two levels of variable B have different means (have significantly different effects).

(c) H_o: $\mu_{1AB} = \mu_{2AB} = \cdots = \mu_{abAB}$

   H_A: At least two of the ab cell means (after removing the effects due to variables A and B) are different. The rejection of this null hypothesis means that there is some combination of levels of the two variables that produces greater effects than the others.

If the third null hypothesis is not rejected (no apparent interactions between levels of A and B), then inferences about the effects of variables A and B apply equally over all levels of B and A, respectively. If interactions do exist, then the proper interpretation of a failure to reject the first and second null hypotheses is that there are no differences in the effects of various levels of variables A and B when averaged over all levels of B and A,

---

[*]Scheffé, H.: The analysis of variance, New York, 1959, John Wiley & Sons, Inc.; Snedecor, G. W.: Statistical methods, Ames, Iowa, 1956, Iowa State University Press.

respectively, but that certain combinations of the two variables have different effects than other combinations.

Step 3. Choose the significance level you will accept for the experiment.

Step 4. Arrange the data as in Table 14-2.

Step 5. Compute the necessary totals for Table 14-2.

Step 6. Compute the total sum of squares (SS_T):

$$SS_T = \text{Grand } \Sigma X^2 - \frac{(\text{Grand total})^2}{\text{Total } N}$$

Step 7. Compute the treatment sum of squares (SS_{Tr}):

$$SS_{Tr} = \frac{\overset{ab}{\underset{ij=11}{\Sigma}} \text{Cell total}_{ij}^2}{n} - \frac{(\text{Grand total})^2}{\text{Total } N}$$

Step 8. Compute the error sum of squares (SS_E):

$$SS_E = SS_T - SS_{Tr}$$

Step 9. Partition the treatment sum of squares (SS_{Tr}) into three parts— variable A sum of squares (SS_A), variable B sum of squares (SS_B), and AB interaction sum of squares (SS_{AB}):

$$SS_A = \frac{\overset{a}{\underset{j=1}{\Sigma}} \text{Row total}_j^2}{bn} - \frac{(\text{Grand total})^2}{\text{Total } N}$$

$$SS_B = \frac{\overset{b}{\underset{i=1}{\Sigma}} \text{Column total}_i^2}{an} - \frac{(\text{Grand total})^2}{\text{Total } N}$$

$$SS_{AB} = SS_{Tr} - SS_A - SS_B$$

Step 10. Compute the mean square for variable A (MS_A):

$$MS_A = \frac{SS_A}{a-1}$$

Step 11. Compute the mean square for variable B (MS_B):

$$MS_B = \frac{SS_B}{b-1}$$

Step 12. Compute the AB interaction mean square (MS_{AB}):

$$MS_{AB} = \frac{SS_{AB}}{(a-1)(b-1)}$$

Step 13. Compute the error mean square (MS_E):

$$MS_E = \frac{SS_E}{ab(n-1)}$$

Step 14. Compute the F-ratio for A effects, B effects, and AB interaction effects:

$$F_A = \frac{MS_A}{MS_E}$$

$$F_B = \frac{MS_B}{MS_E}$$

$$F_{AB} = \frac{MS_{AB}}{MS_E}$$

The error mean square (MS_E) again is an estimate of the population variance (σ^2), whereas MS_A estimates the population variance plus variable A effects, MS_B estimates population variance plus variable B effects, and MS_{AB} estimates the population variance plus AB interaction effects. The three F ratios will increase as the effects of the respective variables increase:

$$F_A = \frac{\text{est. } \sigma^2 + \text{A effects}}{\text{est. } \sigma^2}$$

$$F_B = \frac{\text{est. } \sigma^2 + \text{B effects}}{\text{est. } \sigma^2}$$

$$F_{AB} = \frac{\text{est. } \sigma^2 + \text{AB effects}}{\text{est. } \sigma^2}$$

Step 15. Summarize the results in an analysis of variance table such as Table 14-3.

Table 14-3. Summary of results for two-way analysis of variance

Source of variation	SS	Degrees of freedom	MS	F
Variable A	SS_A	$a - 1$	MS_A	$\dfrac{MS_A}{MS_E}$
Variable B	SS_B	$b - 1$	MS_B	$\dfrac{MS_B}{MS_E}$
AB interaction	SS_{AB}	$(a - 1)(b - 1)$	MS_{AB}	$\dfrac{MS_{AB}}{MS_E}$
Error	SS_E	$ab(n - 1)$	MS_E	
Total	SS_T	$N - 1$		

One problem concerning experimental α levels should be pointed out here. Previously we have computed only one F ratio, but here we compute three. Each of these three F ratios has an α level associated with it. These three α values are usually the same, for example, .05 or .01. However, since we are using the same data to compute three different F ratios, there is some probability greater than α of rejecting one or more of the three null hypotheses when all are true. This overall experimental alpha, α_E, is less than $1 - (1 - \alpha)^3$ when the three hypotheses are each tested with the same α level. When α is .05, the overall experimental alpha is less than .143 and when α is .01, $\alpha_E < .0297$. This overall experimental alpha level should be considered when interpreting the results of a study.

Step 16. Consult a table of the F distribution (Table C-9, Appendix C) to compare the obtained F ratios with those found in the table at the predetermined alpha level and appropriate degrees of freedom. For F_A the degrees of freedom are $a - 1$ and $ab(n - 1)$; for F_B, $b - 1$ and $ab(n - 1)$; and for F_{AB}, $(a - 1)(b - 1)$ and $ab(n - 1)$. As usual, an obtained F ratio greater than the tabled value is interpreted as evidence for rejecting the null hypothesis.

Step 17. If an obtained F ratio is greater than the tabled value, use the Tukey procedure to compare all pairs of means and determine which are significantly different from each other. Differences between the variable A means should be compared with the following:

$$T_A = [q_{\alpha;\, a,\, ab(n-1)}]\, \sqrt{MS_E/bn}$$

Differences between variable B means should be compared with the following:

$$T_B = [q_{\alpha;\, b,\, ab(n-1)}]\, \sqrt{MS_E/an}$$

Differences between cell means (AB interaction effects) should be compared with the following:

$$T_{AB} = [q_{\alpha;\, ab,\, ab(n-1)}]\, \sqrt{MS_E/n}$$

Example of a two-way analysis of variance

Zephyr Flotsam was an assistant gymnastics coach at Driftwood College while working on an advanced degree in the Department of Kinesiology. His particular area of interest was the psychological aspects of highly skilled performance. The gymnastics team practiced in four small rooms and competed in the 4,000 seat Driftwood arena. Zephyr had a feeling that one reason his team performed poorly in competition was the disruptive influence of large crowds compared with that of the small groups that were present in the practice rooms. Since he had learned that high anxiety levels

Table 14-4. Anxiety ratings prior to competition

Variable A \ Variable B	No crowd during competition	Crowd during competition	Row totals	Row means	Row totals²
No crowd during practice	100 145 132 120 115 $\Sigma X = 612$ $\bar{X} = 122.4$	193 187 172 163 181 $\Sigma X = 896$ $\bar{X} = 179.2$	1,508	150.8	2,274,064
Crowd during practice	98 111 103 115 107 $\Sigma X = 534$ $\bar{X} = 106.8$	122 116 103 148 125 $\Sigma X = 614$ $\bar{X} = 122.8$	1,148	114.8	1,317,904
Column totals	1,146	1,510	2,656	-----	3,591,968
Column means	114.6	151.0	-----		
ΣX^2, columns	133,282	237,610	370,892		
Column totals²	1,313,316	2,280,100	3,593,416		

tend to impair motor performance, Zephyr hypothesized that anxiety during competition before crowds was a factor in causing his gymnasts to do poorly, and that the competitors could become "conditioned" to these high anxiety levels by constant exposure to crowd situations in practice.

To test his hypothesis, Zephyr designed an experiment in which half the team practiced in the large arena before crowds and the other half continued to practice in the small rooms. For competition, half of both practice groups performed before a large crowd, whereas the other half performed before three judges in the small rooms. As the dependent variable for the experiment, Zephyr used scores on a paper and pencil test for anxiety that was purported to be very precise. The test was administered just before competition after the gymnasts had seen the spectators present. The two independent variables were spectator presence at practice and during competition. The data are shown in Table 14-4.

Step 1. The assumptions of the analysis of variance seem tenable.

Step 2. Since Zephyr was primarily interested in whether practice before crowds would reduce precompetition anxiety, the primary hypothesis of interest was the hypothesis about interaction effects:

H_o: $\mu_{1AB} = \mu_{2AB} = \mu_{3AB} = \mu_{4AB}$

H_A: At least two of the four cell population means (after removing effects due to A and B variables) are different. In particular, Zephyr suspected that the group which trained before crowds would have lower anxiety levels when performing before crowds than the other groups.

The hypothesis of secondary interest was that the anxiety levels prior to competition in front of crowds would be greater than that before no crowds:

H_o: $\mu_{1B} = \mu_{2B}$

H_A: The mean for crowd during competition is different from the mean for no crowd.

Since the lack of spectators during competition was somewhat artificial, Zephyr was not particularly interested in whether the practice conditions affected the anxiety when performing before only three judges. But since this information might provide support for a broader theory about the transfer of practice anxiety to competition anxiety, he decided to also test the following:

H_o: $\mu_{1A} = \mu_{2A}$

H_A: The mean for no practice crowd is different from the mean for crowd present at practice.

Step 3. Zephyr decided to accept as significant all F ratios exceeding the tabled values at the .05 level. He understood that this implied an overall experimental probability of less than .143 for rejecting one or more of the three null hypotheses when all were correct.

Step 4. The data were arranged in Table 14-4.

Step 5. The necessary totals for Table 14-4 were entered in the table.

Step 6. The total sum of squares was computed:

$$SS_T = \text{Grand } \Sigma X^2 - \frac{(\text{Grand total})^2}{\text{Total } N}$$

$$SS_T = 370{,}892 - \frac{(2{,}656)^2}{20}$$

$$SS_T = 370{,}892 - 352{,}717$$

$$SS_T = 18{,}175$$

Step 7. The treatment sum of squares was computed:

$$SS_{Tr} = \frac{\overset{ab}{\underset{ij=11}{\Sigma}} \text{Cell total}_{ij}^2}{n} - \frac{(\text{Grand total})^2}{\text{Total } N}$$

$$SS_{Tr} = \frac{612^2 + 896^2 + 534^2 + 614^2}{5} - 352{,}717$$

$$SS_{Tr} = \frac{1{,}839{,}512}{5} - 352{,}717$$

$$SS_{Tr} = 367{,}902 - 352{,}717$$

$$SS_{Tr} = 15{,}185$$

Step 8. The error sum of squares was computed:

$$SS_E = SS_T - SS_{Tr}$$

$$SS_E = 18{,}175 - 15{,}185$$

$$SS = 2{,}990$$

Step 9. The treatment sum of squares was partitioned into a sum of squares due to presence or absence of spectators at competition (SS_B), a sum of squares due to presence or absence of spectators during practice (SS_A), and a sum of squares due to the effects of particular combinations of spectators or no spectators at practice and competition (SS_{AB}).

$$SS_A = \frac{\overset{a}{\underset{j=1}{\Sigma}} \text{Row total}_j^2}{bn} - \frac{(\text{Grand total})^2}{\text{Total } N}$$

$$SS_A = \frac{3{,}591{,}968}{2 \times 5} - 352{,}717$$

$$SS_A = 359{,}197 - 352{,}717$$

$$SS_A = 6{,}480$$

$$SS_B = \frac{\overset{b}{\underset{i=1}{\Sigma}} \text{Column total}_i^2}{an} - \frac{(\text{Grand total})^2}{\text{Total } N}$$

$$SS_B = \frac{1{,}146^2 + 1{,}510^2}{2 \times 5} - 352{,}717$$

$$SS_B = \frac{3{,}593{,}416}{10} - 352{,}717$$

$$SS_B = 359{,}342 - 352{,}717$$

$$SS_B = 6{,}625$$

$$SS_{AB} = SS_{Tr} - SS_A - SS_B$$

$$SS_{AB} = 15{,}185 - 6{,}480 - 6{,}625$$

$$SS_{AB} = 2{,}080$$

Step 10. The mean square for practice conditions (variable A) was computed:

$$MS_A = \frac{SS_A}{a-1}$$

$$MS_A = \frac{6{,}480}{2-1}$$

$$MS_A = 6{,}480$$

Step 11. The mean square for competition conditions (variable B) was computed:

$$MS_B = \frac{SS_B}{b-1}$$

$$MS_B = \frac{6{,}625}{2-1}$$

$$MS_B = 6{,}625$$

Step 12. The mean square for practice conditions × competition conditions interactions was computed:

$$MS_{AB} = \frac{SS_{AB}}{(a-1)(b-1)}$$

$$MS_{AB} = \frac{2{,}080}{1 \times 1}$$

$$MS_{AB} = 2{,}080$$

Step 13. The error mean square was computed:

$$MS_E = \frac{SS_E}{ab(n-1)}$$

$$MS_E = \frac{2{,}990}{2 \times 2(5-1)}$$

$$MS_E = \frac{2{,}990}{16}$$

$$MS_E = 187$$

Step 14. The respective F ratios were computed:

$$\text{Practice effects: } F_A = \frac{MS_A}{MS_E} = \frac{6,480}{187} = 34.65$$

$$\text{Competition effects: } F_B = \frac{MS_B}{MS_E} = \frac{6,625}{187} = 35.43$$

Practice $\times$ competition interaction effects:

$$F_{AB} = \frac{MS_{AB}}{MS_E} = \frac{2,080}{187} = 11.12$$

Step 15. The results are summarized in Table 14-5.

Table 14-5. Summary of analysis of variance of anxiety scores

Source of variation	SS	Degrees of freedom	MS	F
Practice conditions	6,480	1	6,480	34.65
Competition conditions	6,625	1	6,625	35.43
Practice $\times$ competition interaction	2,080	1	2,080	11.12
Error	2.990	16	187	
Total	18,175	19		

Step 16. The table of the F distribution (Table C-9, Appendix C) was consulted to obtain the appropriate F ratio at $\alpha = .05$ with the appropriate degrees of freedom.

$$F_A \quad \text{compared to } F_{.05; 1, 16} = 4.49$$

$$F_B \quad \text{compared to } F_{.05; 1, 16} = 4.49$$

$$F_{AB} \quad \text{compared to } F_{.05; 1, 16} = 4.49$$

Step 17. Since all three obtained F ratios were greater than the appropriate tabled value, it was appropriate to compare all A, B, and AB means with the Tukey procedure. However, since both variables A and B had only two levels, there was no need for Tukey comparisons with these variables. The cell-means differences were tabled as in Table 14-6.

Table 14-6. Differences between cell means

Comparison	Comparison − Smallest mean		Comparison − Second smallest mean		Comparison − Second highest mean	
179.2	$179.2 - 106.8 = 72.4$		$179.2 - 122.4 = 56.8$		$179.2 - 122.8 = 56.4$	
122.8	$122.8 - 106.8 = 16.0$		$122.8 - 122.4 = 0.4$		------	
122.4	$122.4 - 106.8 = 15.6$		------		------	
106.8	------		------		------	

The T value with which the differences between cell means should be compared was computed as follows:

$T = [q_{\alpha:\, ab,\, ab(n-1)}] \sqrt{MS_E/n}$ where q is a value
obtained from Table C-6, Appendix C.

$T = [q_{.05;\, 2 \times 2,\, 2 \times 2(5-1)}] \sqrt{187/5}$

$T = [q_{.05;\, 4,\, 16}] \sqrt{187/5}$

$T = (4.05)(6.12)$

$T = 24.79$

Since only one interaction cell mean, "no crowd during practice" $\times$ "crowd during competition" was significantly greater than the others (72.4, 56.8, and 56.4 are the only differences greater than $T = 24.79$), the appropriate conclusion is that greater anxiety levels in response to spectators during competition occur in those who have not practiced before spectators.

Since these interactions were present, the appropriate conclusions about the effects of spectators during practice were that when averaged over both crowd and no crowd competition, anxiety is lower in subjects who have practiced before many spectators. Likewise, the appropriate conclusion about the effects of spectators during competition is that when averaged over both practice conditions, lower anxiety levels were found in those who competed before only a few spectators.

As a practical matter, Zephyr Flotsam concluded that his team would be better off to practice before as many spectators as possible in the large arena. As a theoretical matter, one might postulate that an adaptation to competition anxiety can be brought about by proper anxiety conditioning during precompetition training.

Although we have presented only the procedures for an analysis involving two variables, it should be noted that any number of variables can be handled in a factorial analysis of variance, that is, three-way, four-way, and higher-way designs. Guenther* treats the three factors case.

ANALYSIS OF VARIANCE FOR REPEATED OBSERVATIONS ON THE SAME SUBJECTS—SINGLE-FACTOR MODEL
Purpose

When the effects of individual differences in response to an experimental factor are very large, an investigator may wish to control those effects by designing an experiment in which the same subjects are tested under all levels of the experimental factor. An example of such an experiment is illustrated in Table 14-7. In this experiment the investigator was making an analysis of heart rates when bicycling at a constant speed with three different handlebar positions—high, medium, and low.

Notice that this design looks very similar to the two-way analysis discussed previously; only in this case one factor is "subjects," with the obser-

---

*Guenther, W. C.: Analysis of variance, Englewood Cliffs, N. J., 1964, Prentice-Hall, Inc.

Table 14-7. Heart rates at different handlebar positions

Subject	Handlebar height		
	High	Medium	Low
1	170	167	150
	165	163	152
	168	165	151
2	160	153	142
	158	154	147
	162	152	143
3	188	177	162
	179	170	168
	184	170	163

vations within a cell being repeated observations on those subjects. As a matter of fact, the analysis for this type of design proceeds exactly as that for the two-way analysis except that the denominator of the F ratio for determining experimental factor effects is MS_{AB} rather than MS_E. The reason for this difference is that the subjects under this model are assumed to be a random sample from a very large population of subjects, and the conclusions about subject effects are to be generalized to that large population.

Layout of the data

The layout of the data for this design is exactly as shown in Table 14-2, with subjects as variable A. In the case where there is only one observation per subject under each level of variable B, the layout is the same as that for a randomized blocks design (Table 13-1).

Assumptions of the test

Whereas in the completely randomized model of the two-way analysis the observations were assumed to be independent from each other, the repeated observations on the same subjects will usually be positively correlated with each other; that is, a subject with a high score on one treatment is likely to be high on another because of the unique factors he brings to the experiment with him. Therefore the assumptions underlying the F test are somewhat different. They are as follows:

1. The observations are on at least an interval scale of measurement.
2. The subjects are randomly selected from a large normal population. (The ratio of sample size to population size should approach zero.)
3. The b populations of potential observations under the b experimental treatments are assumed to be normal with equal variances.
4. The populations of potential interactions between subjects and treatments are assumed to be normal.
5. Although subject effects, treatment effects, and subject by treatment interaction effects are each assumed to be normally distributed, some of the variables will usually be correlated.

6. The covariances between all pairs of treatment populations are equal. This homogeneity of covariances assumption can invalidate the F test if the assumption is not satisfied when the data are correlated. A test for this assumption is given by Winer.*

7. Except where learning or carry-over effects are of chief interest, the experimental treatments are assumed to be presented to the subjects in a random order, with adequate time allowed between treatments to dissipate any carry-over effects, for example, fatigue, learning, effect of drug.

When there is doubt about homogeneity of treatment variances and covariances, a conservative F test can be applied to test for significant treatment effects. This F ratio is the same as was indicated previously, MS_{Tr}/MS_{AB} (or MS_{Tr}/MS_E when there is only one observation per cell), but the degrees of freedom are changed to 1 and $n-1$ (number of subjects minus 1) for the numerator and denominator, respectively.

A note of caution should also be registered about possible carry-over effects. Although this design appears attractive because of the smaller number of subjects required than in the one-way completely randomized design, any carry-over effects from one treatment to another may obscure treatment effects. Thus, in an experiment designed to measure physiological or psychological responses to different exercise treatments the investigator must ensure that adequate time is allowed for the subjects to return to their normal states before being exposed to a different treatment. If treatment effects are of primary interest in a study, it is usually wise to use a completely randomized design to avoid carry-over effects; but in a learning or longitudinal experiment one must use the same subjects because the primary interest is in the interaction and carry-over effects. In the usual learning or longitudinal type of experiment in physical education, both trials and exercise or training regimens are of interest, so that the two-factor design with repeated observations is more appropriate than this single-factor design. The two-factor design will be considered in a later section of this chapter.

Analytical procedure

The analysis of the data for the single-factor repeated measures design is done in the same way as that for the two-way completely randomized model, except that the denominator of the F ratio for determining variable B effects is MS_{AB} rather than MS_E. In the special case where there is only one observation per subject per treatment, interaction effects cannot be determined, and the data are analyzed in a manner identical to that for the randomized blocks design, where subjects are considered to be the blocking agents. In this case the interaction effect is lumped into the error term, and the denominator of the F ratio is MS_E, the same as that for the randomized blocks design.

---

*Winer, B. J.: Statistical principles in experimental design, New York, 1962, McGraw-Hill Book Co., pp. 369-374.

ANALYSIS OF VARIANCE FOR REPEATED OBSERVATIONS ON THE SAME SUBJECTS—TWO-FACTOR MODEL
Purpose

One of the most useful experimental designs for investigators in physical education is the design that can be used to test the longitudinal effects or learning effects of two or more experimental treatments, often teaching methods or training programs. Examples of such studies are as follows:

1. Effects of three different teaching methods on learning of a motor skill, e.g., hurdling, basket shooting, ballet movement, javelin throw
2. Effects of regular exercise on body-weight fluctuation
3. Effects of different environmental cues on learning of a perceptual-motor skill
4. Effects of regular exercise on red blood cell counts

Although these studies could all be designed as regular two-way analysis

Table 14-8. Layout of data for a two-factor analysis of variance with repeated observations on the same subjects

Factor A treatments$_j$, where $j = 1, 2, \ldots, a$	Subject$_{jki}$ $j = 1,2,\ldots,a$ $k = 1,2,\ldots,n$	Factor B Trial$_i$, where $i = 1, 2, \ldots, b$ Trial 1	Trial 2	$\cdots$ Trial b	Subject totals	Row totals	Row totals^2
Treatment 1	11 12 $\vdots$ 1n	X_{111} X_{112} $\vdots$ X_{11n}	X_{211} X_{212} $\vdots$ X_{21n}	X_{b11} X_{b12} $\cdots$ $\vdots$ X_{b1n}	ST_{11} ST_{12} $\vdots$ ST_{1n}	RT_1	RT_1^2
	Cell totals Cell means	T_{11} $\overline{X}_{11}$	T_{21} $\overline{X}_{21}$	T_{b1} $\overline{X}_{b1}$	—	—	—
Treatment 2	21 22 $\vdots$ 2n	X_{121} X_{122} $\vdots$ X_{12n}	X_{221} X_{222} $\vdots$ X_{22n}	X_{b21} X_{b22} $\cdots$ X_{b2n}	ST_{21} ST_{22} $\vdots$ ST_{2n}	RT_2	RT_2^2
	Cell totals Cell means	T_{12} $\overline{X}_{12}$	T_{22} $\overline{X}_{22}$	T_{b2} $\overline{X}_{b2}$	—	—	—
$\vdots$	$\vdots$	$\vdots$	$\vdots$ $\vdots$	$\vdots$	$\vdots$	$\vdots$	$\vdots$
Treatment a	a1 a2 $\vdots$ an	X_{1a1} X_{1a2} $\vdots$ $\overline{X}_{1an}$	X_{2a1} X_{2a2} $\vdots$ $\overline{X}_{2an}$	X_{ba1} X_{ba2} $\cdots$ $\vdots$ $\overline{X}_{ban}$	ST_{a1} ST_{a2} $\vdots$ ST_{an}	RT_a	RT_a^2
	Cell totals Cell means	T_{1a} $\overline{X}_{1a}$	T_{2a} $\overline{X}_{2a}$	T_{ba} $\cdots$ $\overline{X}_{ba}$	—	—	—
Column totals		CT_1	CT_2	$\cdots$ CT_b	Grand total	—	$\sum\limits_{j=1}^{a} RT_j^2$
Column totals^2		CT_1^2	CT_2^2	$\cdots$ CT_b^2	$\sum\limits_{i=1}^{b} CT_i^2$	—	
ΣX^2, columns		ΣX_1^2	ΣX_2^2	$\cdots$ ΣX_b^2	Grand ΣX^2	—	

of variance problems, two reasons may be advanced for using repeated measures on the same subjects. First, the variance caused by individual differences in response to the treatments may mask the treatment and longitudinal or learning effects; with the repeated measures design, an attempt is made to remove this variance due to individual differences. Second, a regular two-way design requires independent observations and therefore many more subjects than a repeated measures design, where the observations for each subject are assumed to be correlated.

These two reasons for using the repeated measures design should be evaluated with the knowledge that more restrictive assumptions are required in the repeated measures design than in the regular two-way analysis where independent observations are made. We recommend that the use of the repeated measures design be limited to experiments in which the rate of learning is of primary interest or to experiments that require repeated measures because of insufficient subject availability.

Layout of the data

The data can be depicted in the form of Table 14-8. Note that this layout is essentially the same as that for the regular two-way analysis of variance except that columns for subjects and subject totals have been added, and column and row means have been deleted to save space. In this layout, X_{ijk} is the observation for the kth subject of the jth level of factor A under the ith level of factor B. For example, X_{234} is the observation for the fourth subject for treatment three at trial two.

Assumptions of the test

The assumptions of the two-factor model for repeated measures are similar to those for the single-factor model and are as follows:
1. The observations are on at least an interval scale of measurement.
2. The groups of subjects within each level of factor A are random samples from a common population with an underlying normal distribution.
3. The potential populations of observations under the different levels of factors A and B, and the subject by factor B interaction effects are each assumed to be normally distributed, but there will usually be a correlation between two or more of these variables; that is, all observations are not independent.
4. A homogeneity of variance is assumed to exist between the a groups of subjects and the factor B by subjects interaction effects.
5. There is a homogeneity of covariance between all pairs of columns or a constant correlation between pairs of observations on the same subject, that correlation being the same for all subjects.
6. A special pattern of elements in certain covariance matrices must exist. The latter three assumptions are quite restrictive and may be tested.*

---

*Winer, B. J.: Statistical principles in experimental design, New York, 1962, McGraw-Hill Book Co., pp. 304-305, 364-374.

However, an approximate F test can be used that avoids some of these assumptions. Although this approximate F test (to be discussed under *analytical procedures*) is somewhat conservative, the reader of this text may prefer it to the somewhat involved procedures required to test the assumptions.

Analytical procedure

Most of the now familiar analytical steps are required for the two-factor repeated measures design. They are as follows:

Step 1. Determine whether the assumptions of the test are reasonable. If the covariance assumptions appear untenable, an approximate F test may be used, as explained later in this section.

Step 2. State the hypotheses and alternatives. With a learning type of experiment these are usually as follows:

(a) H_o: $\mu_{11} = \mu_{12} = \cdots = \mu_{ab}$

H_A: At least two of the cell means (after removing the effects due to variables A and B) are different. Rejection of the null hypothesis leads to the conclusion that there is some combination(s) of treatment and trials which produce(s) greater effects than the others.

(b) H_o: $\mu_{1B} = \mu_{2B} = \cdots = \mu_{bB}$

H_A: At least two levels of factor B (usually different trials) have means that are significantly different. Rejection of the null hypothesis leads to the conclusion that one or more learning trials produce greater effects than others when averaged over all levels of factor A. If interaction effects are present, a failure to reject H_o indicates that no trial was significantly different from the others when averaged over all levels of A, but that certain combinations of A and B are different.

(c) H_o: $\mu_{1A} = \mu_{2A} = \cdots = \mu_{aA}$

H_A: At least two levels of factor A have significantly different means. Rejection of H_o leads to the conclusion that at least one treatment (e.g., training method) produced significantly greater effects than the others when averaged over all learning trials or time periods. Remarks made previously for failure to reject the null hypothesis for B effects when interaction effects are present apply equally to A effects.

Step 3. Choose the significance level you will accept.

Step 4. Arrange the data as in Table 14-8.

Step 5. Compute the necessary totals for Table 14-8.

Step 6. Compute the total sum of squares (SS_T):

$$SS_T = \text{Grand } \Sigma X^2 - \frac{(\text{Grand total})^2}{\text{Total } N}$$

Step 7. Compute the factor A (treatment) sum of squares (SS_A):

$$SS_A = \frac{\displaystyle\sum_{j=1}^{a} RT_j^{2*}}{bn} - \frac{(\text{Grand total})^2}{\text{Total } N}$$

Step 8. Compute the factor B (trials) sum of squares (SS_B):

$$SS_B = \frac{\overset{b}{\underset{i=1}{\Sigma}} CT_i{}^2}{an} - \frac{(\text{Grand total})^2}{\text{Total } N}$$

Step 9. Compute the AB interaction sum of squares (SS_{AB}):

$$SS_{AB} = \frac{\overset{ba}{\underset{ij=11}{\Sigma}} T_{ij}{}^2}{n} - SS_A - SS_B - \frac{(\text{Grand total})^2}{\text{Total } N}$$

Step 10. Compute the "between subjects error" sum of squares (SS_{BSE}):

$$SS_{BSE} = \frac{\overset{an}{\underset{jk=11}{\Sigma}} ST_{jk}{}^2}{b} - SS_A - \frac{(\text{Grand total})^2}{\text{Total } N}$$

Step 11. Compute the "within subjects error" sum of squares (SS_{WSE}):

$$SS_{WSE} = SS_T - SS_A - SS_B - SS_{AB} - SS_{BSE}$$

Step 12. Compute the mean square for factor A (MS_A):

$$MS_A = \frac{SS_A}{a-1}$$

This value is an estimate of the error variance (σ^2) plus an amount due to factor A (treatment) effects plus an amount due to individual differences between subjects.

Step 13. Compute the mean square for factor B (MS_B):

$$MS_B = \frac{SS_B}{b-1}$$

This value is an estimate of error variance plus an amount due to factor B (trial) effects plus an amount due to subject by trial interaction effects.

Step 14. Compute the mean square for AB interaction (MS_{AB}):

$$MS_{AB} = \frac{SS_{AB}}{(a-1)(b-1)}$$

This value is an estimate of error variance plus an amount due to AB (treatment $\times$ trial) interaction effects plus an amount due to subject by trial interaction effects.

Step 15. Compute the mean square for "between subjects error" (MS_{BSE}):

$$MS_{BSE} = \frac{SS_{BSE}}{a(n-1)}$$

This value is an estimate of error variance plus an amount due to individual differences between subjects.

Step 16. Compute the mean square for "within subjects error" (MS_{WSE}):

$$MS_{WSE} = \frac{SS_{WSE}}{a(n-1)(b-1)}$$

This value estimates error variance plus subject by trial interaction effects.

Step 17. Compute the F ratio for factor A (treatment) effects:

$$F_{\alpha;\, a-1,\, a(n-1)} = \frac{MS_A}{MS_{BSE}}$$

According to our definitions of the respective mean squares, the F ratio should approach 1.0 with insignificant treatment effects and become larger as treatment effects increase.

Step 18. Compute the F ratio for factor B (trial) effects:

$$F_{\alpha;\, b-1,\, a(n-1)(b-1)} = \frac{MS_B}{MS_{WSE}}$$

As B effects (learning or training) increase, this ratio should also increase in size. A conservative F test for B effects that avoids some of the covariance assumptions required by the regular test simply substitutes 1 and $a(n-1)$ for the degrees of freedom of the numerator and denominator, respectively.

Step 19. Compute the F ratio for AB interaction effects:

$$F_{\alpha;\, (a-1)(b-1),\, a(n-1)(b-1)} = \frac{MS_{AB}}{MS_{WSE}}$$

This ratio will become progressively greater than 1 as treatment by trial interaction effects become greater. A conservative test for AB interaction effects substitutes $a-1$ and $a(n-1)$ for the degrees of freedom of the numerator and denominator. Again with this conservative test, covariance assumptions are avoided, but the test will tend to lead to retention of the null hypothesis too often.

Step 20. Complete an analysis of variance table such as Table 14-9.

Table 14-9. Two-factor, repeated measures analysis of variance table

Source of variation	Sums of squares	Degrees of freedom	Mean squares	F ratios
A (treatments)	SS_A	$a-1$	MS_A	MS_A/MS_{BSE}
Between subjects error	SS_{BSE}	$a(n-1)$	MS_{BSE}	
B (trials)	SS_B	$b-1$	MS_B	MS_B/MS_{WSE}
AB interaction	SS_{AB}	$(a-1)(b-1)$	MS_{AB}	MS_{AB}/MS_{WSE}
Within subjects error	SS_{WSE}	$a(n-1)(b-1)$	MS_{WSE}	
Total	SS_T	$abn-1$		

Step 21. Make the appropriate comparisons between obtained and tabled F ratios at the proper alpha level and with the correct degrees of freedom, as indicated in the analysis of variance table.

Step 22. If a significant F ratio is observed for A, B, or AB effects, complete the usual tables of row, column, and cell mean differences for determining the means that are significantly different from each other. The T values for the Tukey comparisons will be as follows:

(a) For A effects: $T = q_{\alpha;\, a,\, a(n-1)} \sqrt{MS_{\text{BSE}}/bn}$

(b) For B effects: $T = q_{\alpha;\, b,\, a(n-1)(b-1)} \sqrt{MS_{\text{WSE}}/an}$

(c) For AB effects: $T = q_{\alpha;\, ab,\, a(n-1)(b-1)} \sqrt{MS_{\text{WSE}}/n}$

Step 23. Make the appropriate interpretations of the experimental results based on the statistical outcomes and your knowledge of the phenomena under consideration.

Example of a two-factor analysis of variance with repeated measurements on the same subjects*

To test the effects of fatiguing exercise on retention of a motor skill, immediately after learning that skill, two groups of rats were forced to successfully negotiate a maze every other day for 3 weeks. After successfully completing the maze task, one group of animals was immediately exercised to exhaustion on a treadmill, and the other rats were returned to their cages. It was hypothesized that fatigue would reduce the rate of maze learning by the exercised animals. The criterion for maze learning was minutes to successful negotiation.

This experiment illustrates the use of the repeated measures design to test differences in learning as the result of varied exercise programs. Note that carry-over effects of fatigue on learning were avoided by allowing the rats to rest on alternate days. Although data were collected every other day for the course of the experiment, we will consider only the data at the second, fifth, and ninth maze trials. The data are shown in Table 14-10.

Analytical procedure

Step 1. All assumptions seemed tenable with the possible exception of the covariance assumptions. It was decided that the conservative F test would be used rather than the test for covariance assumptions.

Step 2. The main hypothesis of interest was that concerning treatment by trial interaction effects, but the main treatment effects and main trial effects were also tested.

Step 3. Alpha was set at .05.

Steps 4 and 5. See Table 14-10.

Step 6. The total sum of squares was computed:

$$SS_T = \text{Grand } \Sigma X^2 - \frac{(\text{Grand total})^2}{\text{Total } N}$$

$$= 7,688 - \frac{(392)^2}{24}$$

$$= 7,688 - 6,486$$

$$SS_T = 1,202$$

*This example was suggested to us by our colleague, Robert S. Hutton.

Table 14-10. Effects of fatigue on maze learning (minutes)

Treatments	Rats	Maze trials			Rat totals	Row totals	Row totals^2
		Second	Fifth	Ninth			
Sedentary	S1	20	10	5	35	168	28,224
	S2	30	15	7	52		
	S3	18	9	4	31		
	S4	24	18	8	50		
	Cell totals	92	52	24	—	—	—
	Cell means	23	13	6			
Exhausted	E1	23	18	14	55	224	50,176
	E2	30	21	12	63		
	E3	19	13	10	42		
	E4	28	20	16	64		
	Cell totals	100	72	52	—	—	—
	Cell means	25	18	13			
Column totals		192	124	76	392	—	78,300
Column totals^2		36,864	15,376	5,776	58,016	—	—
Σx^2, columns		4,774	2,064	850	7,688	—	—

Step 7. The sum of squares due to factor A (treatments) was computed:

$$SS_A = \frac{\sum\limits_{j=1}^{a} RT_j^2}{bn} - \frac{(\text{Grand total})^2}{\text{Total } N}$$

$$= \frac{78,300}{(3)(4)} - 6,486$$

$$= 6,525 - 6,486$$

$$SS_A = 39$$

Step 8. The sum of squares due to factor B (trials) was computed:

$$SS_B = \frac{\sum\limits_{i=1}^{b} CT_i^2}{an} - \frac{(\text{Grand total})^2}{\text{Total } N}$$

$$= \frac{58,016}{(2)(4)} - 6,486$$

$$= 7,252 - 6,486$$

$$SS_B = 766$$

Step 9. The sum of squares due to AB interaction effects was computed:

$$SS_{AB} = \frac{\sum\limits_{ij=11}^{ba} T_{ij}^2}{n} - SS_A - SS_B - \frac{(\text{Grand total})^2}{\text{Total } N}$$

$$= \frac{92^2 + 52^2 + 24^2 + 100^2 + 72^2 + 52^2}{4} - 39 - 766 - 6{,}486$$

$$= \frac{29{,}632}{4} - 39 - 766 - 6{,}486$$

$$= 7{,}408 - 7{,}291$$

$$SS_{AB} = 117$$

Step 10. The "between subjects error" sum of squares was computed:

$$SS_{BSE} = \frac{\overset{an}{\underset{jk=11}{\Sigma}} ST_{jk}{}^2}{b} - SS_A - \frac{(\text{Grand total})^2}{\text{Total } N}$$

$$= \frac{35^2 + 52^2 + 31^2 + 50^2 + 55^2 + 63^2 + 42^2 + 64^2}{3} - 39 - 6{,}486$$

$$= \frac{20{,}244}{3} - 39 - 6{,}486$$

$$= 6{,}748 - 6{,}525$$

$$SS_{BSE} = 223$$

Step 11. The "within subjects error" sum of squares was computed:

$$SS_{WSE} = SS_T - SS_A - SS_B - SS_{AB} - SS_{BSE}$$

$$= 1{,}202 - 39 - 766 - 117 - 223$$

$$SS_{WSE} = 57$$

Step 12. The appropriate mean squares were computed:

(a) $MS_A = SS_A/a - 1 = 39/1 = 39.0$

(b) $MS_B = SS_B/b - 1 = 766/2 = 383.0$

(c) $MS_{AB} = SS_{AB}/(a-1)(b-1) = 117/(1)(2) = 58.5$

(d) $MS_{BSE} = SS_{BSE}/a(n-1) = 223/2(3) = 37.17$

(e) $MS_{WSE} = SS_{WSE}/a(n-1)(b-1) = 57/(2)(3)(2) = 4.75$

Step 13. The appropriate F ratios were computed:

(a) A effects: $F_{.05; \, a-1, \, a(n-1)} = MS_A/MS_{BSE}$
$F_{.05; \, 1, \, 6} = 39/37.17 = 1.05$

(b) B effects: $F_{.05; \, b-1, \, a(n-1)(b-1)} = MS_B/MS_{WSE}$
$F_{.05; \, 2, \, 12} = 383/4.75 = 80.63$

(c) AB interaction effects:
$F_{.05; \, (a-1)(b-1), \, a(n-1)(b-1)} = MS_{AB}/MS_{WSE}$

$F_{.05; \, 2, \, 12} = 58.5/4.75 = 12.32$

Step 14. An analysis of variance table was completed (Table 14-11).

Step 15. The observed F ratios were compared with tabled values for $F_{.05}$ with the appropriate degrees of freedom. For A effects the degrees of freedom are 1 and 6; for B effects the conservative F test has 1 and 6 degrees of freedom as does the conservative test for AB effects. The critical F ratio for all three tests, there-

Table 14-11. Maze learning analysis of variance table

Source of variation	Sums of squares	Degrees of freedom	Mean squares	F ratios
A (treatments)	39	1	39.00	1.05
Between subjects error	223	6	37.17	
B (trials)	766	2	383.00	80.63
AB interaction	117	2	58.50	12.32
Within subjects error	57	12	4.75	
Total	1,202	23		

fore, is $F_{.05; 1, 6} = 5.99$, and B effects and AB interaction effects are shown to be significant.

Step 16. To determine which of the trial means were significantly different from each other, their differences were computed and analyzed with the Tukey procedure:

Trial$_2$ $\bar{X} = 192/8 = 24$
Trial$_5$ $\bar{X} = 124/8 = 15.5$
Trial$_9$ $\bar{X} = 76/8 = 9.5$

$$\bar{X}_2 - \bar{X}_9 = 14.5, \bar{X}_2 - \bar{X}_5 = 8.5, \bar{X}_5 - \bar{X}_9 = 6.0$$

$$T = q_{\alpha: b, a(n-1)(b-1)} \sqrt{MS_{WSE}/an}$$

$$= q_{.05; 3, 12} \sqrt{4.75/8}$$

$$= 3.77(0.77)$$

$$T = 2.90$$

Since all differences between paired trial means are greater than the computed T value, the appropriate conclusion is that significant learning effects occurred between all three trials.

Step 17. To determine which cell means were significantly different, their paired differences were put into table form (Table 14-12). These differences were then compared to the appropriate Tukey value.

Table 14-12. Differences between paired cell means

Comparison mean (CM)	CM-25	CM-23	CM-18	CM-13	CM-13	CM-6
25	—	2	7*	12*	12*	19*
23	—	—	5	10*	10*	17*
18	—	—	—	5	5	12*
13	—	—	—	—	—	7*
13	—	—	—	—	—	7*
6	—	—	—	—	—	—

$$T = q_{\alpha: ab, a(n-1)(b-1)} \sqrt{MS_{WSE}/n}$$

$$= q_{.05; 6, 12} \sqrt{4.75/4}$$

$$= 4.75(1.09)$$

$$T = 5.18$$

Since only those pairs with mean differences above 5.18 meet the test for significance, only those differences are starred in Table 14-12. The conclusions to be drawn from these tests might be stated as follows:

(a) By the ninth trial the exhausted animals demonstrated significantly inferior maze performances.

(b) This retardation in maze learning appears to be cumulative in nature, with insignificant differences occurring in the early stages of learning.

Problems

1. Analyze the following data with a two-way analysis. First use the completely randomized model and then test the same data with the two-factor repeated measures model.

Effects of diet and exercise on weight loss (pounds)

Dietary treatment	Exercise treatment		
	No exercise	Exercise daily	Exercise twice daily
3 meals daily	2	− 3	− 15
	5	− 10	− 11
	10	− 7	− 5
	7	− 1	− 7
5 meals daily	3	− 5	− 20
	2	− 3	− 16
	5	− 8	− 12
	1	− 12	− 8
1 meal daily	− 4	− 7	− 17
	3	− 8	− 12
	5	− 11	− 8
	− 7	− 2	− 14

Determine (a) whether any exercise program is better than another for losing weight over all three dietary patterns, (b) whether any dietary pattern is better than another over all exercise patterns, and (c) whether any combination of exercise and diet is more effective than another. Set alpha equal to .05.

2. Analyze the results of this experiment to determine the relative effectiveness of weekly testing or monthly testing on volleyball skill at the end of a school term, for groups taught by the whole or part methods.

Effect of test frequency and teaching method on volleyball skill

Teaching method	Test frequency			
	Weekly	Monthly	Weekly	Monthly
Part	80	75	87	80
	75	73	78	69
	83	80	50	48
	92	84	97	90
Whole	72	68	69	68
	75	68	60	52
	68	70	78	71
	75	73	63	40

Chapter **15**

Analysis of covariance

Level - initial differences in subject.

COMPLETELY RANDOMIZED MODEL
Purpose

The analysis of covariance, much like the randomized blocks model of the analysis of variance, is a method of eliminating the effects of an independent variable of no interest, also known as a concomitant variable, so that the denominator of the F test will be smaller and the F test will be more efficient in detecting effects caused by an independent variable of interest.

We might wish, for example, to study the effects of three different methods of circuit training on body weight. Since final body weights depend a great deal on initial body weights, we might use the analysis of covariance to "correct" the final body-weight measures to account for initial weights.

As another example, a track coach who wishes to compare the effects of several different training methods on 220-yard-dash times may wish to use covariance techniques to remove the effects of pretraining sprint times. Again in this case the final 220 times would be highly correlated with the initial times.

In the analysis of covariance a sum of squares for the dependent variable is reduced by removing that portion of the sum of squares which is due to the correlation between the concomitant and dependent variables.

Layout of the data

The data for a completely randomized model of the analysis of covariance can be arranged as in Table 15-1.

In this layout the observations on the concomitant variable (independent variable of no interest) are those in the X columns, and the dependent observations are placed in the Y columns. The value X_{ij} is the jth observation on the concomitant variable for treatment i, where $i = 1, 2, \ldots, r$ and $j = 1, 2, \ldots, n_i$. Notice that a major difference between this layout and the analysis of variance layout is the computation of XY products. These products are used to estimate that part of the Y variance associated with the correlation between the X and Y variables.

Table 15-1. Layout of data for the analysis of covariance

	Treatments												
	1			2			⋯	r			X Grand total	Y Grand total	XY Grand total
	X	Y	XY	X	Y	XY	⋯	X	Y	XY			
Experimental observations	X_{11} X_{12} ⋯ X_{1n_1}	Y_{11} Y_{12} ⋯ Y_{1n_1}	$(X_{11})(Y_{11})$ $(X_{12})(Y_{12})$ ⋯ $(X_{1n_1})(Y_{1n_1})$	X_{21} X_{22} ⋯ X_{2n_2}	Y_{21} Y_{22} ⋯ Y_{2n_2}	$(X_{21})(Y_{21})$ $(X_{22})(Y_{22})$ ⋯ $(X_{2n_2})(Y_{2n_2})$	⋯	X_{r1} X_{r2} ⋯ X_{mn_r}	Y_{r1} Y_{r2} ⋯ Y_{mn_r}	$(X_{r1})(Y_{r1})$ $(X_{r2})(Y_{r2})$ ⋯ $(X_{mn_r})(Y_{mn_r})$			
Totals	T_{1X}	T_{1Y}	T_{1XY}	T_{2X}	T_{2Y}	T_{2XY}	⋯	T_{rX}	T_{rY}	T_{rXY}			
Means	$\bar{X}_1$	$\bar{Y}_1$	—	$\bar{X}_2$	$\bar{Y}_2$	—	⋯	$\bar{X}_r$	$\bar{Y}_r$	—			
Sums of squares	ΣX_1^2	ΣY_1^2	—	ΣX_2^2	ΣY_2^2	—	⋯	ΣX_r^2	ΣY_r^2	—	Grand ΣX^2	Grand ΣY^2	

Assumptions of the test

The assumptions of the completely randomized model of the analysis of covariance are the following:

1. The data are measured on an interval or ratio scale.
2. Each observation on Y represents a random sample of size 1 from each of N populations of combinations of treatment type and concomitant variable value. This requires that subjects are randomly assigned to treatments.
3. Each of the N populations is normal.
4. Each of the N populations has the same variance.
5. The population means within each treatment lie on a straight line. This means that there must be a linear relationship between X and Y within each treatment.
6. The slope of the line in assumption 5 must be the same for each treatment. This requires that for any given increase in X, Y must increase by the same amount for each treatment.

Assumptions 5 and 6 are not found in the one-way analysis of variance, and one should have good reason to believe they are tenable before undertaking a covariance analysis. In the study of the effects of different circuit-training methods on body weight, for example, we can be quite sure that there is a linear relationship between pretraining and posttraining body weights, and we can also feel confident that an increase of 10 pounds in pretraining weight will cause similar increases in posttraining values for all methods. If there is no correlation between the X and Y variables, the scientist would be better off to disregard the X variable and use a one-way analysis of variance on the Y results.

Analytical procedure

The analysis of covariance can be performed according to the following steps:

Step 1. Determine whether the assumptions of the test are tenable.

Step 2. State the hypothesis and its alternative. Usually these will be of the following form:

$$H_o:\ \mu_1^* = \mu_2^* = \cdots = \mu_r^*$$

H_A: At least two of the "corrected" treatment means are different.

Step 3. Choose the level of significance (α) you will accept.

Step 4. Arrange the data as in Table 15-1.

Step 5. Compute the necessary sums and means for Table 15-1.

Step 6. Compute the total sum of squares for the X variable (SS_{T_X}):

$$SS_{T_X} = \text{Grand } \Sigma X^2 - \left[\frac{(\text{Grand total})^2}{\text{Total } N} \right] \quad \text{where } N = \text{number of } (X, Y) \text{ pairs.}$$

Step 7. Compute the treatment sum of squares for X (SS_{Tr_X}):

$$SS_{Tr_X} = \sum_{i=1}^{r} \frac{(X \text{ Column total}_i)^2}{n_i} - \left[\frac{(X \text{ Grand total})^2}{\text{Total } N} \right]$$

Step 8.   Compute the error sum of squares for X (SS_{E_X}):

$$SS_{E_X} = SS_{T_X} - SS_{Tr_X}$$

Step 9.   Compute the total sum of squares for Y (SS_{T_Y}):

$$SS_{T_Y} = \text{Grand } \Sigma Y^2 - \left[\frac{(Y \text{ Grand total})^2}{\text{Total } N} \right]$$

Step 10. Compute the treatment sum of squares for Y (SS_{Tr_Y}):

$$SS_{Tr_Y} = \sum_{i=1}^{r} \frac{(Y \text{ Column total}_i)^2}{n_i} - \left[\frac{(\text{Grand total})^2}{\text{Total } N} \right]$$

Step 11. Compute the error sum of squares for Y (SS_{E_Y}):

$$SS_{E_Y} = SS_{T_Y} - SS_{Tr_Y}$$

Step 12. Compute the total sum of products (SP_T):

$$SP_T = XY \text{ Grand total} - \left[\frac{(X \text{ Grand total})(Y \text{ Grand total})}{\text{Total } N} \right]$$

Step 13. Compute the treatment sum of products (SP_{Tr}):

$$SP_{Tr} = \sum_{i=1}^{r} \frac{(X \text{ Column total}_i)(Y \text{ Column total}_i)}{n_i} - \left[\frac{(X \text{ Grand total})(Y \text{ Grand total})}{\text{Total } N} \right]$$

Step 14. Compute the error sum of products (SP_E):

$$SP_E = SP_T - SP_{Tr}$$

Step 15. Compute the corrected total sum of squares for Y ($SS_{T_Y}^*$):

$$SS_{T_Y}^* = SS_{T_Y} - \frac{(SP_T)^2}{SS_{T_X}}$$

Step 16. Compute the corrected error sum of squares for Y ($SS_{E_Y}^*$):

$$SS_{E_Y}^* = SS_{E_Y} - \frac{(SP_E)^2}{SS_{E_X}}$$

Step 17. Compute the corrected treatment sum of squares for Y ($SS_{Tr_Y}^*$):

$$SS_{Tr_Y}^* = SS_{T_Y}^* - SS_{E_Y}^*$$

Step 18. Compute the corrected treatment mean square for Y ($MS_{Tr_Y}^*$):

$$MS_{Tr_Y}^* = \frac{SS_{Tr_Y}^*}{r-1}$$

Step 19. Compute the corrected error mean square for Y ($MS_{E_Y}^*$):

$$MS_{E_Y}^* = \frac{SS_{E_Y}^*}{N-r-1}$$

Step 20. Compute the F ratio:

$$F = \frac{MS_{Tr_Y}^*}{MS_{E_Y}^*}$$

When the F ratio is large, the null hypothesis is rejected, and the appropriate conclusion is that at least two of the corrected Y treatment means are significantly different.

Step 21. Summarize the results in an analysis of covariance table as in Table 15-2.

Table 15-2. Summary of analysis of covariance results

Source	SS_X	SS_Y	SP	SS_Y^*	Degrees of freedom	MS_Y^*	F
Treatments	SS_{Tr_X}	SS_{Tr_Y}	SP_{Tr}	$SS_{Tr_Y}^*$	$r-1$	$MS_{Tr_Y}^*$	$MS_{Tr_Y}^*$
Error	SS_{E_X}	SS_{E_Y}	SP_E	$SS_{E_Y}^*$	$N-r-1$	$MS_{E_Y}^*$	$MS_{E_Y}^*$
Total	SS_{T_X}	SS_{T_Y}	SP_T	$SS_{T_Y}^*$			

Step 22. Consult a table of the F distribution (Table C-9, Appendix C) to compare the obtained F ratio with that found in the table at the predetermined alpha level having the appropriate degrees of freedom, $r-1$ and $N-r-1$. If the obtained F ratio is greater than the tabled value, reject the null hypothesis and conclude that at least two of the treatment means for Y, corrected to remove the effects of the correlation between X and Y, are different from each other. If the obtained F is smaller than the tabled F, conclude that there is not enough evidence to reject the null hypothesis.

Step 23. If the obtained F ratio is greater than the tabled value, use the Scheffé procedure to discover which means are significantly different from each other. The Scheffé procedure requires that the following values be computed:

(a) The differences between all possible pairs of Y treatment means, $(\bar{Y}_i - \bar{Y}_{i'})$, and the corresponding differences between all pairs of X treatment means $(\bar{X}_i - \bar{X}_{i'})$.

(b) $S = \quad (r-1) F_{\alpha:\, r-1,\, N-r-1}$

(c) $W = \dfrac{\left[(\bar{Y}_i - \bar{Y}_{i'}) - \dfrac{SP_E}{SS_{E_X}} (\bar{X}_i - \bar{X}_{i'}) \right]^2}{MS_{E_Y}^* \left[\dfrac{1}{n_i} + \dfrac{1}{n_{i'}} + \dfrac{(\bar{X}_i - \bar{X}_{i'})^2}{SS_{E_X}} \right]}$

computed for each pair of treatments.

If W is greater than S, then the two treatment means in question are significantly different. There is a probability, alpha, that one or more false statements of differences will be made.

There are other models of the analysis of covariance, which we will not discuss in this text. The model we have presented is probably the one most frequently encountered in physical education research, where final scores are corrected for initial scores or for some other variable highly correlated to final scores.

Example of the analysis of covariance

Experimental design. A physical activity specialist, Neon Argyle, believed that people engage in vigorous physical activity more often if there is social interaction involved in the activity in which they are skilled. To study this possibility, Neon decided to compare the activity patterns of subjects skilled in single-participant activities with those of subjects skilled in activities requiring the participation of others. He studied subjects who had just received extensive training in one of three forms of activity and who had no particular ability or training in other types of physical activity. All subjects were paid and were randomly assigned to one of the three groups—weight lifting, tennis, or volleyball. After their training, all subjects were given weekly bulletins describing the sports programs available every day. There was no problem of equipment or other participants, since team members and opponents were always available at reserved facilities.

The dependent variable of interest was the average number of times a person participated in vigorous physical activity every week. The study was carried on for two years after the training program. Since there was good evidence to indicate that participation in vigorous physical activity was also dependent on an innate "activity drive," Neon recorded the average number of times the subjects participated in vigorous physical activity for 6 months prior to the training period and used these data as an estimate of "activity drive." The physical activity of all subjects was filmed from an orbiting satellite, since Neon had convinced the Air Force that this was a vital research project. The Air Force had donated 6.8 billion dollars to finance the study.

Thus data were obtained on an independent (concomitant) variable (pretraining frequency of activity) and on a dependent variable (posttraining frequency of activity). An analysis of covariance was used to compare the effects of training in a nonsocial skill (weight lifting), a skill requiring some social interaction (tennis), and a skill requiring much social interaction (volleyball). If the volleyball players participated more than the other groups and the tennis players more than the weight lifters, then Neon felt he would have some evidence to support his belief that frequency of participation in physical activity is partly determined by the amount of social interaction involved in the activity in which one is skilled. The data are presented in Table 15-3.

Analytical procedure

Step 1. Neon had conducted several pilot studies and found evidence which led him to conclude that the analysis of covariance assumptions were not violated.

Step 2. Following are the test hypothesis and its alternative:

H_o: μ^* weight lifting $= \mu^*$ tennis $= \mu^*$ volleyball

H_A: At least two of the means for posttraining frequency of participation in physical activity are different when corrected for pretraining frequency of participation, a measure of "activity drive."

Table 15-3. Frequency of participation in physical activity before and after training

	Treatments										
	Weight lifting			Tennis			Volleyball				
	Pre	Post	Pre × Post	Pre	Post	Pre × Post	Pre	Post	Pre × Post		
Average frequency of weekly participation per subject	0.0	0.8	0.00	1.0	4.1	4.10	0.3	1.0	0.30		
	7.0	7.0	49.00	1.0	3.0	3.00	0.0	1.4	0.00		
	0.0	1.2	0.00	0.2	2.8	0.56	5.0	5.0	25.00		
	2.5	3.1	7.75	0.0	2.1	0.00	0.0	2.0	0.00		
	1.3	2.0	2.60	4.1	6.0	24.60	1.0	3.0	3.00		
	0.0	0.9	0.00	1.0	3.6	3.60	2.0	2.5	5.00		
	0.4	1.5	0.60	0.0	2.5	0.00	3.5	4.0	14.00		
	0.0	1.3	0.00	2.0	4.8	9.60	0.0	1.0	0.00		
Totals	11.20	17.80	59.95	9.30	28.90	45.46	11.80	19.90	47.30	32.30	66.60	152.71
Means	1.40	2.23	—	1.16	3.61	—	1.48	2.49	—	—	
Column sums of squares	57.10	69.44	—	23.85	116.31	—	42.34	64.21	—	123.29	249.96

Step 3.   Since a rejection of the test hypothesis would mean massive federal pressure to teach only those types of activities that proved most apt to cause greater participation, Neon wanted to make sure that such a rejection had little chance for error. Therefore he chose the .01 level of significance as acceptable.

Step 4.   The layout of the data is found in Table 15-3.

Step 5.   The necessary sums and means were computed and entered in Table 15-3.

Step 6.   The total sum of squares for pretraining data was computed:

$$SS_{T_X} = \text{Grand } \Sigma X^2 - \left[\frac{(X \text{ Grand total})^2}{\text{Total } N} \right]$$

$$SS_{T_X} = 123.29 - \frac{(32.30)^2}{24}$$

$$SS_{T_X} = 79.82$$

Step 7.   The treatment sum of squares for pretraining data was computed:

$$SS_{Tr_X} = \sum_{i=1}^{r} \frac{(X \text{ Column total}_i)^2}{n_i} - \left[\frac{(X \text{ Grand total})^2}{\text{Total } N} \right]$$

$$= \frac{(11.20)^2}{8} + \frac{(9.30)^2}{8} + \frac{(11.80)^2}{8} - \frac{(32.30)^2}{24}$$

$$SS_{Tr_X} = 0.43$$

Step 8.   The error sum of squares for pretraining data was computed:

$$SS_{E_X} = SS_{T_X} - SS_{Tr_X}$$

$$= 79.82 - 0.43$$

$$SS_{E_X} = 79.39$$

Step 9.   The total sum of squares for posttraining data was computed:

$$SS_{T_Y} = \text{Grand } \Sigma Y^2 - \left[\frac{(Y \text{ Grand total})^2}{\text{Total } N} \right]$$

$$= 249.96 - \frac{(66.60)^2}{24}$$

$$SS_{T_Y} = 65.14$$

Step 10. The treatment sum of squares for posttraining data was computed:

$$SS_{Tr_Y} = \sum_{i=1}^{r} \frac{(Y \text{ Column total}_i)^2}{n_i} - \left[\frac{(Y \text{ Grand total})^2}{\text{Total } N} \right]$$

$$= \frac{(17.80)^2}{8} + \frac{(28.90)^2}{8} + \frac{(19.90)^2}{8} - \frac{(66.60)^2}{24}$$

$$SS_{Tr_Y} = 8.69$$

Step 11. The error sum of squares for posttraining data was computed:

$$SS_{E_Y} = SS_{T_Y} - SS_{Tr_Y}$$

$$= 65.14 - 8.69$$

$$SS_{E_Y} = 56.45$$

Step 12. The total sum of products was computed:

$$SP_T = XY \text{ Grand total} - \left[\frac{(X \text{ Grand total})(Y \text{ Grand total})}{\text{Total } N} \right]$$

$$= 152.71 - \frac{(32.30)(66.60)}{24}$$

$$SP_T = 63.08$$

Step 13. The treatment sum of products was computed:

$$SP_{Tr} = \sum_{i=1}^{r} \frac{(X \text{ Column total}_i)(Y \text{ Column total}_i)}{n_i} - \left[\frac{(X \text{ Grand total})(Y \text{ Grand total})}{\text{Total } N} \right]$$

$$= \frac{(11.20)(17.80)}{8} + \frac{(9.30)(28.90)}{8} + \frac{(11.80)(19.90)}{8} - \frac{(32.30)(60.60)}{24}$$

$$SP_{Tr} = -1.76$$

Note here that sums of products, unlike sums of squares, are not always positive.

Step 14. The error sum of products was computed:

$$SP_E = SP_T - SP_{Tr}$$

$$= 63.08 - (-1.76)$$

$$SP_E = 64.84$$

Step 15. The corrected total sum of squares for Y was computed:

$$SS_{T_Y}^* = SS_{T_Y} - \frac{(SP_T)^2}{SS_{T_X}}$$

$$= 65.14 - \frac{(63.08)^2}{79.82}$$

$$SS_{T_Y}^* = 15.29$$

Step 16. The corrected error sum of squares for Y was computed:

$$SS_{E_Y}^* = SS_{E_Y} - \frac{(SP_E)^2}{SS_{E_X}}$$

$$= 56.45 - \frac{(64.84)^2}{79.39}$$

$$SS_{E_Y}^* = 3.49$$

Step 17. The corrected treatment sum of squares for Y was computed:

$$SS_{Tr_Y}^* = SS_{T_Y}^* - SS_{E_Y}^*$$

$$= 15.29 - 3.49$$

$$SS_{Tr_Y}^* = 11.80$$

Step 18. The corrected treatment mean square for Y was computed:

$$MS^*_{\text{Tr}_Y} = \frac{SS^*_{\text{Tr}_Y}}{r-1}$$

$$= \frac{11.80}{3-1}$$

$$MS^*_{\text{Tr}_Y} = 5.90$$

Step 19. The corrected error mean square for Y was computed:

$$MS^*_{\text{E}_Y} = \frac{SS^*_{\text{E}_Y}}{N-r-1}$$

$$= \frac{3.49}{24-3-1}$$

$$MS^*_{\text{E}_Y} = 0.174$$

Step 20. The F ratio was computed:

$$F = \frac{MS^*_{\text{Tr}_Y}}{MS^*_{\text{E}_Y}}$$

$$= \frac{5.90}{.174}$$

$$F = 33.91$$

Step 21. The results were summarized in an analysis of covariance table (Table 15-4).

Table 15-4. Summary of analysis of covariance results

Source	SS_{Pre}	SS_{Post}	SP	SS^*_{Post}	Degrees of freedom	MS^*_{Post}	F
Treatments	0.43	8.69	−1.76	11.80	2	5.90	33.91
Error	79.39	56.45	64.84	3.49	20	0.174	
Total	79.82	65.14	63.08	15.29			

Step 22. The obtained F ratio, 33.91, was compared with the tabled value at $\alpha = .01$ with 2 and 20 degrees of freedom. This value is 5.85. Therefore Neon concluded that at least two of the training groups had significantly different frequencies of post-training physical activity when these values were corrected for pretraining physical activity.

Step 23. To determine which of the groups were significantly different from each other, Neon performed a Scheffé comparison between the three means as follows:

(a) The differences between posttraining means were tabulated, as well as the corresponding differences between pretraining means (Table 15-5).

Table 15-5. Differences between pairs of means

	a Tennis— weight lifting	b Tennis— volleyball	c Volleyball— weight lifting
$\bar{Y}_i - \bar{Y}_{i'}$ Posttraining	$3.61 - 2.23 = 1.38$	$3.61 - 2.49 = 1.12$	$2.49 - 2.23 = 0.26$
$\bar{X}_i - \bar{X}_{i'}$ Pretraining	$1.16 - 1.40 = -0.24$	$1.16 - 1.48 = -0.32$	$1.48 - 1.40 = 0.08$

(b) The S value was computed:

$$S = (r-1)\, F_{\alpha;\, r-1,\, N-r-1}$$
$$= (3-1)\, F_{.01;\, 3-1,\, 24-3-1}$$
$$S = 11.70$$

(c) The W value was computed for each pair of treatments:

$$W = \frac{\left[(\bar{Y}_i - \bar{Y}_{i'}) - \dfrac{SP_E}{SS_{E_X}} (\bar{X}_i - \bar{X}_{i'}) \right]^2}{MS^*_{E_Y} \left[\dfrac{1}{n_i} + \dfrac{1}{n_{i'}} + \dfrac{(\bar{X}_i - \bar{X}_{i'})^2}{SS_{E_X}} \right]}$$

(1) Tennis—weight lifting

$$W = \frac{\left[1.38 - \dfrac{64.84}{79.39}(-0.24) \right]^2}{0.174 \left[1/8 + 1/8 + \dfrac{(-0.24)^2}{79.39} \right]}$$

$$W = \frac{(1.18)^2}{0.174(0.25)}$$

Tennis—weight lifting $W = 32.01$

(2) Tennis—volleyball

$$W = \frac{\left[1.12 - \dfrac{64.84}{79.39}(-0.32) \right]^2}{0.174 \left[1/8 + 1/8 + \dfrac{(-0.32)^2}{79.39} \right]}$$

$$W = \frac{(.86)^2}{0.174(0.25)}$$

Tennis—volleyball $W = 17.00$

(3) Volleyball—weight lifting

$$W = \frac{\left[0.26 - \dfrac{64.84}{79.39}(0.08) \right]^2}{0.174 \left[1/8 + 1/8 + \dfrac{(0.08)^2}{79.39} \right]}$$

$$W = \frac{(.19)^2}{0.174(.25)}$$

Volleyball—weight lifting $W = 0.83$

Conclusions. Since the W value for tennis—weight lifting (32.01) and tennis—volleyball (17.00) were greater than the S value (11.70), Neon concluded that participation in physical activity was more frequent after training in tennis than in either weight lifting or volleyball. However, the

W value (0.83) for volleyball—weight lifting was not greater than the S value so he had no evidence to conclude that volleyball training resulted in more participation in physical activity than the other groups.

Consequently, Neon could draw little support for his proposition that persons participate more often in sports if the sport in which they are particularly skilled involves a high degree of social interaction. However, the data did provide a clue to Neon for further study. Since tennis is thought of as an upper-class sport, Neon's new hypothesis was that people participate in sports more frequently if their skill is in a sport that tends to be more acceptable in the upper strata of society. He is currently submitting an enlarged supplementary research grant request to investigate this possibility.

Problems

1. A teacher taught the mechanical principles of ice skating to two different groups of students. One group was taught solely by lecture and discussion methods, whereas the other group was also exposed to a loop film illustrating correct and incorrect mechanics in ice skaters. At the end of the school term both groups were given a test to evaluate their knowledge of mechanics. To control variability caused by differences in skating experience, the teacher performed an analysis of covariance on the test results, with years of experience serving as a concomitant variable. Analyze these data.

Effect of teaching method on knowledge of mechanics

Film		No film		Film		No film	
Experience	Grade	Experience	Grade	Experience	Grade	Experience	Grade
5.0	90	1.0	63	5.0	97	2.5	83
3.5	85	0.5	74	3.0	88	5.5	90
1.0	79	4.0	88	1.0	70	0.5	79
0.5	63	2.0	75	1.5	78	0.5	55
0.5	74	0.5	78				

2. In an experiment to test the effects of exercise on blood cholesterol levels, Barney Klarb used body weight as a concomitant variable, since it was known that a linear relationship existed between body weight and cholesterol levels. Analyze Barney's data on the effects of single and repeated bouts of exercise on blood cholesterol.

Effect of single and repeated bouts of exercise on blood cholesterol (mg./100 ml.)

No exercise		Single bout		Repeated bouts	
Body weight	Cholesterol	Body weight	Cholesterol	Body weight	Cholesterol
150	120	256	240	170	112
175	200	167	165	230	115
163	140	149	123	149	120
148	170	154	140	228	208
150	112	158	178	164	117
205	250	170	132	158	110
147	115	162	115	139	109
190	120	140	125	164	112

Chapter **16**

Multiple regression and multiple and partial correlation

PURPOSE OF MULTIVARIATE TECHNIQUES

All those who have an interest in physical education and athletics or other types of physical performance are at one time or another drawn to making predictions of an individual's success in some type of performance, athletic or otherwise, based upon certain characteristics they have observed in that individual. For instance, one may be inclined to predict that a trackman who is fairly tall, fast, and limber should make a good high-hurdler or that a strong, heavy, and quick athlete could probably be a good football tackle. It would save athletic coaches a good deal of time and frustration if they were able to accurately predict an untrained individual's chances of future success in an athletic event given only his scores on four or five tests administered to him. These types of predictions can be put on a mathematical basis through the techniques described in this section.

As a specific example of a problem for which these methods would be useful, consider the task of predicting, on the basis of various measurements made on twenty untrained college track candidates, the success in the 440-yard dash of future track candidates. The first part of the problem is to decide what pretraining measurements should be made. Assuming that running speed, oxygen debt capacity, and oxygen consumption capacity are among the most important factors in determining ultimate 440 speed, let us use as pretraining variables (1) 100-yard-dash times, (2) oxygen debt capacity, and (3) maximum oxygen uptake capacity as determined in the exercise physiology laboratory. Next, the three measurements must be obtained on each of the twenty 440-yard-dash candidates. After 15 weeks of training, final 440 times are recorded for all subjects. Data are now available on four variables, one of which (final 440 times) is considered to be the dependent variable, whereas the other three are thought of as independent variables.

Questions that might then be answered with these data are the following: (1) What is the best linear estimate or prediction of final 440 time (the dependent variable) given the scores on the other three tests (independent variables)? The solution of this problem requires multiple regression techniques. (2) How much of the total variance of final 440 times can be explained by the effects of all three independent variables acting together? Another way of asking this question is, "How good is the prediction of final 440 times based on the other tests?" These questions can be answered by computing a multiple correlation coefficient. (3) Is one or more of the independent variables of little or no value in prediction of final 440 times? Interpretation of multiple correlation coefficients and regression equations gives the answer to this question. (4) What is the linear relationship between final 440 times and each of the independent variables taken separately when that relationship is adjusted for the linear effects of the other three variables on the dependent variable? This question can be answered by computing partial correlation coefficients.

Before presenting the computing formulas used in answering these questions, a small amount of theory for the general case of multiple regression and multiple and partial correlation will be presented.

MULTIPLE REGRESSION PREDICTION EQUATIONS

Assume that we have tabulated values of a dependent variable, Y (e.g., 440-yard-dash time), for many combinations of several independent variables, $X_1, X_2, \ldots, X_k$ (e.g., 100-yard-dash time, oxygen debt capacity, and so on). For instance, we might have scores for 100 individuals with 100 combinations of values for the independent variables and 100 values for the dependent variable. There may be several individuals who have the same values for the independent variables; for example, eight of 100 trackmen may have 100-yard-dash times of 10.0 seconds, oxygen debt capacities of 14 liters, and identical scores in several other tests. If the 440-yard-dash times (the dependent variable) of these eight individuals were likewise identical, and if other groups with like scores on the independent variables had like scores on the dependent variable, then it would be possible to predict 440 times perfectly by knowing only the scores on the independent variables.

However, it is rare that those with the same combination of scores on the independent variables will have exactly the same scores on the dependent variable. For example, the eight subjects with identical scores on independent measures may have a distribution of 440 times of 50.0, 50.2, 53.5, 48.6, 58.0, 57.8, 51.2, and 49.9 seconds. Therefore it would be impossible to predict 440 times from the scores on other variables with perfect accuracy. However, we should be able to predict 440 times with more accuracy than if we had no information at all about the subjects.

Multiple regression equations describe the path of the *mean* values of the dependent variable, Y, for all combinations of the independent variables, $X_1, X_2, \ldots, X_k$. The greater the variability in Y values for combinations of X values, the smaller the chance that any particular Y score will be near the mean Y value and the less accurate will be the multiple regression equation as a technique for predicting a Y value when the X values are known.

Assumptions of multiple linear regression and correlation analysis

The population distribution of Y values for each combination of X values will have some true mean and standard deviation. The path of these means will be a surface in a many dimensional space (rather than a line in two-dimensional space as was the case for simple linear regression). The following assumptions are made:

1. The observations on all variables are on at least an interval scale.
2. The distributions of Y values are all normal.
3. The standard deviations of the Y distributions are equal.
4. The path of the Y distributions' means assumes a simple, linear-type form, analogous to the linear form of the two-variable case studied in Chapter 8.

More advanced statistics texts give tests for assumptions (2) and (3), but in most cases of physical education research these two assumptions are probably valid. The assumption of a linear-type path of means is a good first estimate for most physical education problems, but one must remember that a failure to find a strong linear-type relation between variables does not mean that there is no relation between them. The relation could possibly be completely described by another type of curvilinear equation, but such equations are beyond the scope of this text.

Form of the multiple linear regression equation

In simple linear regression, the form of the predicted path of the means for the Y distribution at given X values was the following:

$$Y = \alpha + \beta X$$

In multiple linear regression we will assume a predicted path of Y means analogous to that of the simple case, namely,

$$Y = \alpha + \beta_1 X_1 + \beta_2 X_2 + \cdots + \beta_k X_k$$

where α is a constant, $\beta_1, \beta_2, \ldots + \beta_k$ are constants known as partial regression coefficients, Y is the variable taken to be dependent, and X_1, X_2, $\ldots X_k$ are the independent variables.

It should be noted here that any of the variables can be thought of as the dependent or Y variable. Therefore it is not surprising that sometimes the regression equation is expressed as

$$X_1 = \alpha + \beta_2 X_2 + \beta_3 X_3 + \cdots + \beta_k X_k$$

where any of the variables can be considered as the dependent variable X_1. This is the form we will consider for the rest of this chapter. In some cases, however, it would make no sense to consider a variable dependent; for example, height is obviously not dependent on 440 times.

Computational methods for multiple regression prediction equations

Since the α and the β's of the regression equation refer to population constants and we are to compute this equation only from sample values, we must estimate the α and β's with "a" and "b's" as follows:

$$\text{Predicted } X_1 = a + b_2 X_2 + b_3 X_3 + \cdots b_k X_k$$

$$\text{where } a = \bar{X}_1 - S_1 \left(\frac{\beta_2^* \bar{X}_2}{S_2} + \frac{\beta_3^* \bar{X}_3}{S_3} + \cdots + \frac{\beta_k^* \bar{X}_k}{S_k} \right),$$

$$b_2 = \beta_2^* \left(\frac{S_1}{S_2} \right), b_3 = \beta_3^* \left(\frac{S_1}{S_3} \right), \cdots, b_k = \beta_k^* \left(\frac{S_1}{S_k} \right)$$

In these equations the "β^*'s" are known as *"beta weights"* and are not the same as the "β's" of the regression equation. The "S's" are the standard deviations of the sample values for each variable; for example, $S_1 =$ standard deviation of the X_1 values. We will call the "b's" the *estimated partial regression coefficients.*

For small numbers of independent variables, up to about $k=5$, the computation of the beta weights can be done by hand without too much difficulty, but for larger numbers of variables the beta weight computations become extremely tedious without the use of an electronic computer. Therefore we present a method for solving regression equations with only four or fewer variables and recommend that problems with more variables be handled with the aid of a computer. The following method is patterned after the Doolittle method.* Although given here for only four variables, the method can be used for any number by repeating the systematic patterns established.

The Doolittle method requires the prior computation of the simple Pearson product-moment correlation coefficients between all pairs of variables. These values can be tabulated as in Table 16-1. We have listed the hypothetical correlations found between 440 time, oxygen debt capacity, 100-yard-dash time, and maximum oxygen consumption capacity in 100 freshman track candidates.

These intercorrelations are next inserted into Table 16-2 for determination of the beta weights. The instructions for the use of this table are included in the far-left column, and the column at the far right should help the user to avoid mathematical errors.

Once the beta weights have been calculated, it is a simple matter to calculate the a and b_j constants for the regression equation. As an example of this calculation, we will continue to analyze the data obtained from the 440-yard-dash candidates, where $X_1 =$ final 440 times, $X_2 =$ oxygen debt capacities, $X_3 = 100$ times, and $X_4 =$ maximum oxygen consumption values. The important data are summarized in Table 16-3.

---

*See, for example, Peters, C. C., and Wykes, E. C.: Simplified methods for computing regression coefficients and partial and multiple correlations, Journal of Educational Research, May, 1931.

Table 16-1. Table of intercorrelations for 100 track candidates

		X_2 O_2 debt	X_3 100 time	X_4 O_2 consumption	(Y) X_1 440 time
O_2 debt	X_2	$r_{22} = 1$	$r_{23} = -.20$	$r_{24} = .40$	$r_{21} = -.80$
100 time	X_3		$r_{33} = 1$	$r_{34} = -.10$	$r_{31} = .50$
O_2 consumption	X_4			$r_{44} = 1$	$r_{41} = -.30$
440 time	X_1				$r_{11} = 1$

Table 16-2. Doolittle method for determining beta weights in 440 prediction problem

Row	X_2	X_3	X_4	X_1 (or Y)	Row sums for math check
1. Insert values for r_{2j} $j = 2, 3, 4, 1$	r_{22} 1	r_{23} $-.20$	r_{24} .40	$-r_{21}$ .80	A. Sum of row 1 2.00
2. Divide row 1 entries by -1	-1	.20	$-.40$	$-.80$	B. Sum of row 2 or $-A$ -2.00
3. Insert values for r_{3j} $j = 3, 4, 1$		r_{33} 1	r_{34} $-.10$	$-r_{31}$ $-.50$	C. Sum of row 3 .40
4. Multiply columns X_3, X_4, X_1 of row 1 by $-r_{23}$		$-.04$	.08	.16	D. Sum of row 4 .20
5. Add rows 3 and 4 by columns		.96	$-.02$	$-.34$	E. Sum of row 5 or $C + D$ .60
6. Divide row 5 entries by negative of item in row 5, column X_3		-1	.0208	.3542	
7. Insert values for r_{4j} $j = 4, 1$			r_{44} 1	$-r_{41}$ .30	F. Sum of row 7 1.30
8. Multiply columns X_4 and X_1 of row 1 by $-r_{24}$			$-.16$	$-.32$	G. Sum of row 8 $-.48$
9. Multiply columns X_4 and X_1 of row 5 by item in row 6, column X_4			$-.0004$	$-.0071$	H. Sum of row 9 $-.0075$
10. Add rows 7, 8, 9 by columns			.8396	$-.0271$	I. Sum of row 10 or $F + G + H$ .8125
11. Divide row 10 by negative of item in row 10, column X_4			-1	.0323	J. Sum of row 11 or $I \div$ item in row 10, column X_4 $-.9677$

12. $\beta_4^* =$ Item in row 11, column X_1 [i.e., .0323]

13. $\beta_3^* = (\beta_4^* \times$ item in row 6, column X_4) $+$ item in row 6, column X_1
[i.e., .0323(.0208) + .3542 = .3549]

14. $\beta_2^* = (\beta_4^* \times$ item in row 2, column X_4) $+$ ($\beta_3^* \times$ item in row 2, column X_3) $+$ item in row 2, column X_1
[i.e., .0323($-.40$) + .3549(.20) + ($-.80$) = $-.7419$]

15. Check for beta weight errors: $\beta_2^* r_{24} + \beta_3^* r_{34} + \beta_4^* = r_{41}$
[i.e., ($-.7419$)(.40) + (.3549)($-.10$) + .0323 = $-.30$]

Table 16-3. Means and standard deviations of 440 data ($n = 100$)

	X_1 440 time	X_2 O_2 debt	X_3 100 time	X_4 O_2 consumption
Means	$\overline{X}_1 = 50.0$ sec.	$\overline{X}_2 = 15$ L.	$\overline{X}_3 = 10.5$ sec.	$\overline{X}_4 = 4.9$ L./min.
Standard deviations	$S_1 = 4.2$ sec.	$S_2 = 2$ L.	$S_3 = 1.2$ sec.	$S_4 = 0.8$ L./min.

The best estimate we can make for predicting 440-yard-dash times from other data is described by the regression equation

$$X_1 = a + b_2\, X_2 + b_3\, X_3 + b_4\, X_4$$

where

$$a = \overline{X}_1 - S_1 \left(\frac{\beta_2^* \overline{X}_2}{S_2} + \frac{\beta_3^* \overline{X}_3}{S_3} + \frac{\beta_4^* \overline{X}_4}{S_4} \right)$$

and

$$b_2 = \beta_2^* \left(\frac{S_1}{S_2}\right),\, b_3 = \beta_3^* \left(\frac{S_1}{S_3}\right),\, b_4 = \beta_4^* \left(\frac{S_1}{S_4}\right)$$

Substituting the appropriate values is done as follows:

$$a = 50.0 - 4.2 \left[\frac{(-.7419)(15)}{2} + \frac{(.3549)(10.5)}{1.2} + \frac{(.0323)(4.9)}{0.8} \right]$$

$$a = 59.4962$$

$$b_2 = -.7419 \left(\frac{4.2}{2}\right) \qquad b_3 = .3549 \left(\frac{4.2}{1.2}\right) \qquad b_4 = .0323 \left(\frac{4.2}{0.8}\right)$$

$$b_2 = -1.5580 \qquad\qquad b_3 = 1.2422 \qquad\qquad b_4 = .1696$$

$$X_1 = 59.4962 - 1.5580\, X_2 + 1.2422\, X_3 + .1696\, X_4$$

or

Predicted 440 time $= 59.4962 - 1.5580 \times O_2$ debt capacity $+ 1.2422 \times 100$ time $+ .1696$ maximum O_2 consumption capacity

If a coach now wished to estimate a 440-yard-dash candidate's potential, he could test him for 100-yard-dash time, O_2 debt capacity, and maximum O_2 intake capacity and predict what that candidate's time would be after 15 weeks of training. Assume, for example, that candidate Moose Kretzer had initial scores of 12.0 seconds in the 100-yard dash, 10.0 liters O_2 debt, and 3.0 liters per minute maximum O_2 consumption capacity. His predicted potential for the 440 would then be calculated as follows:

Predicted 440 time $= 59.4962 - 1.5580 \times 10.0 + 1.2422 \times 12.0 + .1696 \times 3.0$
Predicted 440 time $= 59.3$ seconds

After examining the potential of Moose to run the 440, the coach would surely suggest that he train for some other event such as the hammer throw, where his magnificent physique would be an asset.

Interpretation of the prediction equation

The estimated partial regression coefficients (the b's) can be interpreted as constants that tell how much the "dependent" variable increases or decreases for every change in a particular "independent" variable, with the effects of the other variables held constant. In our example with $b_2 = -1.5580$, for each liter increase in O_2 debt capacity, predicted 440 time is faster by 1.5580 seconds. To more fully evaluate the effectiveness of the prediction equation, one must have some familiarity with multiple correlation.

MULTIPLE CORRELATION

Purpose of multiple correlation

Once a multiple regression equation has been calculated, the next logical step is to find out how good the equation is in prediction, or stated another way, what proportion of the variance in the "dependent" variable can be explained by the effects of the other variables working together. In our example we would like to find out how much of the variance in 440 times is explained by the other variables so we can judge whether the regression equation is useful, or whether other variables are more important in predicting potential for this event. To do this we must compute R^2, the square of the multiple correlation coefficient R.

Computation of R^2

The squared multiple correlation coefficient or *coefficient of multiple determination*, R^2, can be determined by several methods. Since we have already used the Doolittle method to develop a regression equation, we will use the beta weights computed with that method to assist us in calculating R^2. We will use the following formula:

$$R^2_{1 \cdot 23 \cdots k} = \beta^*_2 r_{21} + \beta^*_3 r_{31} + \cdots + \beta^*_k r_{k1}$$

Note that this formula uses only the beta weights computed for the regression equation and the zero-order correlation coefficients between the dependent (X_1) and the $k-1$ other variables of the problem. The dot after the first subscript of R^2 indicates that the computation is for determining the proportion of variance in variable 1 attributed to the $k-1$ other variables working together. If we continue our study of 440-yard-dash candidates, we can compute the following:

$$
\begin{aligned}
R^2_{1 \cdot 234} &= \beta^*_2 r_{21} + \beta^*_3 r_{31} + \beta^*_4 r_{41} \\
&= -7419(-.80) + .3549(.50) + .0323(-.30) \\
&= .5935 + .1774 - .0037 \\
R^2_{1 \cdot 234} &= .7613
\end{aligned}
$$

The coefficient of multiple correlation, R, is obviously $\sqrt{R^2}$ or the following:

$$R_{1 \cdot 234 \cdots k} = \sqrt{\beta^*_2 r_{21} + \beta^*_3 r_{31} + \cdots + \beta^*_k r_{k1}}$$

In our example, $R_{1 \cdot 234} = \sqrt{.7613} = .8725$. Although R is almost always reported in multiple correlation studies, R^2 is usually a more meaningful value.

Correction of R^2 for small samples

The method used to arrive at R^2 assures a maximum value of R^2 for the sample data used. In fact, the method tends to be biased toward high

R^2 values, particularly for small samples. Therefore, when determining R^2 for samples of less than 100, a corrected value should be computed to minimize this bias as follows:

$$R^2_{\text{corr.}} = 1 - (1 - R^2)\left(\frac{N-1}{N-k}\right)$$

where R^2 = the uncorrected R^2, N = the number of cases in the sample, and k = the number of variables correlated.

In our example, $R^2_{\text{corr.}} = 1 - (1 - .7613)\left(\frac{100-1}{100-4}\right) = .7588$. Since our sample was fairly large, the correction did little to affect the R^2, but let us assume that we had sampled only twenty track candidates instead of 100. In that case, $R^2_{\text{corr.}} = 1 - (1 - .7613)\left(\frac{20-1}{20-4}\right) = .7166$. Thus, when the number of cases is quite small, it is very important to make a correction for the probable bias of the method used to obtain R^2.

Interpretation of R^2 and R

The coefficient of multiple determination, R^2, is usually interpreted as the proportion of variance in the "dependent" variable (X_1 or Y) due to the effects of whatever is measured by the independent variables acting together, not including duplicate effects that the independent variables might produce in common. Once again using the 440-yard-dash example, the R^2 of .76 indicates that 76% of the variance in 440 times after 15 weeks of training is due to whatever is measured by oxygen debt capacity, 100-yard-dash time, and maximum oxygen consumption capacity combined, without considering twice the effects that two or more of the variables have in common. In this instance we would conclude that the three "independent" variables taken together in a multiple regression equation give us a very good predictive measure of potential for the 440.

As a general rule of thumb it can be said that an absolute value of R less than .40 shows a low relationship between the dependent variable and the independent variables taken together, whereas an absolute value of R between .40 and .69 indicates a moderate relationship, an R between .69 and .89 shows a high relationship, and an absolute value of R between .90 and 1.00 shows a very strong relationship.

Significance test for multiple R

When a high multiple R is obtained from a set of sample data, one must remember that this R may be a result of chance or sampling error. With large samples we should have more confidence in the obtained R than with small samples. An analysis of variance significance test for R can be computed that will help to establish confidence in an obtained R by indicating the probability of obtaining such an R even when there is no linear-type relationship between the dependent variable and the independent variables working together. In other words, this test is also a test of the hypothesis that the true R may be zero or that there is no linear-type relationship present.

Since R^2 represents the proportion of the variance (ΣX_1^2) of the X_1 variable due to the assumed linear-type relationship, $1 - R^2$ represents the proportion of ΣX_1^2 unexplained by linearity. Therefore an F test of

$$\frac{R_2 \, \Sigma X_1^2}{(1 - R^2) \, \Sigma X_1^2}$$

with the appropriate degrees of freedom for both numerator and denominator should be the test of significance needed. Since the ΣX_1^2 drop out of the ratio, the actual test is

$$F_{\alpha; \, k, \, N-k-1} = \frac{R^2}{1 - R^2} \times \frac{N - k - 1}{k}$$

where $k =$ the number of variables correlated, and $N =$ the number of cases tested.

Returning to the 440-yard-dash example for illustration, and setting $\alpha = .05$,

$$F_{05; \, 4, \, (100-4-1)} = \frac{.76}{1 - .76} \times \frac{100 - 4 - 1}{4} = \frac{72.20}{.96} = 75.2$$

which is obviously very significant when compared to $F_{.95; \, 4, \, 95} = 2.4$.

When the obtained F ratio is insignificant, we can have little confidence that our obtained R is meaningful. An R of .90 for a sample $N = 3$ explains 81% of the total variance in X_1 just as would an R of .90 for a sample of $N = 300$, but very little confidence could be placed in the value computed from the small sample.

At this point a note of caution should be inserted concerning the meaning of a multiple R when large numbers of variables and a small number of cases are being considered. As the number of variables approaches the number of cases, R approaches 1, and when the number of variables correlated equals the number of cases studied, the R is automatically 1. This problem usually arises only when very small samples are considered, and a multiple R in that situation probably should not be computed in the first place.

Relative contribution of independent variables to variance of dependent variable

The relative contribution of each of the independent variables to the total variance in X_1 can be estimated by examining the components of the R^2 formula. (See p. 164.) In our example, $R^2 = .7613 = .5935 + .1774 - .0037$.

We can conclude that about 59% of the X_1 variance is contributed by oxygen debt capacity when what it has in common with 100 time and oxygen consumption capacity are held constant. In the same manner, 100-yard time contributes about 18% of the X_1 variance, and oxygen consumption capacity almost nothing. It appears that the oxygen consumption measure contributes very little to the prediction of 440 times, probably because it measures many things in common with oxygen debt capacity. (Recall that these two measures had a zero-order correlation coefficient of

.40.) As a general rule, one should attempt to include in a multiple regression problem those independent variables that have a fairly high correlation with the dependent variable but very low intercorrelations with the other independent variables. In our example it appears that the maximum oxygen consumption test could just as well be eliminated from the regression equation. This would save both time and expense at the loss of little predictive power.

Significance of a difference between multiple R's

One can easily run a test to determine whether the inclusion of a greater number of independent variables results in a significantly greater R than with a small number of variables. The test is as follows:

$$F_{\alpha;\,(k_1-k_2),\,(N-k_1-1)} = \frac{(R_1^2 - R_2^2)(N - k_1 - 1)}{(1 - R_1^2)(k_1 - k_2)}$$

If, for example, an R^2 with three independent variables and a sample size of 100 were .800 and an R^2 computed after eliminating one variable were .798, the F ratio would be (with $\alpha = .01$)

$$F_{.01;\,(4-3),\,(100-4-1)} = \frac{(.800 - .798)(100 - 4 - 1)}{(1 - .80)(4 - 3)} = .95$$

which is not significant when compared to $F_{.01;\,3,\,95} = 6.9$.

In this case the investigator would feel justified in eliminating that one variable from his test battery. The techniques of estimating the relative contribution of each independent variable to the variance of the dependent variable and testing the significance of the difference between two multiple R's can be used in physical education to eliminate extraneous tests from batteries purporting to measure physical fitness, athletic aptitude, and so on.

PARTIAL CORRELATION COEFFICIENTS
Purpose of partial correlation coefficients

Often when those in physical education research examine a relationship between variables, that relationship is obviously influenced by one or more other variables. If one were to study the relationship between leg strength and body weight, for instance, that relationship would be lower in a group of boys of the same age than it would if the boys were of all ages. The reason is that both weight and strength tend to be correlated with age so that age tends to increase the degree of relationship between weight and leg strength.

If some method were desired to find the relationship between leg strength and body weight uncomplicated by the age factor, two alternatives would be open. The most obvious would be to correlate results only on boys in the same age groups. A more efficient method would be to calculate a partial correlation coefficient. A partial correlation coefficient is a measure of the degree of association between two variables when the effects of one or more other variables are adjusted for or held constant.

Computation of partial correlation coefficients

Computation of partial correlation coefficients is not too tedious unless more than four variables are involved. Although partial correlations with more than four variables are rarely used in physical education research, their computation when necessary is made quite simple with computers. We shall present only the computation formulas for first-order partial correlation coefficients (one variable controlled) and second-order partials (two variables controlled).

The formula for a first-order partial correlation coefficient $r_{ij \cdot k}$ is

$$r_{ij \cdot k} = \frac{r_{ij} - (r_{ik})(r_{jk})}{\sqrt{1 - r^2_{ik}} \ \sqrt{1 - r^2_{jk}}}$$

where $r_{ij \cdot k} =$ the partial correlation coefficient expressing the correlation between variables i and j when the effects of variable k are controlled.

As an illustration, let us assume we have tested several hundred school boys on leg strength and body weight and have also recorded their ages. We could now compute the simple, zero-order intercorrelations between the three variables and might end up with a table such as Table 16-4.

Table 16-4. Intercorrelations between leg strength, body weight, and age

		Leg strength X_1	Body weight X_2	Age X_3
Leg strength	X_1	1	.60	.40
Body weight	X_2		1	.70
Age	X_3			1

To compute the correlation between leg strength and body weight with the effects of age "partialed out" or held constant, we would compute $r_{12 \cdot 3}$ as follows:

$$r_{12 \cdot 3} = \frac{r_{12} - (r_{13})(r_{23})}{\sqrt{1 - r^2_{13}} \ \sqrt{1 - r^2_{23}}} = \frac{.60 - (.40)(.70)}{\sqrt{1 - (40)^2} \ \sqrt{1 - (.70)^2}} = .49$$

As expected, the correlation is much lower when the effects of age are controlled. Instead of an r of .60, we now have an r of .49.

Similarly, the formula for a second-order partial correlation coefficient $r_{ij \cdot kl}$ is

$$r_{ij \cdot kl} = \frac{r_{ij \cdot k} - (r_{jl \cdot k})(r_{jl \cdot k})}{\sqrt{1 - r^2_{il \cdot k}} \ \sqrt{1 - r^2_{jl \cdot k}}}$$

where $r_{ij \cdot kl} =$ the coefficient expressing the correlation between variables i and j when the effects of variables k and l are controlled.

Note that we must compute three first-order partial correlation coefficients in order to compute a second-order coefficient. Since this formula is a straightforward extension of the first-order formula, we will not illustrate its use. It may be helpful to compute the needed first-order partials and then solve all the possible second-order partials for the 440-yard inter-correlation data in Table 16-1.

Problems

1. Dr. Crank had just developed a comprehensive motor performance inventory, the Crank test (C.T.), and wished to gather information that might help him determine factors influencing scores on the C.T. so that he might be able to predict C.T. scores from other information. He chose to study the relationship between age, ear lobe length, and shoe size with C.T. scores. The data are presented below. Compute the equation for predicting C.T. scores from the other scores; also compute the multiple correlation coefficient, the coefficient of multiple determination, and the second-order partial correlation coefficient expressing the correlation between C.T. score and shoe size when the effects of age and ear lobe length are controlled. Interpret the results.

Means and standard deviations of Crank data ($n = 100$)

	C.T. score	Age	Shoe size	Ear lobe length
Means	75	15	8	4
Standard deviations	20	5	3	2

Intercorrelations for data on 100 Crank subjects

	Age	Shoe size	Ear lobe length	CT. score
Age	1	.60	.20	.30
Shoe size		1	−.10	.60
Ear lobe length			1	.70
C.T. score				1

2. Test the significance of the multiple R computed in problem 1 and determine whether the elimination of the ear lobe variable would have any significant effect on R.

Chapter **17**

Other statistical methods

FACTOR ANALYSIS

For many years physical educators have been attempting to describe and measure such general characteristics as physical fitness, athletic ability, motor ability, and athletic aptitude. To measure these characteristics the usual procedure is to administer a large battery of tests, each of which supposedly measures some component or components of the general characteristic. Underlying each of the tests are basic physical or mental abilities required for high test scores. Physical educators should know which basic abilities are measured by various test batteries, such as those involved in fitness tests and motor ability tests, so that they do not waste valuable time using multiple tests that measure the same basic ability or that measure an ability having no relationship to fitness or motor performance.

Factor analysis is a statistical procedure that can be used to identify the underlying basic abilities or factors measured by a large group of tests. For instance, if a physical-fitness test battery included tests of pull-ups, push-ups, and dips on the parallel bars, one might suspect that results on these three tests would be highly correlated because each of the three tests probably measures some common factor or ability involving the repeated, intense contractions of local muscle groups. Factor analysis procedures could be used to attempt to confirm the hypothesis that the three tests do measure a common factor or ability.

If this common factor were discovered and could be given a meaningful name such as "dynamic arm strength," then the factor analysis would have been useful for developing a meaningful concept of what the push-ups, pull-ups, and dips actually measured.

There are two basic uses of factor analysis in physical education that have already been alluded to. First, factor analysis is most often used simply to describe or identify underlying basic abilities or factors measured by a large battery of performance tests. Once the factors have been isolated by factor analysis, they can often be named so that a few meaningful underlying factors can be used to explain the results of many not so meaningful tests. Second, factor analysis is sometimes used to test hypotheses about predicted underlying abilities in a battery of tests.

170

Basically, factor analysis utilizes correlation techniques to interrelate test results in a battery of tests. For example, if five of ten tests are highly correlated with each other but not with the remaining five, which are also highly correlated, it might be concluded that the ten tests measure two underlying factors. The variance of the scores for each test can be classified into a variance common to the other tests, a variance specific to the test in question (something not measured by the other tests), and a variance caused by error and lack of control. Depending on how much variance each test has in common with others, factor analysis will help the scientist determine which common basic factors are measured by the test battery.

The actual procedures of factor analysis are too involved to be included in a book of this scope. The interested student will find an elementary exposition of these procedures in Fruchter's *Introduction to Factor Analysis.** An example of a comprehensive factoral analysis of physical fitness tests can be found in Fleishman's *The Structure and Measurement of Physical Fitness.*†

NONPARAMETRIC METHODS

In Chapter 2 the concept of measurement was discussed, and it was pointed out that the level of measurement—nominal, ordinal, interval, or ratio—in a research study should be considered when deciding what type of statistical analysis is appropriate for the data obtained. One reason for this is that certain kinds of arithmetical operations are necessary to estimate many test statistics, such as mean and standard deviation, and these operations are meaningless with data at a certain measurement level. For example, if the only data of a study were classifications of athletes at ten schools by sport of participation (e.g., football, basketball, or track), it would be meaningless to try to compute a mean sport value—the average of three basketball players and ten football players has no meaning. Likewise, when measurements are on an ordinal scale where it is known that one score is "better" than another but it is not known exactly how much better (e.g., judges' ratings in gymnastics or diving competition), means and standard deviations are not properly computed for such scores because the intervals between scores are not necessarily equal (the distance between a "5.0" and a "7.0" diving rating is probably much shorter than the distance between an "8.0" and a "10.0" rating). Any hypothesis tests of such statistics at the ordinal level must lead to conclusions of indefinite value, since the data probably do not accurately measure real values (i.e., "gymnastics ability," "intelligence") in the population on an interval scale.

Another reason for considering the question of level of measurement of sample data is that many statistical tests are based upon assumptions about the form of the population distribution of the variable under consideration, and conclusions reached when these assumptions are not met may well be invalid. For instance, the analysis of variance techniques assume that the

---

*Fruchter, B.: Introduction to factor analysis, Princeton, N. J., 1954, D. Van Nostrand Co., Inc.
†Fleishman, E. A.: The structure and measurement of physical fitness, Englewood Cliffs, N. J., 1964, Prentice-Hall, Inc.

populations sampled have normal distributions and equal variances, and if a significant F ratio is calculated for sample data from grossly nonnormal populations, the validity of any conclusions reached may be questionable. (If slight nonnormality is the only violation of the analysis of variance assumptions, little harm will result, since this technique is quite "robust" or resistant to small deviations from normality when large samples are available.) In some cases, data obtained may grossly appear to be on an interval scale but upon closer inspection may show evidence of nonnormality, or the investigator may hesitate to assume a true interval scale of measurement. In cases such as these it may be wise to seriously question the use of the usual statistical treatments because the conclusions reached may not have validity.

The judgement about whether a departure from statistical assumptions requires the use of special statistical techniques has been a topic of controversy in recent years. One school of thought (as espoused by Siegel*) emphasizes the need for special techniques, whereas another (see, for example, Games and Klare†) suggests that the use of statistics need not depend on the way numbers are obtained. This second school of thought maintains that it is foolhardy to worry about whether test scores represent "true" values for some variable such as motor educability or diving proficiency. They say that scientists should study only the observable test scores for such variables and make conclusions only about those scores. Since addition, subtraction, and other numerical operations can be carried out on any numerical scores, these statisticians conclude that means and standard deviations computed from such numerical data are perfectly acceptable and meaningful. We find the arguments of both groups equally appealing. To give the readers of this text some idea of the special techniques developed to treat data that obviously do not satisfy the assumptions of the usual statistical techniques, we have included this brief introduction to nonparametric methods.

Parametric and nonparametric techniques

The most common statistical techniques in physical education, the t tests, F tests, and correlation methods, all require fairly restrictive assumptions about the form of the population distributions and about certain parameters (i.e., means and standard deviations) of those distributions and have become known as *parametric* tests. Other techniques do not require such restrictive assumptions about the form of the distributions or about parameters and are known as *nonparametric* methods. One should realize that nonparametric methods are not free of all assumptions, and in many cases the reason for not using parametric methods may be cause enough to invalidate nonparametric methods. A failure to select random samples, for instance, invalidates both parametric and nonparametric methods in most instances.

---

*Siegel, S.: Nonparametric statistics for the behavioral sciences, New York, 1956, McGraw-Hill Book Co.

†Games, Paul A., and Klare, George R.: Elementary statistics: data analysis for the behavioral sciences, New York, 1967, McGraw-Hill Book Co., p. 474.

Selection of nonparametric techniques

It would be beyond the scope of this book to summarize the methods for all the nonparametric techniques that might be useful in physical education research, especially when a very readable book* containing most of the important nonparametric methods is already available. We suggest that Chapter 18 of our book, dealing with experimental design, be used as a rough guideline for determining which parametric or nonparametric methods may be applicable to a given research problem. If a nonparametric method is selected, Siegel's book can then be consulted for details of the method.

When not to use nonparametric methods

Since some statisticians believe that nonparametric tests need never be utilized with numerical data, it is difficult to state succinctly when such methods should be used, except in the case of nonnumerical (i.e., nominal) data. However, some statements can be made about when such methods should *not* be used.

1. Nonparametric methods should not be used if it is known that the population variable distribution meets all the assumptions for a parametric method. The reason for this is that nonparametric methods require greater sample sizes than do parametric methods to achieve the same degree of efficiency in rejecting the null hypothesis when it is false.
2. Nonparametric methods should not be used in place of an F or t test when the only reason for objecting to F or t tests is an apparently slight deviation from normality of the population or an apparent inequality among variances. With large sample sizes ($n > 10$) of equal size, such deviations are of little importance for these tests.
3. Do not use nonparametric methods to avoid responsibility for sloppy data collection or sampling procedures. Any statistical test is only as good as the data it treats.

---

*Siegel, S.: Nonparametric statistics for the behavioral sciences, New York, 1956, McGraw-Hill Book Co.

Chapter 18

Typical research paradigms and statistical treatments for physical education

Scheme n
design

Although nearly every conceivable type of research design and statistical analysis has been used at one time or another by physical education researchers, a number of these designs and analyses are far more prevalent and useful than others. In this chapter we have outlined typical designs and suggest statistical treatments that may be appropriate for each design. The statistical methods are explained either in this text, or, in the case of nonparametric methods, in Siegel.* Siegel presents extremely lucid explanations of the nonparametric methods, and the reader of the present text should have little difficulty with those explanations.

Again, it should be emphasized that this section does not attempt to examine all possible designs† and that some of the analyses suggested herein may not be appropriate to a particular set of data. However, as a first resource this chapter should prove very useful to the novice researcher.

I. SINGLE GROUP DESIGNS
A. SINGLE VARIABLE, ONE OBSERVATION PER SUBJECT
(Could this sample have come from a specified population?)

Subject	Observations
1	X_1
2	X_2
⋮	⋮
n	X_n

Examples: Elbow flexor strength of ninth-grade boys; 600-yard-run times for obese girls; number of successful trials in balancing skill.

---

*Siegel, S.: Nonparametric statistics, New York, 1956, McGraw-Hill Book Co.
†For other designs, see Winer, B. J.: Statistical principles in experimental design, New York, 1962, McGraw-Hill Book Co.

1. Data measured on interval scale
   a. t test assumptions tenable (**use t test of difference between sample and theoretical means**)
   b. t test assumptions untenable (**use Kolmogorov-Smirnov one-sample test**)
2. Data measured on ordinal scale (**use Kolmogorov-Smirnov one-sample test**)
3. Data measured on nominal scale
   a. Data in two categories (**use binomial test**)
   b. Data in at least two categories (**use χ^2 one-sample test**)
B. SINGLE VARIABLE, TWO OBSERVATIONS PER SUBJECT, THAT IS, PRETEST AND POSTTEST EXPERIMENTS
(Could this sample have come from a specified population?)

Subject	Pretest observation	Posttest observation
1	X_{11}	X_{12}
2	X_{21}	X_{22}
$\vdots$	$\vdots$	$\vdots$
n	X_{n1}	X_{n2}

Examples: Pretraining and posttraining body weights, arm strength, running speed, heart rate, skill rating, blood cholesterol level, aggression index.
1. Data measured on interval scale
   a. t test assumptions tenable (***t test of difference between $\bar{X}_1 - \bar{X}_2$ and hypothesized $\mu_1 - \mu_2$***)
   b. t test assumptions untenable
      (1) Sample $n < 10$ (**randomization test for matched pairs**)
      (2) Sample $n > 9$ and < 15 (**Walsh test**)
      (3) Sample $n > 14$ (**Wilcoxon matched-pairs signed ranks test**)
2. Data measured on ordinal scale
   a. Sample $n < 7$ (**sign test**)
   b. Sample $n > 6$ (**Wilcoxon matched-pairs signed ranks test**)
3. Data measured on nominal scale (**McNemar test**)
C. SINGLE VARIABLE, $r > 2$ TREATMENTS OR OBSERVATIONS PER SUBJECT, FOR EXAMPLE, r DIFFERENT TREATMENTS ON THE SAME INDIVIDUALS.
(Could these r samples have come from the same population?)

Subject	Treatment 1	Treatment 2	$\cdots$	Treatment r
1	X_{111}	X_{121}		X_{1r1}
	X_{112}	X_{122}	$\cdots$	X_{1r2}
	$\vdots$	$\vdots$		$\vdots$
	X_{11k}	X_{12k}		X_{1rk}
2	X_{211}	X_{221}		X_{2r1}
	X_{212}	X_{222}	$\cdots$	X_{2r2}
	$\vdots$	$\vdots$		$\vdots$
	X_{21k}	X_{22k}		X_{2rk}
$\vdots$	$\vdots$	$\vdots$	$\cdots$	$\vdots$
n	X_{n11}	X_{n21}		X_{nr1}
	X_{n12}	X_{n22}	$\cdots$	X_{nr2}
	$\vdots$	$\vdots$		$\vdots$
	X_{n1k}	X_{n2k}		X_{nrk}

Examples: Effects of r different diets on endurance to a treadmill run; effects of r different work tasks on blood lactic acid levels; effects of r different environmental conditions on motor performance test results.

1. Data measured on interval scale
   a. Analysis of variance assumptions tenable **(analysis of variance for repeated observations on the same subjects—single factor model)**
   b. Analysis of variance assumptions untenable **(Friedman two-way analysis of variance by ranks on mean cell scores)**
2. Data measured on ordinal scale **(Friedman two-way analysis of variance by ranks on mean cell scores)**
3. Data measured on nominal scale **(Cochran Q test)**

D. TWO VARIABLES, ONE PAIR OF OBSERVATIONS PER SUBJECT

(What is the degree of relationship between these two variables, and how well can one be predicted with prior knowledge of the second?)

Subject	Observations on variable 1	Observations on variable 2
1	X_1	Y_1
2	X_2	Y_2
$\vdots$	$\vdots$	$\vdots$
n	X_n	Y_n

Examples: Relationship between leg strength and high-jump performance, body weight and mile-run performance, heart rate and work intensity.

1. Data measured on interval scale
   a. Pearson product-moment assumptions tenable **(Pearson product-moment correlation coefficient, r, and simple linear regression)**
   b. Pearson product-moment assumptions untenable **(Spearman rank correlation coefficient, r_s; Kendall rank correlation coefficient, T)**
2. Data measured on ordinal scale **(Spearman rank correlation coefficient, r_s; Kendall rank correlation coefficient, T)**
3. Data measured on nominal scale **(contingency coefficient, C)**

E. $r > 2$ VARIABLES, ONE OBSERVATION ON EACH VARIABLE FOR EACH SUBJECT

Subject	Observations on variable 1	Observations on variable 2	$\cdots$	Observations on variable r
1	X_{11}	X_{12}		X_{1r}
2	X_{21}	X_{22}		X_{2r}
$\vdots$	$\vdots$	$\vdots$		$\vdots$
n	X_{n1}	X_{n2}	$\cdots$	X_{nr}

Examples: Scores on a battery of r different fitness tests or skills tests for each subject, scores on r different physiological variables or psychological tests.

E_1. Determining the degree of relationship between the combined effects of two or more variables and a criterion variable, for example, relationship between combined effects of height, weight, and arm strength on performance of a military press in weight lifting (**multiple correlation coefficient, R**)

E_2. Predicting scores on a criterion variable from scores on two or more other variables (**multiple linear regression**)

E_3. Determining common factors underlying the relationship between two or more variables and a criterion variable, for example, a common "dynamic strength" factor underlying the positive relationship between performance on push-up tests, parallel-bar dips, and arm curls on ability to perform pull-ups (**factor analysis**)

E_4. Determining degree of relationship between two variables with a third held constant, for example, relationship between height and weight with age held constant

    1. Data measured on interval scale

        a. Pearson product-moment assumptions tenable

          (Partial product-moment correlation coefficient)

        b. Pearson product-moment assumptions untenable

          (Kendall partial rank correlation coefficient, $T_{XY \cdot Z}$)

    2. Data measured on ordinal scale

        (Kendall partial rank correlation coefficient, $T_{XY \cdot Z}$)

II. TWO-GROUP DESIGNS

A. SINGLE VARIABLE, ONE OBSERVATION PER SUBJECT

(Could these two samples have come from the same population?)

Observations for treatment or group 1	Observations for treatment or group 2
X_{11}	X_{21}
X_{12}	X_{22}
$\vdots$	$\vdots$
X_{1n}	X_{2n}

Examples: Heart rates of trained and untrained groups of subjects, attitudes towards sport of upper- and lower-class individuals, pain tolerance in trained and untrained subjects.

A_1. Independent observations

    1. Data measured on interval scale

        a. t test assumptions tenable (**t test of means**)

        b. t test assumptions untenable

          (1) Sample $n < 10$ (**randomization test of means for two independent samples**)

          (2) Sample $n > 9$ (**Mann-Whitney U test of central tendency**)

    2. Data measured on ordinal scale

        a. Sample $n < 9$ (**Kolmogorov-Smirnov two-sample test**)

        b. Sample $n > 8$ (**Mann-Whitney U test of central tendency; median test**)

    3. Data measured on nominal scale

        a. Data in two categories, sample $n < 10$ (**Fisher exact probability test**)

        b. Sample $n > 9$, or data in more than two categories (**chi-square test for two independent samples**)

A_2. Correlated observations, that is, two matched groups (e.g., effects of two methods of weight training when subjects are matched on body weight)

    1. Data measured on interval scale

        a. t test assumptions tenable (**t test of difference between $[\overline{X}_1 - \overline{X}_2]$ and $[\mu_1 - \mu_2]$**)

b. t test assumptions untenable
   (1) Sample $n < 10$ **(randomization test for matched pairs)**
   (2) Sample $n > 9$ and < 15 **(Walsh test)**
   (3) Sample $n > 14$ **(Wilcoxon matched-pairs signed ranks test)**
2. Data measured on ordinal scale
  a. Sample $n > 7$ **(sign test)**
  b. Sample $n < 6$ **(Wilcoxon matched-pairs signed ranks test)**
3. Data measured on nominal scale **(McNemar test)**

B. SINGLE VARIABLE, TWO OBSERVATIONS PER SUBJECT, THAT IS, PRETEST-POSTTEST EXPERIMENTS

Observations for treatment or group 1		Observations for treatment or group 2	
Pretest	Posttest	Pretest	Posttest
X_{111}	X_{121}	X_{211}	X_{221}
X_{112}	X_{122}	X_{212}	X_{222}
$\vdots$	$\vdots$	$\vdots$	$\vdots$
X_{11n_1}	X_{12n_1}	X_{21n_2}	X_{22n_2}

Examples: Effects of two methods of training on heart rate, skill performance, or weight loss.
1. Data measured on interval scale
  a. t test assumptions tenable (***t* test of difference between sample means of pretest-posttest differences and hypothetical difference between population means of pretest-posttest differences)**
  b. t test assumptions untenable **(analyze pretest-posttest differences according to II A$_1$1b or II A$_2$1b)**
2. Data measured on ordinal scale **(analyze pretest-posttest differences according to II A$_1$2 or II A$_2$2)**
3. Data measured on nominal scale **(analyze pretest-posttest differences according to II A$_1$3 or II A$_2$3)**

C. TWO CORRELATED VARIABLES, ONE PAIR OF OBSERVATIONS PER SUBJECT **(analysis of covariance)**

Observations on treatment or group 1		Observations on treatment or group 2	
Variable X	Variable Y	Variable X	Variable Y
X_{11}	Y_{11}	X_{21}	Y_{21}
X_{12}	Y_{12}	X_{22}	Y_{22}
$\vdots$	$\vdots$	$\vdots$	$\vdots$
X_{1n}	Y_{1n}	X_{2n}	Y_{2n}

Examples: Effects of two exercise regimens on strength (Y) when pretraining body weight (X) is taken into account; effects of two methods of training on 880-yard-run time (Y) when pretraining maximum oxygen consumption capacity (X) is taken into account.

III. r-GROUP DESIGNS, WHERE $r > 2$
  A. SINGLE VARIABLE MANIPULATED, ONE OBSERVATION PER SUBJECT
  (Could these r samples have come from the same population?)

Observations for treatment or group 1	Observations for treatment or group 2	$\cdots$	Observations for treatment or group r
X_{11}	X_{21}	$\cdots$	X_{r1}
X_{12}	X_{22}	$\cdots$	X_{r2}
$\vdots$	$\vdots$		$\vdots$
X_{1n_1}	X_{2n_2}	$\cdots$	X_{rn_r}

Examples: Effects of r different exercise programs on body composition, effects of r methods of teaching on skill improvement, effects of r types of diet on endurance.
  1. Independent observations, that is, subjects randomly assigned to treatments or groups
    a. Data measured on interval scale
      (1) Analysis of variance assumptions tenable **(one-way, fixed effects, completely randomized model of analysis of variance)**
      (2) Analysis of variance assumptions untenable **(Kruskal-Wallis one-way analysis of variance by ranks)**
    b. Data measured on ordinal scale **(Kruskal-Wallis one-way analysis of variance by ranks)**
    c. Data measured on nominal scale **(chi-square test for k independent samples)**
  2. Correlated observations (n matched groups of subjects, r subjects per group)
    a. Data measured on interval scale
      (1) Analysis of variance assumptions tenable **(one-way, fixed effects, randomized blocks model of analysis of variance)**
      (2) Analysis of variance assumptions untenable **(Friedman two-way analysis of variance by ranks)**
    b. Data measured on ordinal scale **(Friedman two-way analysis of variance by ranks)**
    c. Data measured on nominal scale **(Cochran Q test)**
  B. ONE VARIABLE MANIPULATED, ONE PAIR OF OBSERVATIONS PER SUBJECT IN EACH OF r TREATMENTS OR GROUPS
  (Could these r samples have come from the same population?) **(analysis of covariance)**

Observations for treatment or group 1		Observations for treatment or group 2		$\cdots$	Observations for treatment or group r	
Variable X	Variable Y	Variable X	Variable Y		Variable X	Variable Y
X_{11}	Y_{11}	X_{21}	Y_{21}	$\cdots$	X_{r1}	Y_{r1}
X_{12}	Y_{12}	X_{22}	Y_{22}	$\cdots$	X_{r2}	Y_{r2}
$\vdots$	$\vdots$	$\vdots$	$\vdots$		$\vdots$	$\vdots$
X_{1n}	Y_{1n}	X_{2n}	Y_{2n}	$\cdots$	X_{rn}	Y_{rn}

Examples: Effects of r different types of training on body weight when pretraining body weight is considered; effects of r methods of teaching on high-jump performance when leg strength is considered; effects of r methods of training on maze performance when pretraining maze performance is considered.

C. FACTORIAL DESIGNS—MORE THAN ONE INDEPENDENT VARIABLE MANIPULATED, INTERACTION EFFECTS OF INTEREST

(Could these samples have come from the same population?)

1. One observation per subject (two- or higher way, fixed effects completely randomized analysis of variance)
2. Repeated observations on the same subjects (two-factor analysis of variance with repeated measurements on the same subjects)

		Levels of factor A			
		Observations for level 1 of factor A	Observations for level 2 of factor A	...	Observations for level r of factor A
	Observations for level 1 of factor B	X_{111} X_{112} $\vdots$ X_{11n}	X_{211} X_{212} $\vdots$ X_{21n}	...	X_{a11} X_{a12} $\vdots$ X_{a1n}
Levels of factor B	Observations for level 2 of factor B	X_{121} X_{122} $\vdots$ X_{12n}	X_{221} X_{222} $\vdots$ X_{22n}	...	X_{a21} X_{a22} $\vdots$ X_{a2n}
	$\vdots$	$\vdots$	$\vdots$	...	$\vdots$
	Observations for level b of factor B	X_{1b1} X_{1b2} $\vdots$ X_{1bn}	X_{2b1} X_{2b2} $\vdots$ X_{2bn}	...	X_{ab1} X_{ab2} $\vdots$ X_{abn}

Examples: Effects of a different exercise programs and b different diets on serum cholesterol levels; effects of a different teaching methods and b different class period lengths on motor learning or knowledge test results.

Appendix **A**

Tests and testing
in physical education

In physical education, as in any other academic area, the teacher is faced with the necessity of evaluating his students' performances in as objective a manner as possible. The problems inherent in evaluation are greatly minimized if the teacher has a knowledge of available tests, the way these tests are scored, to whom the tests are applicable, and how they are most efficiently administered. An equally important aspect is for the teacher to possess the necessary skills to enable him to evaluate tests found in the physical education literature. In this Appendix we will attempt to establish the criteria used in evaluating tests and also direct the reader to some tests widely used in various aspects of physical education programs.

EVALUATION OF TESTS

It is obvious that not all tests do the job of evaluation in a satisfactory manner. To intelligently select tests the teacher must be sure the test will measure those items he wishes to measure and not be influenced by other factors in which he has no interest. He must also be sure that the test results are not influenced by any personal factors that the tester introduces into the testing situation. Next, the teacher should be sure that the test will produce results that are consistent when the test is administered a number of times. The value and meaning of a test is also enhanced when it has tables that allow the teacher to compare the scores of his students with those of others. Finally, a test may possess all the above qualities and still be useless if the time or equipment required for administration of the test is beyond the available limits of a given situation. These factors should all be considered in evaluating a test to be used in the teaching situation.

Validity

The concept of validity in a test situation denotes the degree to which the test actually measures what it is designed to measure. For instance, it is obvious that a weight-lifting test could not be used to test for football playing ability. Although strength is certainly an important factor in playing football, it is only a part of the total picture. Many other factors also play

181

an important role, such as speed, agility, endurance, intelligence, and desire. Therefore a test of weight lifting would not be appropriate. It would not measure what we wish to measure. It would therefore not be a valid test of football playing ability.

Another example might concern a test of speed as measured by the time required to cover a certain distance. A common example might be the 220-yard dash. This is agreed upon as a test of speed. However, suppose we were to use the same starting procedures (starting blocks and gun) for a 2-yard dash. Would this still be a valid test of speed? The answer is obviously no. The winner of a 2-yard dash, because of the very small distance involved, would owe a far larger share of his credit for winning such a race to reaction time than to speed. Therefore it would not be valid to consider a 2-yard dash a measure of speed.

The validity of a test is usually determined by comparing its results to the results of a test known to be valid, or to the evaluations of a panel of experts in the area. If the results of the test in question correlate highly with the results of the known test or with the experts' ratings, the test is considered valid.

Objectivity

The objectivity of a test refers to its ability to produce consistent results when administered by different people. In other words, the results obtained on a given test should not reflect the attitudes or personality of the person giving the test. For example, if running time on a treadmill is used as a test of endurance, the test directions should be explicit as to the amount of encouragement to be given to the runner. A great amount of vocal encouragement can push the runner to greater endurance than would be shown if no encouragement were given. If no directions are given to the tester, the outgoing, highly vocal tester may cause results that differ from those obtained by a calmer, quieter tester, thus impairing the objectivity of the test.

Reliability

The reliability of a test refers to its ability to produce consistent results when administered to one group a number of times. If a test of cardiovascular fitness is given to a group of students on 2 successive days, the scores should be the same both times for the various students. Actually, almost all tests involve some degree of learning so that the scores might be expected to improve from test to test. However, the relative ranking of each student should remain the same.

The reliability of a particular test may be established by means of a coefficient of correlation. The r is obtained using the scores from two administrations of the test to a single group of students. The value thus produced is often referred to as a reliability coefficient. Clarke's review indicates that this reliability coefficient may be roughly interpreted as follows:

.95 to .99   Very high: rarely found among present tests
.90 to .94   High: equaled by a few of the best tests

.80 to .89   Fairly high: fairly adequate for individual measurements
.70 to .79   Rather low: adequate for group measurement but not very satisfactory for individual measurement
Below .70   Low: entirely inadequate for individual measurement, although useful for group averages and school surveys

Norms

Norms, or percentile tables as they are often called, are standards derived from repeated administrations of a test to a large number of subjects. Norms are generally listed in terms of percentiles. A percentile tells us what percentage of the individuals to whom the test was administered fell below a given score. For example, let us look at the data in Table A-1.

Table A-1

Handgrip norms*												
Boys' ages						Percentile	Girls' ages					
13	14	15	16	17	18		13	14	15	16	17	18
105	125	139	157	165	163	99th	65	83	84	90	99	101
102	120	130	149	156	156	98th	63	78	79	86	93	98
100	118	128	147	149	149	97th	62	76	77	83	90	96
95	115	121	140	144	144	95th	60	67	74	79	86	91
85	108	115	130	134	138	90th	58	60	69	76	79	86
80	105	111	126	129	134	85th	57	57	66	71	77	80
78	96	108	121	125	129	80th	55	56	62	69	75	78
75	93	106	118	120	125	75th	53	54	60	67	72	76
70	89	103	115	118	120	70th	50	52	59	66	69	73
67	84	98	110	115	117	60th	45	48	57	63	67	70
65	78	93	106	109	114	50th	42	43	55	59	63	67
57	75	88	101	106	109	40th	35	40	52	57	59	64
52	65	85	97	101	105	30th	33	38	49	55	57	59
50	59	81	93	98	101	25th	30	37	47	51	56	57
46	55	78	89	96	98	20th	28	36	46	49	56	56
43	50	76	86	92	96	15th	26	35	42	47	50	53
41	46	69	81	88	90	10th	24	32	39	45	47	49
39	41	61	76	82	86	5th	20	25	36	38	43	46
37	39	56	71	78	83	3rd	17	23	32	35	38	41
35	37	48	68	76	81	2nd	15	20	28	34	37	39
33	34	36	62	69	77	1st	10	15	20	31	31	37

Scores are in "pounds pressure."
*From Fleishman, Edwin A.: The structure and measurement of physical fitness, Englewood Cliffs, N. J., 1964, Prentice-Hall, Inc., by permission of the publishers.

The 80th percentile for a 14-year-old boy for the handgrip is 96 pounds pressure. This means that 80% of the 14-year-old boys tested, whose scores constitute the basis for these norms, were able to exert less than 96 pounds of pressure. Conversely, only 20% of the 14-year-old boys tested were able to exert more than 96 pounds of pressure. Therefore, as the percentile rises, the score improves, and as the percentile falls, the score worsens.

The advantage of norms should be obvious to the reader. If you test a 16-year-old boy on his handgrip and he exerts 130 pounds of pressure, this score by itself has little meaning to you or to the boy. However, if the norms are available, they provide a standard that indicates how good or bad a particular score is. In this case a score of 130 falls at the 90th percentile, which then places the score in focus.

Unfortunately, norms for many tests are not often available. However, the teacher can easily construct his own norms from data generated by his own students. These procedures were discussed in Chapter 4.

Feasibility

A final consideration in the selection and administration of tests involves the cost in terms of both time and money. It is obvious that a test may be valid, objective, reliable, have norms, and not be at all usable in a teaching situation because it takes too long or because the equipment needed is too expensive. The type of test used should also consider the subjects who are being tested. The testing situation should have meaning for the pupils. The test results should be interpreted in a manner that is clear and meaningful. Remember that tests are not given simply as a means of determining grades but are invaluable in determining needs, setting goals and objectives, and measuring progress.

SOME AVAILABLE TESTS

Since the emphasis of this text is on the quantitative aspects of physical education, we will not deal at length with the tests that are available in terms of the way they are administered and scored. However, the reader should find this Appendix, which lists some of the many individual tests, and tests and measurements books, which deal extensively and in detail with specific tests and their administration, helpful.

The references listed below are indicative of those to be found by the physical education teacher. These references are grouped into specific categories for convenience. The reader is strongly urged to consult the original references for the most thorough understanding of the various tests.

Knowledge

Bridges, F.: Health knowledge test for college women, Chicago, 1956, Psychometric Affiliates.

Broer, M., and Miller, D.: Achievement tests for beginning and intermediate tennis, Research Quarterly **21:** 303, Oct., 1950.

Deitz, D., and Frech, B.: Hockey knowledge test for girls, Journal of Health Physical Education and Recreation **11:** 366, June, 1940.

Fox, K.: Beginning badminton written examination, Research Quarterly **24:** 135, May, 1953.

French, F.: The construction of knowledge tests in selected professional courses in physical education, Research Quarterly **14:** 406, Dec., 1943.

Gershon, E.: Apparatus gymnastics knowledge test for college men in professional physical education, Research Quarterly **28:** 332, Dec., 1957.

Heath, M., and Rodgers, E.: A study in the use of knowledge and skill tests in soccer, Research Quarterly **3:** 33, Dec., 1932.

Hennis, G.: Construction of knowledge tests in selected physical education activities for college women, Research Quarterly **27:** 310, Oct., 1956.

Hewitt, J.: Hewitt's comprehensive tennis knowledge test—form A and B revised, Research Quarterly **35:** 147, May, 1964.

Kelly, E., and Brown, J.: The construction of a field hockey test for women physical education majors, Research Quarterly **23:** 322, Oct., 1952.

Kilander, F.: Kilander health knowledge test for college students, ed. 5, Staten Island, 1966, Wagner College.

Langston, D.: Standardization of a volleyball knowledge test for college men physical education majors, Research Quarterly **26:** 60, March, 1955.

Miller, W.: Achievement levels in tennis knowledge and skill for women physical education major students, Research Quarterly **24:** 81, May, 1953.

Phillips, M.: Standardization of a badminton knowledge test for college women, Research Quarterly **17:** 48, March, 1946.

Scott, G.: Achievement examinations for elementary and intermediate swimming classes, Research Quarterly **11:** 100, May, 1940.

Scott, G.: Achievement examinations for elementary and intermediate tennis classes, Research Quarterly **12:** 40, March, 1941.

Scott, G.: Achievement examinations in badminton, Research Quarterly **12:** 242, May, 1941.

Waglow, I., and Rehling, C.: A golf knowledge test, Research Quarterly **24:** 463, Dec., 1953.

Waglow, I., and Stephens, F.: A softball knowledge test, Research Quarterly **26:** 234, May, 1955.

Skills

Bassett, G., Glassow, R., and Locke, M.: Studies in testing volleyball skills, Research Quarterly **8:** 60, Dec., 1937.

Boyd, C., McCachren, J., and Waglow, I.: Predictive ability of a selected basketball test, Research Quarterly **26:** 364, Oct., 1955.

Brady, G.: Preliminary investigations of volleyball playing ability, Research Quarterly **16:** 14, March, 1945.

Cornish, C.: A study of measurement of ability in handball, Research Quarterly **20:** 215, May, 1949.

Dyer, J.: Revision of the backboard test of tennis ability, Research Quarterly **9:** 25, March, 1938.

French, E., and Cooper, B.: Achievement tests in volleyball for high school girls, Research Quarterly **8:** 150, May, 1937.

French, E., and Stalter, E.: Study of skill tests in badminton for college women, Research Quarterly **20:** 257, Oct., 1949.

Fox, M.: Swimming power test, Research Quarterly **28:** 233, Oct., 1957.

Glassow, R., and Broer, M.: Measuring achievement in physical education, Philadelphia, 1938, W. B. Saunders Co.

Hewitt, J.: Achievement scale scores for high school swimming, Research Quarterly **20:** 170, May, 1949.

Hewitt, J.: Swimming achievement scale scores for college men, Research Quarterly **19:** 282, Dec., 1949.

Hyde, E.: An achievement scale in archery, Research Quarterly **8:** 109, May, 1937.

Kelson, R.: Baseball classification plan for boys, Research Quarterly **24:** 304, Oct., 1953.

Lehsten, C.: A measure of basketball skills in high school boys, The Physical Educator **5:** 103, Dec., 1948.

Lockhart, A., and McPherson, F.: The development of a test of badminton playing ability, Research Quarterly **20:** 402, Dec., 1949.

Martin, J., and Keogh, J.: Bowling norms for college students in elective physical education classes, Research Quarterly **35:** 325, Oct., 1964.

Martin, J.: Bowling norms for college men and women, Research Quarterly **31:** 113, March, 1960.

Miller, F.: A badminton wall volley test, Research Quarterly **22:** 208, May, 1951.

Miller, W.: Achievement levels in basketball skills for women physical education majors, Research Quarterly **25:** 450, Dec., 1954.

Phillips, M., and Summers, D.: Bowling norms and learning curves for college women, Research Quarterly **21:** 377, Dec., 1950.

Russell, N., and Lange, E.: Achievement tests in volleyball for junior high school girls, Research Quarterly **11:** 33, Dec., 1940.

Stroup, F.: Game results as a criterion for validating basketball skill tests, Research Quarterly **26:** 353, Oct., 1955.

Fitness

AAHPER youth fitness test manual, rev. ed., Washington, 1965, AAHPER.

Bookwalter, K.: Test manual for Indiana University motor fitness indices for high school and college men, Research Quarterly **14**: 356, Dec., 1943.

Brouha, L.: The step test: a simple method of measuring physical fitness for muscular work in young men, Research Quarterly, **14**: 31, March, 1943.

Carlson, H.: Fatigue curve test, Research Quarterly **16**: 169, Oct., 1945.

Clarke, H.: A manual: cable-tension strength tests, Chicopee, Mass., 1953, Brown-Murphy.

Clarke H., and Carter, G.: Oregon simplification of the strength and physical fitness indices for upper elementary, junior high, and senior high school boys, Research Quarterly **30**: 3, March, 1959.

Consolazio, F., Johnson, R., and Pecora, L.: Physiological measurements of metabolic functions in man, New York, 1963, McGraw-Hill Book Co.

Cureton, T.: Physical fitness appraisal and guidance, St. Louis, 1947, The C. V. Mosby Co.

Gallagher, J., and Brouha, L.: A simple method of testing the physical fitness of boys, Research Quarterly **14**: 23, March, 1943.

Kraus, H., and Hirschland, R.: Minimum muscular fitness tests in school children, Research Quarterly **25**: 178, May, 1954.

Larson, L.: Some findings resulting from the army air forces physical training program, Research Quarterly **17**: 144, May, 1946.

Phillips, B.: The JCR test, Research Quarterly **18**: 12, March, 1947.

Phillips, M., et. al.: Analysis of results from the Kraus-Weber test of minimum muscular fitness in children, Research Quarterly **26**: 314, Oct., 1955.

Skubic, V., and Hodgkins, J.: Cardiovascular efficiency test scores for girls and women in the United States, Research Quarterly **34**: 454, Dec., 1963.

Slater-Hammel, A., and Butler, L.: Accuracy in securing pulse rates by palpation, Research Quarterly **11**: 18, May, 1940.

Taylor, C.: A maximal pack test of exercise tolerances, Research Quarterly **15**: 291, Dec., 1944.

Tuttle, W., and Dickenson, R.: A simplification of the pulse-ratio technique for rating physical efficiency and present condition, Research Quarterly **9**: 73, May, 1938.

Motor ability

Barrow, H.: Test of motor ability for college men, Research Quarterly **25**: 253, Oct., 1954.

Hatlestad, L.: Motor educability tests for women college students, Research Quarterly **13**: 10, March, 1942.

Henry, F.: Influence of motor and sensory sets on reaction latency and speed of discrete movements, Research Quarterly **31**: 459, Oct., 1960.

Humiston, D.: A measurement of motor ability in college women, Research Quarterly **8**: 181, May, 1937.

Larson, L.: A factor analysis of motor ability variables and tests, with tests for college men, Research Quarterly **12**: 499, Oct., 1941.

Latchaw, M.: Measuring selected motor skills in fourth, fifth, and sixth grades, Research Quarterly **25**: 439, Dec., 1954.

McCloy, C.: A preliminary study of factors in motor educability, Research Quarterly **11**: 28, May, 1940.

Metheny, E.: Studies of the Johnson test as a test of motor educability, Research Quarterly **9**: 105, Dec., 1938.

Powell, E., and Howe, E.: Motor ability tests for high school girls, Research Quarterly **10**: 81, Dec., 1939.

Scott, G.: Motor ability tests for college women, Research Quarterly **14**: 402, Dec., 1943.

Body mechanics

Cureton, T.: Bodily posture as an indicator of fitness, supplement to the Research Quarterly **12**: 348, May, 1941.

Davies, E.: Relationship between selected postural divergencies and motor ability, Research Quarterly **28:** 1, March, 1957.

Flint, M.: Lumbar posture: a study of roentgenographic measurement and the influence of flexibility and strength, Research Quarterly **34:** 15, March, 1963.

Fox, M., and Young, O.: Placement of the gravital line in anteroposterior standing posture, Research Quarterly **25:** 277, Oct., 1954.

Goldthwaite, J.: Body mechanics, ed. 5, Philadelphia, 1952, J. B. Lippincott Co.

Kelly, E.: A comparative study of structure and function of normal, pronated, and painful feet among children, Research Quarterly **18:** 291, Dec., 1947.

Lee, M., and Wagner, M.: Fundamentals of body mechanics and conditioning, Philadelphia, 1949, W. B. Saunders Co.

McCloy, C.: X-ray studies of innate differences in straight and curved spines, Research Quarterly **9:** 50, May, 1938.

Massey, W.: A critical study of objective measures for measuring anterior-posterior posture with a simplified technique, Research Quarterly **14:** 3, March, 1943.

Moriarity, M., and Irwin, L.: A study of the relationship of certain physical and emotional factors to habitual poor posture among school children, Research Quarterly **23:** 221, May, 1952.

Attitudes

Adams, R.: Two scales for measuring attitude toward physical education, Research Quarterly **34:** 91, March, 1963.

Blanchard, B.: A behavior frequency rating scale for the measurement of character and personality in physical education classroom situations, Research Quarterly **7:** 56, May, 1936.

Breck, S.: A sociometric measurement of status in physical education classes, Research Quarterly **21:** 75, May, 1950.

Clarke, H., and Greene, W.: Relationships between personal-social measures applied to 10-year-old boys, Research Quarterly **34:** 288, Oct., 1963.

Cowell, C.: Validating and index of social adjustment for high school use, Research Quarterly **29:** 7, March, 1958.

Isenberger, W.: Self-attitudes of women physical education major students and of women physical education teachers, Research Quarterly **30:** 44, March, 1959.

McGee, R.: Comparison of attitudes toward intensive competition for high school girls, Research Quarterly **27:** 60, March, 1956.

O'Neel, F.: A behavior frequency rating scale for the measurement of character and personality in high school physical education for boys, Research Quarterly **7:** 67, May, 1936.

Todd, F.: Sociometry in physical education, Journal of Health Physical Education and Recreation **24:** 23, May, 1953.

Wear, C.: The evaluation of attitude toward physical education as an activity course, Research Quarterly **22:** 114, March, 1951.

Additional sources of tests

Barrow, H., and McGee, R.: A practical approach to measurement in physical education, Philadelphia, 1964, Lea and Febiger.

Clarke, H.: Application of measurement to health and physical education, ed. 4, Englewood Cliffs, N. J., 1967, Prentice-Hall, Inc.

Fleishman, E.: The structure and measurement of physical fitness, Englewood Cliffs, N. J., 1964, Prentice-Hall, Inc.

Latchaw, M., and Brown, C.: The evaluation process in health education, physical education and recreation, Englewood Cliffs, N. J., 1962, Prentice-Hall, Inc.

Mathews, D.: Measurement in physical education, ed. 3, Philadelphia, 1968, W. B. Saunders Co.

Meyers, C., and Blesh, T.: Measurement in physical education, New York, 1962, The Ronald Press Co.

Scott, G., and French, E.: Measurement and evaluation in physical education, Dubuque, Iowa, 1959, Wm. C. Brown Co., Publishers.

Appendix **B**

A review of mathematics skills

In Chapter 1 we discussed the need to be able to handle simple arithmetic processes as being basic to the understanding of statistics. It should be emphasized that these processes are elementary and extend only through simple algebra. The beginning statistics student is often plagued by unfamiliarity with the arithmetic of a statistical process. As a result he often becomes so involved with an item such as taking a square root, clearing a fraction, or solving for an unknown in an equation that he loses sight of the meaning and value of the entire procedure. In most cases the student is not totally unfamiliar with the process but has simply not used his arithmetic skills in a long time. Another problem is haste and sloppiness. Remember that arithmetic and statistics are both precise and orderly processes. To successfully deal with them the student's work should also be precise and orderly.

This review of fundamental processes is presented to refamiliarize the student with the mechanics and rules needed for computations of the kind that are treated in this text.

READING SYMBOLIC DIRECTIONS

Arithmetic operations are indicated by the use of appropriate symbols that direct the user. The symbols of addition $(+)$, subtraction $(-)$, multiplication $(\times)$, and division $(\div)$ are thoroughly familiar. In addition, these processes are sometimes indicated by other means. Multiplication may be indicated by parentheses or by placing values in juxtaposition to each other. Division may be indicated by separating the quantities by a bar. For example, if we want to write "multiply 8 by 12" we may write this as 8×12, $(8)(12)$, or $8(12)$. If we want to write "multiply a by c" we may write $a \times c$, $(a)(c)$, $a(c)$, or $a\,c$. In indicating the process of division, 84 divided by 21 may be written $84 \div 21$, $21\overline{)84}$, $84/21$, or $\frac{84}{21}$. In most cases the specific sign of multiplication or division is not used. We may consider that this is part of the shorthand notation of statistics, which, when learned, simplifies our calculations.

The symbols $<$ and $>$ mean "is less than" and "is greater than," respectively. The statement "the product of m and r is greater than 60" is more simply written $m\,r > 60$. When either of these symbols is placed over a single bar, it means "is less than or equal to" or "is greater than or equal to." If we wish to say "24 divided by X is less than or equal to 9" it is written $24/X \leq 9$.

Another symbol often encountered is Σ, the Greek capital letter sigma. This is the symbol for summation or the process of adding. In dealing with a variable, or a quantity which may assume different values or which varies, we may wish to indicate that we want to find the sum of these values. If there are n values of our variable X and we want to add these, we state this as ΣX, which is equal to $X_1 + X_2 + X_3 + X_4 + X_5 + \cdots + X_n$. As a specific example let us consider the variable of height (measured to the nearest inch) of 21-year-old males. If the heights of ten men constitute the values of X available to us, and we wish to find the sum of these heights: $\Sigma X = X_1 + X_2 + X_3 + X_4 + X_5 + X_6 + X_7 + X_8 + X_9 + X_{10}$.

FRACTIONS

Dealing with fractions will be greatly simplified if one simple rule is remembered: Both the numerator (upper term) and denominator (lower term) of a fraction may be *multiplied* or *divided* by the same term without changing the value of the fraction. Note that this is *not* true of addition or subtraction of the same term to the numerator and denominator. If both the numerator and denominator of the fraction 3/6 are multiplied by 2, we get 6/12, which is an equivalent fraction. If both the numerator and denominator of the fraction 3/6 are divided by 3, we get 1/2, which is an equivalent fraction. Likewise, if we subtract 2 from both the numerator and denominator of the fraction 3/6, we get 1/4, which is not an equivalent fraction.

To add or subtract fractions we must first transform them to equivalent fractions having a common denominator. To do this we make use of our primary rule. For example, if we wish to add 1/6 and 2/7 we must transform these fractions so that they both have the same denominator. We normally choose the smallest value by which all our denominators can be evenly divided. This is known as the lowest common denominator. In this case, 42 is the lowest common denominator. Thus:

$$\frac{1}{6} + \frac{1}{7} = \frac{1}{6}\left(\frac{7}{7}\right) + \frac{1}{7}\left(\frac{6}{6}\right) = \frac{7}{42} + \frac{6}{42} = \frac{13}{42}$$

Note that when we have transformed our original fractions to equivalent fractions with a common denominator, we add or subtract only the numerators and place the answer over the common denominator. If we wish to subtract 5/6 from 7/8, we determine that the lowest common denominator is 24. Thus:

$$\frac{7}{8} - \frac{5}{6} = \frac{7}{8}\left(\frac{3}{3}\right) - \frac{5}{6}\left(\frac{4}{4}\right) = \frac{21}{24} - \frac{20}{24} = \frac{1}{24}$$

To multiply fractions we multiply all the numerators and place their product over the product of all the denominators. Thus:

$$\frac{1}{6} \times \frac{1}{7} = \frac{1}{42} \qquad\qquad \frac{7}{8} \times \frac{5}{6} = \frac{35}{48}$$

$$\frac{1}{6} \times \frac{1}{7} \times \frac{7}{8} \times \frac{5}{66} \times \frac{35}{2016} = \frac{5}{288} \qquad \frac{a}{b} + \frac{b}{c} + \frac{c}{d} = \frac{abc}{bcd} = \frac{a}{d}$$

To divide fractions we simply invert the divisor and multiply as above. Thus:

$$\frac{5}{6} \div \frac{1}{4} = \frac{5}{6} \times \frac{4}{1} = \frac{20}{6} = 3\frac{1}{3}$$

$$3\frac{1}{4} \div \frac{2}{3} = \frac{13}{4} \times \frac{3}{2} = \frac{39}{8} = 4\frac{7}{8}$$

$$\frac{r}{s} \div \frac{x}{y} = \frac{r}{s} \times \frac{y}{x} = \frac{ry}{sx}$$

DECIMALS

When adding or subtracting decimals, be sure that the decimal point in each value is aligned precisely below that of the number above it. This procedure will greatly minimize errors that commonly occur when dealing with decimals. To add 86.134, 19.6 and 7.63:

$$\begin{array}{r} 86.134 \\ 19.6 \\ 7.63 \\ \hline 113.364 \end{array}$$

To subtract 28.0845 from 452.1:

$$\begin{array}{r} 452.1 \\ 28.0845 \\ \hline 424.0155 \end{array}$$

When multiplying decimals, the answer will have as many decimal points as the sum of the number of decimal points in the multiplicand and multiplier. Thus:

$$\begin{array}{r} 23.2 \\ \times .07 \\ \hline 1.624 \end{array} \qquad \begin{array}{r} 232 \\ \times .07 \\ \hline 16.24 \end{array} \qquad \begin{array}{r} .232 \\ \times .07 \\ \hline .01624 \end{array} \qquad \begin{array}{r} 232 \\ \times .7 \\ \hline 162.4 \end{array}$$

When dividing decimals, the answer will have as many decimal points as the number of decimal points in the dividend (numerator) minus the number of decimal points in the divisor (denominator). Thus:

$$\frac{2.16}{.36} = 6 \qquad\qquad \frac{2.16}{3.6} = .6 \qquad\qquad \frac{2.16}{36} = .06$$

If there are fewer decimal places in the dividend than in the divisor, we must add 0's to right of the decimal point in the dividend. Thus:

$$\frac{21.6}{.36} = \frac{21.60}{.36} = 60. \qquad\qquad \frac{216}{.36} = \frac{216.00}{.36} = 600.$$

ROUNDING

Regardless of how many places we are rounding to, the usual rule is that if the last digit >5, the digit preceding it is raised to the next highest digit. If the last digit <5, it is dropped. When the last digit $=5$, it is treated as >5 if the digit preceding it is an odd number. If the digit preceding the 5 is an even number, we treat the 5 as <5. Thus:

To the nearest thousandth	18.9847 = 18.985
	6.2183 = 6.218
	142.6525 = 142.652
To the nearest hundredth	1.088 = 1.09
	15.464 = 15.46
	11.197 = 11.20
To the nearest tenth	157.75 = 157.8
	44.44 = 44.4
	9.37 = 9.4
To the nearest whole number	37.8 = 39
	452.3 = 452
	68.5 = 68

Understanding the mechanics of rounding still often leaves a large unanswered question, namely, "How do we decide to how many places to round a number?" We may basically consider that an answer should not have more than one digit more than exists in our original untreated data. For example, if we are recording running times for boys in the 100-yard dash to the nearest tenth of a second, we could express the average of these times to the nearest hundredth. Although it is mathematically possible to report the average to five, six, or more decimal places, no further accuracy is gained by doing this. Actually, an attempt to express such an average running time to five or six decimal places would almost seem to be deliberately misleading of the accuracy inherent in the original measurements.

PROPORTIONS AND PERCENTS

A proportion is a given part of a whole expressed as a decimal. This proportion is derived by dividing the number of interest by the total number. For example, if we know that sixteen boys in a class of forty can chin one or more times, the proportion of those who can chin in this class is 16/40, 2/5, or .40. If, in the following class of fifty, eighteen boys can chin one or more times, the proportion is 18/50, 9/25, or .36.

A proportion is transformed into a percent by simply multiplying the proportion by 100. In the first case the percentage of chinners is 40%. In the second case the percentage is 36%.

We may also determine the number in a given category by multiplying the proportion by the total number. For instance, if the proportion of boys who can chin in a third class is .40 and we know there are thirty boys in the class, the number who can chin is 30 (.40) = 12.

Finally, a qualitative statement is in order. Often percentages are reported in order to make a particular point seem more important than it really is. An example might be an advertisement for a new type of bowling aid that "raised bowlers' averages 50% in only 3 weeks of use." It must be noted that if the total number is small, small changes will reflect relatively large percentage changes. Thus the manufacturer may neglect to mention that the bowlers who used the product had no previous bowling experience and started with a bowling average of approximately 50. After 3 weeks the bowlers' averages climbed to 75, which would be expected as a result of learning even without the bowling aid. This is obviously far different than a 50% rise in average for an experienced bowler who begins with an average of 150. Generally, when percentages are reported, the number of cases on which they are based should also be reported.

POSITIVE AND NEGATIVE NUMBERS

Negative numbers can be used to indicate values below some given reference point. Commonly this reference point is zero, as in the case of temperature. However, the reference point may be something like an average. For instance, if the average weight in a class is 150 pounds, a boy who weighs 160 pounds and another who weighs 140 pounds would each be 10 pounds from the average. The first boy's weight might be considered a *deviation* from the average, since it is different than the average. His weight might be scored as $+10$ or 10, with the positive sign being understood, since it is above the average. The second boy's weight is also deviant from the average and might be scored as -10, since it is below the average.

To add numbers, all of which have the same sign, take the sum and attach the common sign. Thus:

$$8+4+12+11+9+13+16=73$$
$$(-9)+(-5)+(-5)+(-12)+(-7)=-38$$

To add two numbers with different signs, take the difference and attach the sign of the larger of the two values. Thus:

$$
\begin{array}{rrrr}
-21 & 21 & 43 & -84 \\
\underline{18} & \underline{-18} & \underline{-27} & \underline{11} \\
-3 & 3 & 16 & -73 \\
\end{array}
$$

To add many numbers with different signs, add the positive numbers, add the negative numbers, and add these two sums according to the rule directly above. Thus:

$$8-4-12-11+9+13-16=30+(-43)=-13$$
$$-11+3+6-8+20-15+12=41+(-34)=7$$

To subtract one number from another, regardless of the signs, change the sign of the subtrahend and add according to the rules above. Thus:

$$
\begin{array}{rrrr}
52 & 52 & -20 & -20 \\
\underline{-12} & \underline{-(-12)} & \underline{-9} & \underline{-(-9)} \\
40 & 64 & -29 & -11 \\
\end{array}
$$

When multiplying, the product of numbers with the same sign has a positive sign. The product of numbers with different signs has a negative sign. Thus:

$$
\begin{array}{rrrr}
9 & 9 & -9 & -9 \\
\underline{\times 3} & \underline{\times -3} & \underline{\times 3} & \underline{\times -3} \\
27 & -27 & -27 & 27 \\
\end{array}
$$

When dividing, if both the dividend and divisor have the same sign, the quotient will be positive. If the dividend and divisor have different signs, the quotient will be negative. Thus:

$$\frac{9}{3}=3 \qquad \frac{9}{-3}=-3 \qquad \frac{-9}{3}=-3 \qquad \frac{-9}{-3}=3$$

ZERO

Adding or subtracting zero to any number, the number is not changed. Thus:

$$123+0=123 \qquad\qquad 123-0=123$$

Multiplying any number by zero equals zero. Thus:

$$31(0)=0 \qquad\qquad (18)(24)(19)(.0238)(0)(41)=0$$

Zero divided by any number equals zero. Thus:

$$\frac{0}{2}=0 \qquad\qquad \frac{0}{43,865}=0$$

A number cannot be divided by zero.

THE ORDER OF OPERATIONS

Usually the order in which operations are to be carried out is indicated by parentheses or brackets. All the terms within parentheses or brackets should be treated as a single value and then the remaining operations should be performed. Thus:

$$(8+7)+9=15+9=24$$
$$(6-3)-(4+8)+(5-2)=3-12+3=-6$$
$$8(4-2)+16=8(2)+16=16+16=32$$
$$[5(8+6)]-4[3(5-2)]=5(14)-4[3(3)]=70-4(9)=70-36=34$$

SQUARES AND SQUARE ROOTS

Tables C-1 and C-2, Appendix C, may be used for finding squares (the value of a number multiplied by itself) and square roots (a number which, when multiplied by itself, gives us our original value). Be sure to check with your instructor if you are unfamiliar with the operation of these tables.

EQUATIONS

In solving equations for an unknown, only one basic rule must be remembered: What is done on one side of the equation must also be done on the other side. This includes addition, subtraction, multiplication, division, squaring, and taking the square root. In the following examples we shall solve for X and illustrate these procedures:

(a) $X-Y=3+Y$
    adding Y to both sides:
    $X-Y+Y=3+Y+Y$
    $\qquad X=3+2Y$

(b) $X + 3 = Y$
subtracting 3 from both sides:
$X + 3 - 3 = Y - 3$
$\quad X = Y - 3$

(c) $\dfrac{X}{Y} = 3$
multiplying both sides by Y:

$$Y\left(\frac{X}{Y}\right) = 3Y$$
$$X = 3Y$$

(d) $3X = Y$
dividing both sides by 3:

$$\frac{3X}{3} = \frac{Y}{3}$$

$$X = \frac{Y}{3}$$

(e) $\sqrt{X} = 3Y$
squaring both sides:
$$(\sqrt{X})^2 = (3Y)^2$$
$$X = 9Y^2$$

(f) $X^2 = 3Y$
taking the square root of both sides:
$$\sqrt{X^2} = \sqrt{3Y}$$
$$X = \sqrt{3Y}$$

In the following we will see how a series of such steps can be taken in solving an equation.

$$\sqrt{\frac{3XY - Z}{4}} = 8$$

squaring both sides:

$$\left(\sqrt{\frac{3XY - Z}{4}}\right)^2 = 8^2$$

$$\frac{3XY - Z}{4} = 64$$

multiplying both sides by 4:

$$4\left(\frac{3XY - Z}{4}\right) = 64(4)$$

$$3XY - Z = 256$$
adding Z to both sides:
$$3XY - Z + Z = 256 + Z$$
$$3XY = 256 + Z$$
dividing both sides by $3Y$:

$$\frac{3XY}{3Y} = \frac{256 + Z}{3Y}$$

$$X = \frac{256 + Z}{3Y}$$

Examples

1. Read each of the following aloud:

   (a) $3+4=8-1$
   (b) $18-3>27-15$
   (c) $24+6-X-Y$
   (d) $\sqrt{100}=22+(10-4)$
   (e) $120/6<16+5$

   (f) $\Sigma X = X_1 + X_2 + \cdots X_n$
   (g) $Y<X+B$
   (h) $2(5)=\sqrt{144}-2$
   (i) $2[3(4-1)]>4^2$
   (j) $XY=(\sqrt{X})^2\,(\sqrt{Y})^2$

2. Perform the following operations:

   (a) $2/8+1/8$
   (b) $3/7+4/5$
   (c) $4/7+3/a$
   (d) $5/6-2/3$
   (e) $6/11+3/8$
   (f) $4/5+3/5+5/7$
   (g) $1/3 \times 1/3$
   (h) $1/3 \times 3/1$
   (i) $1/3 \times 4/5$
   (j) $5/6 \div 3/4$

   (k) $8/10 \div 1/2$
   (l) $8/10 - 1/2$
   (m) $16/23 \div 2/3$
   (n) $5/8 \times 4\ 1/2$
   (o) $7/11-8/15$
   (p) $4/9 \div 4/7$
   (q) $9/13-2/11$
   (r) $16/18 \div 8/9$
   (s) $14/16-7/8$
   (t) $12/13 \times 9/16$

3. Perform the following operations:

   (a) $1.38 \times .04$
   (b) $16.3 \div 1.40$
   (c) $9.6 \times .468$
   (d) $113 \div .045$
   (e) $18 \times .086$

   (f) $137.2/13.72$
   (g) $(11.21)(11.21)$
   (h) $4.60/23$
   (i) $(.4052)(13.5)$
   (j) $9.100/13$

4. Round the following numbers:

   (a) 18.0462
   (b) 9.31
   (c) 185.786
   (d) 73.4
   (e) 85.625

   (f) 96.214
   (g) 9.6215
   (h) 87.1
   (i) 89.9
   (j) 412.63

5. Add the following:

   (a) $\begin{array}{r} 8 \\ -3 \\ \hline \end{array}$
   (e) $\begin{array}{r} 47 \\ -15 \\ \hline \end{array}$
   (i) $\begin{array}{r} -71 \\ -50 \\ \hline \end{array}$

   (b) $\begin{array}{r} -19 \\ 13 \\ \hline \end{array}$
   (f) $\begin{array}{r} -8 \\ -5 \\ \hline \end{array}$
   (j) $\begin{array}{r} 50 \\ 50 \\ \hline \end{array}$

   (c) $\begin{array}{r} 61 \\ -40 \\ \hline \end{array}$
   (g) $\begin{array}{r} -18 \\ 11 \\ \hline \end{array}$

   (d) $\begin{array}{r} -52 \\ -18 \\ \hline \end{array}$
   (h) $\begin{array}{r} 36 \\ -9 \\ \hline \end{array}$

6. Subtract each of the following:

(a) $\begin{array}{r} -16 \\ -12 \\ \hline \end{array}$ (e) $\begin{array}{r} -9 \\ -4 \\ \hline \end{array}$ (i) $\begin{array}{r} 65 \\ -(-9) \\ \hline \end{array}$

(b) $\begin{array}{r} 0 \\ -5 \\ \hline \end{array}$ (f) $\begin{array}{r} 16 \\ -(-8) \\ \hline \end{array}$ (j) $\begin{array}{r} -46 \\ -23 \\ \hline \end{array}$

(c) $\begin{array}{r} -41 \\ -(-20) \\ \hline \end{array}$ (g) $\begin{array}{r} -16 \\ -5 \\ \hline \end{array}$

(d) $\begin{array}{r} -11 \\ -(-8) \\ \hline \end{array}$ (h) $\begin{array}{r} 33 \\ -16 \\ \hline \end{array}$

7. Perform the following operations:

(a) (3)(6)   (f) $-22/11$
(b) (3)(-6)   (g) $63/-9$
(c) (-18)(4)   (h) $46/23$
(d) (-23)(-9)   (i) $-85/-17$
(e) (-5)(2)   (j) $-213/71$

8. Find the following using the appropriate tables:

(a) $\sqrt{21}$ (f) 66^2
(b) 7.3^2 (g) $\sqrt{490}$
(c) $\sqrt{293}$ (h) 37.3^2
(d) 6.05^2 (i) $\sqrt{14.4}$
(e) $\sqrt{2.864}$ (j) 8.21^2

9. Solve the following:

(a) $(9+3)+6=$ (f) $(4)(3)-[3(6-1)]=$
(b) $3(9)+4(5)=$ (g) $[4(6/3)-(4)(2)]^2=$
(c) $8(3+6)=$ (h) $(3)(-4)=$
(d) $8(4-2)+3^2=$ (i) $5[4(3+5)]^2=$
(e) $4[3(6-2)+(3+2)]=$ (j) $(8-6)(4-2)^2[2(4-3)]=$

10. Solve for X in the following equations:

(a) $3X=9$ (f) $X-4=Y+3$
(b) $X^2=Y+8$ (g) $XY=75Y$
(c) $\sqrt{X+Y}=5$ (h) $(X+3)^2=Y+6X$
(d) $\dfrac{4X+Y}{5}=6$ (i) $\sqrt{X}=Y$
                              (j) $\dfrac{X}{Y}=3$
(e) $X-Y=16$

Appendix C

Tables

Table C-1. Squares*

	0	1	2	3	4	5	6	7	8	9
0	0	1	4	9	16	25	36	49	64	81
1	100	121	144	169	196	225	256	289	324	361
2	400	441	484	529	576	625	676	729	784	841
3	900	961	1024	1089	1156	1225	1296	1369	1444	1521
4	1600	1681	1764	1849	1936	2025	2116	2209	2304	2401
5	2500	2601	2704	2809	2916	3025	3136	3249	3364	3481
6	3600	3721	3844	3969	4096	4225	4356	4489	4624	4761
7	4900	5041	5184	5329	5476	5625	5776	5929	6084	6241
8	6400	6561	6724	6889	7056	7225	7396	7569	7744	7921
9	8100	8281	8464	8649	8836	9025	9216	9409	9604	9801
10	10000	10201	10404	10609	10816	11025	11236	11449	11664	11881
11	12100	12321	12544	12769	12996	13225	13456	13689	13924	14161
12	14400	14641	14884	15129	15376	15625	15876	16129	16384	16641
13	16900	17161	17424	17689	17956	18225	18496	18769	19044	19321
14	19600	19881	20164	20449	20736	21025	21316	21609	21904	22201
15	22500	22801	23104	23409	23716	24025	24336	24649	24964	25281
16	25600	25921	26244	26569	26896	27225	27556	27889	28224	28561
17	28900	29241	29584	29929	30276	30625	30976	31329	31684	32041
18	32400	32761	33124	33489	33856	34225	34596	34969	35344	35721
19	36100	36481	36864	37249	37636	38025	38416	38809	39204	39601
20	40000	40401	40804	41209	41616	42025	42436	42849	43264	43681
21	44100	44521	44944	45369	45796	46225	46656	47089	47524	47961
22	48400	48841	49284	49729	50176	50625	51076	51529	51984	52441
23	52900	53361	53824	54289	54756	55225	55696	56169	56644	57121
24	57600	58081	58564	59049	59536	60025	60516	61009	61504	62001
25	62500	63001	63504	64009	64516	65025	65536	66049	66564	67081
26	67600	68121	68644	69169	69696	70225	70756	71289	71824	72361

n	0	1	2	3	4	5	6	7	8	9
27	72900	73441	73984	74529	75076	75625	76176	76729	77284	77841
28	78400	78961	79524	80089	80656	81225	81796	82369	82944	83521
29	84100	84681	85264	85849	86436	87025	87616	88209	88804	89401
30	90000	90601	91204	91809	92416	93025	93636	94249	94864	95481
31	96100	96721	97344	97969	98596	99225	99856	100489	101124	101761
32	102400	103041	103684	104329	104976	105625	106276	106929	107584	108241
33	108900	109561	110224	110889	111556	112225	112896	113569	114244	114921
34	115600	116281	116964	117649	118336	119025	119716	120409	121104	121801
35	122500	123201	123904	124609	125316	126025	126736	127449	128164	128881
36	129600	130321	131044	131769	132496	133225	133956	134689	135424	136161
37	136900	137641	138384	139129	139876	140625	141376	142129	142884	143641
38	144400	145161	145924	146689	147456	148225	148996	149769	150544	151321
39	152100	152881	153664	154449	155236	156025	156816	157609	158404	159201
40	160000	160801	161604	162409	163216	164025	164836	165649	166464	167281
41	168100	168921	169744	170569	171396	172225	173056	173889	174724	175561
42	176400	177241	178084	178929	179776	180625	181476	182329	183184	184041
43	184900	185761	186624	187489	188356	189225	190096	190969	191844	192721
44	193600	194481	195364	196249	197136	198025	198916	199809	200704	201601
45	202500	203401	204304	205209	206116	207025	207936	208849	209764	210681
46	211600	212521	213444	214369	215296	216225	217156	218089	219024	219961
47	220900	221841	222784	223729	224676	225625	226576	227529	228484	229441
48	230400	231361	232324	233289	234256	235225	236196	237169	238144	239121
49	240100	241081	242064	243049	244036	245025	246016	247009	248004	249001
50	250000	251001	252004	253009	254016	255025	256036	257049	258064	259081
51	260100	261121	262144	263169	264196	265225	266256	267289	268324	269361
52	270400	271441	272484	273529	274576	275625	276676	277729	278784	279841
53	280900	281961	283024	284089	285156	286225	287296	288369	289444	290521
54	291600	292681	293764	294849	295936	297025	298116	299209	300304	301401

*From Fisher, Sir Ronald A., and Yates, Frank: Statistical tables for biological, agricultural, and medical research, ed. 6, Edinburgh, 1963, Oliver & Boyd Ltd.; by permission of the authors and publishers.

Continued.

Table C-1. Squares—cont'd

	0	1	2	3	4	5	6	7	8	9
55	302500	303601	304704	305809	306916	308025	309136	310249	311364	312481
56	313600	314721	315844	316969	318096	319225	320356	321489	322624	323761
57	324900	326041	327184	328329	329476	330625	331776	332929	334084	335241
58	336400	337561	338724	339889	341056	342225	343396	344569	345744	346921
59	348100	349281	350464	351649	352836	354025	355216	356409	357604	358801
60	360000	361201	362404	363609	364816	366025	367236	368449	369664	370881
61	372100	373321	374544	375769	376996	378225	379456	380689	381924	383161
62	384400	385641	386884	388129	389376	390625	391876	393129	394384	395641
63	396900	398161	399424	400689	401956	403225	404496	405769	407044	408321
64	409600	410881	412164	413449	414736	416025	417316	418609	419904	421201
65	422500	423801	425104	426409	427716	429025	430336	431649	432964	434281
66	435600	436921	438244	439569	440896	442225	443556	444889	446224	447561
67	448900	450241	451584	452929	454276	455625	456976	458329	459684	461041
68	462400	463761	465124	466489	467856	469225	470596	471969	473344	474721
69	476100	477481	478864	480249	481636	483025	484416	485809	487204	488601
70	490000	491401	492804	494209	495616	497025	498436	499849	501264	502681
71	504100	505521	506944	508369	509796	511225	512656	514089	515524	516961
72	518400	519841	521284	522729	524176	525625	527076	528529	529984	531441
73	532900	534361	535824	537289	538756	540225	541696	543169	544644	546121
74	547600	549081	550564	552049	553536	555025	556516	558009	559504	561001

	0	1	2	3	4	5	6	7	8	9
75	562500	564001	565504	567009	568516	570025	571536	573049	574564	576081
76	577600	579121	580644	582169	583696	585225	586756	588289	589824	591361
77	592900	594441	595984	597529	599076	600625	602176	603729	605284	606841
78	608400	609961	611524	613089	614656	616225	617796	619369	620944	622521
79	624100	625681	627264	628849	630436	632025	633616	635209	636804	638401
80	640000	641601	643204	644809	646416	648025	649636	651249	652864	654481
81	656100	657721	659344	660969	662596	664225	665856	667489	669124	670761
82	672400	674041	675684	677329	678976	680625	682276	683929	685584	687241
83	688900	690561	692224	693889	695556	697225	698896	700569	702244	703921
84	705600	707281	708964	710649	712336	714025	715716	717409	719104	720801
85	722500	724201	725904	727609	729316	731025	732736	734449	736164	737881
86	739600	741321	743044	744769	746496	748225	749956	751689	753424	755161
87	756900	758641	760384	762129	763876	765625	767376	769129	770884	772641
88	774400	776161	777924	779689	781456	783225	784996	786769	788544	790321
89	792100	793881	795664	797449	799236	801025	802816	804609	806404	808201
90	810000	811801	813604	815409	817216	819025	820836	822649	824464	826281
91	828100	829921	831744	833569	835396	837225	839056	840889	842724	844561
92	846400	848241	850084	851929	853776	855625	857476	859329	861184	863041
93	864900	866761	868624	870489	872356	874225	876096	877969	879844	881721
94	883600	885481	887364	889249	891136	893025	894916	896809	898704	900601
95	902500	904401	906304	908209	910116	912025	913936	915849	917764	919681
96	921600	923521	925444	927369	929296	931225	933156	935089	937024	938961
97	940900	942841	944784	946729	948676	950625	952576	954529	956484	958441
98	960400	962361	964324	966289	968256	970225	972196	974169	976144	978121
99	980100	982081	984064	986049	988036	990025	992016	994009	996004	998001

Table C-2. Square roots*

	0	1	2	3	4	5	6	7	8	9	1	2	3	4	5
10	10000	10050	10100	10149	10198	10247	10296	10344	10392	10440	5	10	15	20	24
	31623	31780	31937	32094	32249	32404	32558	32711	32863	33015	15	31	46	62	77
11	10488	10536	10583	10630	10677	10724	10770	10817	10863	10909	5	9	14	19	23
	33166	33317	33466	33615	33764	33912	34059	34205	34351	34496	15	30	44	59	74
12	10954	11000	11045	11091	11136	11180	11225	11269	11314	11358	4	9	13	18	22
	34641	34785	34928	35071	35214	35355	35496	35637	35777	35917	14	28	43	57	71
13	11402	11446	11489	11533	11576	11619	11662	11705	11747	11790	4	9	13	17	22
	36056	36194	36332	36469	36606	36742	36878	37014	37148	37283	14	27	41	55	68
14	11832	11874	11916	11958	12000	12042	12083	12124	12166	12207	4	8	13	17	21
	37417	37550	37683	37815	37947	38079	38210	38341	38471	38601	13	26	39	53	66
15	12247	12288	12329	12369	12410	12450	12490	12530	12570	12610	4	8	12	16	20
	38730	38859	38987	39115	39243	39370	39497	39623	39749	39875	13	25	38	51	64
16	12649	12689	12728	12767	12806	12845	12884	12923	12961	13000	4	8	12	16	20
	40000	40125	40249	40373	40497	40620	40743	40866	40988	41110	12	25	37	49	62
17	13038	13077	13115	13153	13191	13229	13266	13304	13342	13379	4	8	11	15	19
	41231	41352	41473	41593	41713	41833	41952	42071	42190	42308	12	24	36	48	60
18	13416	13454	13491	13528	13565	13601	13638	13675	13711	13748	4	7	11	15	18
	42426	42544	42661	42778	42895	43012	43128	43243	43359	43474	12	23	35	47	58
19	13784	13820	13856	13892	13928	13964	14000	14036	14071	14107	4	7	11	14	18
	43589	43704	43818	43932	44045	44159	44272	44385	44497	44609	11	23	34	45	57
20	14142	14177	14213	14248	14283	14318	14353	14387	14422	14457	4	7	10	14	18
	44721	44833	44944	45056	45166	45277	45387	45497	45607	45717	11	22	33	44	55
21	14491	14526	14560	14595	14629	14663	14697	14731	14765	14799	3	7	10	14	17
	45826	45935	46043	46152	46260	46368	46476	46583	46690	46797	11	22	32	43	54
22	14832	14866	14900	14933	14967	15000	15033	15067	15100	15133	3	7	10	13	17
	46904	47011	47117	47223	47329	47434	47539	47645	47749	47854	11	21	32	42	53
23	15166	15199	15232	15264	15297	15330	15362	15395	15427	15460	3	7	10	13	16
	47958	48062	48166	48270	48374	48477	48580	48683	48785	48888	10	21	31	41	52

Main tabulated values (each argument has two lines):

Arg										
24	15492	15524	15556	15588	15620	15652	15684	15716	15748	15780
	48990	49092	49193	49295	49396	49497	49598	49699	49800	49900
25	15811	15843	15875	15906	15937	15969	16000	16031	16062	16093
	50000	50100	50200	50299	50398	50498	50596	50695	50794	50892
26	16125	16155	16186	16217	16248	16279	16310	16340	16371	16401
	50990	51088	51186	51284	51381	51478	51575	51672	51769	51865
27	16432	16462	16492	16523	16553	16583	16613	16643	16673	16703
	51962	52058	52154	52249	52345	52440	52536	52631	52726	52820
28	16733	16763	16793	16823	16852	16882	16912	16941	16971	17000
	52915	53009	53104	53198	53292	53385	53479	53572	53666	53759
29	17029	17059	17088	17117	17146	17176	17205	17234	17263	17292
	53852	53944	54037	54129	54222	54314	54406	54498	54589	54681
30	17321	17349	17378	17407	17436	17464	17493	17521	17550	17578
	54772	54863	54955	55045	55136	55227	55317	55408	55498	55588
31	17607	17635	17664	17692	17720	17748	17776	17804	17833	17861
	55678	55767	55857	55946	56036	56125	56214	56303	56391	56480
32	17889	17916	17944	17972	18000	18028	18055	18083	18111	18138
	56569	56657	56745	56833	56921	57009	57096	57184	57271	57359
33	18166	18193	18221	18248	18276	18303	18330	18358	18385	18412
	57446	57533	57619	57706	57793	57879	57966	58052	58138	58224
34	18439	18466	18493	18520	18547	18574	18601	18628	18655	18682
	58310	58395	58481	58556	58652	58737	58822	58907	58992	59076
35	18708	18735	18762	18788	18815	18841	18868	18894	18921	18947
	59161	59245	59330	59414	59498	59582	59666	59749	59833	59917
36	18974	19000	19026	19053	19079	19105	19131	19157	19183	19209
	60000	60083	60166	60249	60332	60415	60498	60581	60663	60745
37	19235	19261	19287	19313	19339	19365	19391	19416	19442	19468
	60828	60910	60992	61074	61156	61237	61319	61400	61482	61563
38	19494	19519	19545	19570	19596	19621	19647	19672	19698	19723
	61644	61725	61806	61887	61968	62048	62129	62210	62290	62370

Proportional parts (upper value for the first function, lower value for the second function):

Arg					
24	16 / 51	13 / 40	10 / 30	6 / 20	3 / 10
25	16 / 50	13 / 40	9 / 30	6 / 20	3 / 10
26	15 / 49	12 / 39	9 / 29	6 / 19	3 / 10
27	15 / 48	12 / 38	9 / 29	6 / 19	3 / 10
28	15 / 47	12 / 38	9 / 28	6 / 19	3 / 9
29	15 / 46	12 / 37	9 / 28	6 / 18	3 / 9
30	14 / 45	11 / 36	9 / 27	6 / 18	3 / 9
31	14 / 45	11 / 36	8 / 27	6 / 18	3 / 9
32	14 / 44	11 / 35	8 / 26	6 / 18	3 / 9
33	14 / 43	11 / 35	8 / 26	5 / 17	3 / 9
34	14 / 43	11 / 34	8 / 26	5 / 17	3 / 9
35	13 / 42	11 / 34	8 / 25	5 / 17	3 / 8
36	13 / 41	10 / 33	8 / 25	5 / 17	3 / 8
37	13 / 41	10 / 33	8 / 25	5 / 16	3 / 8
38	13 / 40	10 / 32	8 / 24	5 / 16	3 / 8

Continued.

Table C-2. Square roots—cont'd

	0	1	2	3	4	5	6	7	8	9	1	2	3	4	5
39	19748	19774	19799	19824	19849	19875	19900	19925	19950	19975	3	5	8	10	13
	62450	62530	62610	62690	62769	62849	62929	62008	63087	63166	8	16	24	32	40
40	20000	20025	20050	20075	20100	20125	20149	20174	20199	20224	2	5	7	10	12
	63246	63325	63403	63482	63561	63640	63718	63797	63875	63953	8	16	24	31	39
41	20248	20273	20298	20322	20347	20372	20396	20421	20445	20469	2	5	7	10	12
	64031	64109	64187	64265	64343	64420	64498	64576	64653	64730	8	16	23	31	39
42	20494	20518	20543	20567	20591	20616	20640	20664	20688	20712	2	5	7	10	12
	64807	64885	64962	65038	65115	65192	65269	65345	65422	65498	8	15	23	31	38
43	20736	20761	20785	20809	20833	20857	20881	20905	20928	20952	2	5	7	10	12
	65574	65651	65727	65803	65879	65955	66030	66106	66182	66257	8	15	23	30	38
44	20976	21000	21024	21048	21071	21095	21119	21142	21166	21190	2	5	7	10	12
	66332	66408	66483	66558	66633	66708	66783	66858	66933	67007	8	15	22	30	38
45	21213	21237	21260	21284	21307	21331	21354	21378	21401	21424	2	5	7	9	12
	67082	67157	67231	67305	67380	67454	67528	67602	67676	67750	7	15	22	30	37
46	21448	21471	21494	21517	21541	21564	21587	21610	21633	21656	2	5	7	9	12
	67823	67897	67971	68044	68118	68191	68264	68337	68411	68484	7	15	22	29	37
47	21679	21703	21726	21749	21772	21794	21817	21840	21863	21886	2	5	7	9	12
	68557	68629	68702	68775	68848	68920	68993	69065	69138	69210	7	15	22	29	36
48	21909	21932	21954	21977	22000	22023	22045	22068	22091	22113	2	5	7	9	11
	69282	69354	69426	96498	69570	69642	69714	69785	69857	69929	7	14	22	29	36
49	22136	22159	22181	22204	22226	22249	22271	22293	22316	22338	2	4	7	9	11
	70000	70071	70143	70214	70285	70356	70427	70498	70569	70640	7	14	21	28	36
50	22361	22383	22405	22428	22450	22472	22494	22517	22539	22561	2	4	7	9	11
	70711	70781	70852	70922	70993	71063	71134	71204	71274	71344	7	14	21	28	35
51	22583	22605	22627	22650	22672	22694	22716	22738	22760	22782	2	4	7	9	11
	71414	71484	71554	71624	71694	71764	71833	71903	71972	72042	7	14	21	28	35
52	22804	22825	22847	22869	22891	22913	22935	22956	22978	23000	2	4	7	9	11
	72111	72180	72250	72319	72388	72457	72526	72595	72664	72732	7	14	21	28	34

No.	0	1	2	3	4	5	6	7	8	9					
53	23022	23043	23065	23087	23108	23130	23152	23173	23195	23216	2	4	6	9	11
	72801	72870	72938	73007	73075	73144	73212	73280	73348	73417	7	14	21	27	34
54	23238	23259	23281	23302	23324	23345	23367	23388	23409	23431	2	4	6	9	11
	73485	73553	73621	73689	73756	73824	73892	73959	74027	74095	7	14	20	27	34
55	23452	23473	23495	23516	23537	23558	23580	23601	23622	23643	2	4	6	8	11
	74162	74229	74297	74364	74431	74498	74565	74632	74699	74766	7	13	20	27	34
56	23664	23685	23707	23728	23749	23770	23791	23812	23833	23854	2	4	6	8	11
	74833	74900	74967	75033	75100	75166	75233	75299	75366	75432	7	13	20	27	33
57	23875	23896	23917	23937	23958	23979	24000	24021	24042	24062	2	4	6	8	10
	75408	75565	75565	75631	75697	75763	75829	75895	75961	76026	7	13	20	26	33
58	24083	24104	24125	24145	24166	24187	24207	24228	24249	24269	2	4	6	8	10
	76158	76223	76289	76354	76420	76485	76551	76616	76681	76746	7	13	20	26	33
59	24290	24310	24331	24352	24372	24393	24413	24434	24454	24474	2	4	6	8	10
	76811	76877	76942	77006	77071	77136	77201	77266	77330	77395	6	13	19	26	32
60	24495	24515	24536	24556	24576	24597	24617	24637	24658	24678	2	4	6	8	10
	77460	77524	77589	77653	77717	77782	77846	77910	77974	78038	6	13	19	26	32
61	24698	24718	24739	24759	24779	24799	24819	24839	24860	24880	2	4	6	8	10
	78102	78166	78230	78294	78358	78422	78486	78549	78613	78677	6	13	19	26	32
62	24900	24920	24940	24960	24980	25000	25020	25040	25060	25080	2	4	6	8	10
	78740	78804	78867	78930	78994	79057	79120	79183	79246	79310	6	13	19	25	32
63	25100	25120	25140	25159	25179	25199	25219	25239	25259	25278	2	4	6	8	10
	79373	79436	79498	79561	79624	79687	79750	79812	79875	79937	6	13	19	25	31
64	25298	25318	25338	25357	25377	25397	25417	25436	25456	25475	2	4	6	8	10
	80000	80062	80125	80187	80250	80312	80374	80436	80498	80561	6	12	19	25	31
65	25495	25515	25534	25554	25573	25593	25612	25632	25652	25671	2	4	6	8	10
	80623	80685	80747	80808	80870	80932	80994	81056	81117	81179	6	12	19	25	31
66	25690	25710	25729	25749	25768	25788	25807	25826	25846	25865	2	4	6	8	10
	81240	81302	81363	81425	81486	81548	81609	81670	81731	81792	6	12	28	25	31
67	25884	25904	25923	25942	25962	25981	26000	26019	26038	26058	2	4	6	8	10
	81854	81915	81976	82037	82098	82158	82219	82280	82341	82401	6	12	18	24	30
68	26077	26096	26115	26134	26153	26173	26192	26211	26230	26249	2	4	6	8	10
	82462	82523	82583	82644	82704	82765	82825	82885	82946	83006	6	12	18	24	30

Continued.

Table C-2. Square roots—cont'd

	0	1	2	3	4	5	6	7	8	9	1	2	3	4	5
69	26268 83066	26287 83126	26306 83187	26325 83247	26344 83307	26363 83367	26382 83427	26401 83487	26420 83546	26439 83606	2 6	4 12	6 18	8 24	10 30
70	26458 83666	26476 83726	26495 83785	26514 83845	26533 83905	26552 83964	26571 84024	26589 84083	26608 84143	26627 84202	2 6	4 12	6 18	8 24	9 30
71	26646 84261	26665 84321	26683 84380	26702 84439	26721 84499	26739 84558	26758 84617	26777 84676	26796 84735	26814 84794	2 6	4 12	6 18	7 24	9 30
72	26833 84853	26851 84912	26870 84971	26889 85029	26907 85088	26926 85147	26944 85206	26963 85264	26981 85323	27000 85381	2 6	4 12	6 18	7 23	9 29
73	27019 85440	27037 85499	27055 85557	27074 85615	27092 85674	27111 85732	27129 85790	27148 85849	27166 85907	27185 85965	2 6	4 12	6 17	7 23	9 29
74	27203 86023	27221 86081	27240 86139	27258 86197	27276 86255	27295 86313	27313 86371	27331 86429	27350 86487	27368 86545	2 6	4 12	5 17	7 23	9 29
75	27386 86603	27404 86660	27423 86718	27441 86776	27459 86833	27477 86891	27495 86948	27514 87006	27532 87063	27550 87121	2 6	4 12	5 17	7 23	9 29
76	27568 87178	27586 87235	27604 87293	27622 87350	27641 87407	27659 87464	27677 87521	27695 87579	27713 87636	27731 87693	2 6	4 11	5 17	7 23	9 29
77	27749 87750	27767 87807	27785 87864	27803 87920	27821 87977	27839 88034	27857 88091	27875 88148	27893 88204	27911 88261	2 6	4 11	5 17	7 23	9 28
78	27928 88318	27946 88374	27964 88431	27982 88487	28000 88544	28018 88600	28036 88657	28054 88713	28071 88769	28089 88826	2 6	4 11	5 17	7 23	9 28
79	28107 88882	28125 88938	28142 88994	28160 89051	28178 89107	28196 89163	28213 89219	28231 89275	28249 89331	28267 89387	2 6	4 11	5 17	7 22	9 28
80	28284 89443	28302 89499	28320 89554	28337 89610	28355 89666	28373 89722	28390 89778	28408 89833	28425 89889	28443 89944	2 6	4 11	5 17	7 22	9 28
81	28460 90000	28478 90056	28496 90111	28513 90167	28531 90222	28548 90277	28566 90333	28583 90388	28601 90443	28618 90499	2 6	4 11	5 17	7 22	9 28
82	28636 90554	28653 90609	28671 90664	28688 90719	28705 90774	28723 90830	28740 90885	28758 90940	28775 90995	28792 91049	2 6	3 11	5 16	7 22	9 28

N	0	1	2	3	4	5	6	7	8	9			PP		
83	28810	28827	28844	28862	28879	28896	28914	28931	28948	28965	2	3	5	7	9
	91104	91159	91214	91269	91324	91378	91433	91488	91542	91597	5	11	16	22	27
84	28983	29000	29017	29034	29052	29069	29086	29103	29120	29138	2	3	5	7	9
	91652	91706	91761	91815	91869	91924	91978	92033	92087	92141	5	11	16	22	27
85	29155	29172	29189	29206	29223	29240	29257	29275	29292	29309	2	3	5	7	9
	92195	92250	92304	92358	92412	92466	92520	92574	92628	92682	5	11	16	22	27
86	29326	29343	29360	29377	29394	29411	29428	29445	29462	29479	2	3	5	7	8
	92736	92790	92844	92898	92952	93005	93059	93113	93167	93220	5	11	16	22	27
87	29496	29513	29530	29547	29563	29580	29597	29614	29631	29648	2	3	5	7	8
	93274	93327	93381	93434	93488	93541	93595	93648	93702	93755	5	11	16	21	27
88	29665	29682	29698	29715	29732	29749	29766	29783	29799	29816	2	3	5	7	8
	93808	93862	93915	93968	94021	94074	94128	94181	94234	94287	5	11	16	21	27
89	29833	29850	29866	29883	29900	29917	29933	29950	29967	29983	2	3	5	7	8
	94340	94393	94446	94499	94552	94604	94657	94710	94763	94816	5	11	16	21	26
90	30000	30017	30033	30050	30067	30083	30100	30116	30133	30150	2	3	5	7	8
	94868	94921	94974	95026	95079	95131	95184	95237	95289	95341	5	11	16	21	26
91	30166	30183	30199	30216	30232	30249	30265	30282	30299	30315	2	3	5	7	8
	95394	95446	95499	95551	95603	95656	95708	95760	95812	95864	5	10	16	21	26
92	30332	30348	30364	30381	30397	30414	30430	30447	30463	30480	2	3	5	7	8
	95917	95969	96021	96073	96125	96177	96229	96281	96333	96385	5	10	16	21	26
93	30496	30512	30529	30545	30561	30578	30594	30610	30627	30643	2	3	5	7	8
	96437	96488	96540	96592	96644	96695	96747	96799	96850	96902	5	10	16	21	26
94	30659	30676	30692	30708	30725	30741	30757	30773	30790	30806	2	3	5	7	8
	96954	97005	97057	97108	97160	97211	97263	97314	97365	97417	5	10	15	21	26
95	30822	30838	30854	30871	30887	30903	30919	30935	30952	30968	2	3	5	6	8
	97468	97519	97570	97622	97673	97724	97775	97826	97877	97929	5	10	15	21	26
96	30984	31000	31016	31032	31048	31064	31081	31097	31113	31129	2	3	5	6	8
	97980	98031	98082	98133	98184	98234	98285	98336	98387	98438	5	10	15	20	26
97	31145	31161	31177	31193	31209	31225	31241	31257	31273	31289	2	3	5	6	8
	98489	98539	98590	98641	98691	98742	98793	98843	98894	98944	5	10	15	20	25
98	31305	31321	31337	31353	31369	31385	31401	31417	31432	31448	2	3	5	6	8
	99045	99096	99146	99197	99247	99298	99348	99398	99448	99499	5	10	15	20	25
99	31464	31480	31496	31512	31528	31544	31559	31575	31591	31607	2	3	5	6	8
	99499	99549	99599	99649	99700	99750	99800	99850	99900	99950	5	10	15	20	25

Table C-3. Random numbers*

03	47	43	73	86	36	96	47	36	61	46	98	63	71	62	33	26	16	80	45	60	11	14	10	95
97	74	24	67	62	42	81	14	57	20	42	53	32	37	32	27	07	36	07	51	24	51	79	89	73
16	76	62	27	66	56	50	26	71	07	32	90	79	78	53	13	55	38	58	59	88	97	54	14	10
12	56	85	99	26	96	96	68	27	31	05	03	72	93	15	57	12	10	14	21	88	26	49	81	76
55	59	56	35	64	38	54	82	46	22	31	62	43	09	90	06	18	44	32	53	23	83	01	30	30
16	22	77	94	39	49	54	43	54	82	17	37	93	23	78	87	35	20	96	43	84	26	34	91	64
84	42	17	53	31	57	24	55	06	88	77	04	74	47	67	21	76	33	50	25	83	92	12	06	76
63	01	63	78	59	16	95	55	67	19	98	10	50	71	75	12	86	73	58	07	44	39	52	38	79
33	21	12	34	29	78	64	56	07	82	52	42	07	44	38	15	51	00	13	42	99	66	02	79	54
57	60	86	32	44	09	47	27	96	54	49	17	46	09	62	90	52	84	77	27	08	02	73	43	28
18	18	07	92	46	44	17	16	58	09	79	83	86	19	62	06	76	50	03	10	55	23	64	05	05
26	62	38	97	75	84	16	07	44	99	83	11	46	32	24	20	14	85	88	45	10	93	72	88	71
23	42	40	64	74	82	97	77	77	81	07	45	32	14	08	32	98	94	07	72	93	85	79	10	75
52	36	28	19	95	50	92	26	11	97	00	56	76	31	38	80	22	02	53	53	86	60	42	04	53
37	85	94	35	12	83	39	50	08	30	42	34	07	96	88	54	42	06	87	98	35	85	29	48	39
70	29	17	12	13	40	33	20	38	26	13	89	51	03	74	17	76	37	13	04	07	74	21	19	30
56	62	18	37	35	96	83	50	87	75	97	12	25	93	47	70	33	24	03	54	97	77	46	44	80
99	49	57	22	77	88	42	95	45	72	16	64	36	16	00	04	43	18	66	79	94	77	24	21	90
16	08	15	04	72	33	27	14	34	09	45	59	34	68	49	12	72	07	34	45	99	27	72	95	14
31	16	93	32	43	50	27	89	87	19	20	15	37	00	49	52	85	66	60	44	38	68	88	11	80
68	34	30	13	70	55	74	30	77	40	44	22	78	84	26	04	33	46	09	52	68	07	97	06	57
74	57	25	65	76	59	29	97	68	60	71	91	38	67	54	13	58	18	24	76	15	54	55	95	52
27	42	37	86	53	48	55	90	65	72	96	57	69	36	10	96	46	92	42	45	97	60	49	04	91
00	39	68	29	61	66	37	32	20	30	77	84	57	03	29	10	45	65	04	26	11	04	96	67	24
29	94	98	94	24	68	49	69	10	82	53	75	91	93	30	34	25	20	57	27	40	48	73	51	92
16	90	82	66	59	83	62	64	11	12	67	19	00	71	74	60	47	21	29	68	02	02	37	03	31
11	27	94	75	06	06	09	19	74	66	02	94	37	34	02	76	70	90	30	86	38	45	94	30	38
35	24	10	16	20	33	32	51	26	38	79	78	45	04	91	16	92	53	56	16	02	75	50	95	98
38	23	16	86	38	42	38	97	01	50	87	75	66	81	41	40	01	74	91	62	48	51	84	08	32
31	96	25	91	47	96	44	33	49	13	34	86	82	53	91	00	52	43	48	85	27	55	26	89	62

66	67	40	67	14	64	05	71	95	86	11	05	65	09	68	76	83	20	37	90	57	16	00	11	66
14	90	84	45	11	75	73	88	05	90	52	27	41	14	86	22	98	12	22	08	07	52	74	95	80
68	05	51	18	00	33	96	02	75	19	07	60	62	93	55	59	33	82	43	90	49	37	38	44	59
20	46	78	73	90	97	51	40	14	02	04	02	33	31	08	39	54	16	49	36	47	95	93	13	30
64	19	58	97	79	15	06	15	93	20	01	90	10	75	06	40	78	78	89	62	02	67	74	17	33
05	26	93	70	60	22	35	85	15	13	92	03	51	59	77	59	56	78	06	83	52	91	05	70	74
07	97	10	88	23	09	98	42	99	64	61	71	62	99	15	06	51	29	16	93	58	05	77	09	51
68	71	86	85	85	54	87	66	47	54	73	32	08	11	12	44	95	92	63	16	29	56	24	29	48
26	99	61	65	53	58	37	78	80	70	42	10	50	67	42	32	17	55	85	74	94	44	67	16	94
14	65	52	68	75	87	59	36	22	41	26	78	63	06	55	13	08	27	01	50	15	29	39	39	43
17	53	77	58	71	71	41	61	50	72	12	41	94	96	26	44	95	27	36	99	02	96	74	30	83
90	26	59	21	19	23	52	23	33	12	96	93	02	18	39	07	02	18	36	07	25	99	32	70	23
41	23	52	55	99	31	04	49	69	96	10	47	48	45	88	13	41	43	89	20	97	17	14	49	17
60	20	50	81	69	31	99	73	68	68	35	81	33	03	76	24	30	12	48	60	18	99	10	72	34
91	25	38	05	90	94	58	28	41	36	45	37	59	03	09	90	35	57	29	12	82	62	54	65	60
34	50	57	74	37	98	80	33	00	91	09	77	93	19	82	74	94	80	04	04	45	07	31	66	49
85	22	04	39	43	73	81	53	94	79	33	62	46	86	28	08	31	54	46	31	53	94	13	38	47
09	79	13	77	48	73	82	97	22	21	05	03	27	24	83	72	89	44	05	60	35	80	39	94	88
88	75	80	18	14	22	95	75	42	49	39	32	82	22	49	02	48	07	70	37	16	04	61	67	87
90	96	23	70	00	39	00	03	06	90	55	85	78	38	36	94	37	30	69	32	90	89	00	76	33
53	74	23	99	67	61	32	28	69	84	94	62	67	86	24	98	33	41	19	95	47	53	53	38	09
63	38	06	86	54	99	00	65	26	94	02	82	90	23	07	79	62	67	80	60	75	91	12	81	19
35	30	58	21	46	06	72	17	10	94	25	21	31	75	96	49	28	24	00	49	55	65	79	78	07
63	43	36	82	69	65	51	18	37	88	61	38	44	12	45	32	92	85	88	65	54	34	81	85	35
98	25	37	55	26	01	91	82	81	46	74	71	12	94	97	24	02	71	37	07	03	92	18	66	75
02	63	21	17	69	71	50	80	89	56	38	15	70	11	48	43	40	45	86	98	00	83	26	91	03
64	55	22	21	82	48	22	28	06	00	61	54	13	43	91	82	78	12	23	29	06	66	24	12	27
85	07	26	13	89	01	10	07	82	04	59	63	69	36	03	69	11	15	83	80	13	29	54	19	28
58	54	16	24	15	51	54	44	82	00	62	61	65	04	69	38	18	65	18	97	85	72	13	49	21
34	85	27	84	87	61	48	64	56	26	90	18	48	13	26	37	70	15	42	57	65	65	80	39	07

*From Fisher, Sir Ronald A., and Yates, Frank: Statistical tables for biological, agricultural, and medical research, ed. 6, Edinburgh, 1963, Oliver & Boyd Ltd.; by permission of the authors and publishers.

Continued.

Table C-3. Random numbers—cont'd

```
03 92 18 27 46 57 99 16 96 56 30 33 72 85 22 84 64 38 56 98 99 01 30 98 64
62 95 30 27 59 37 75 41 66 48 86 97 80 61 45 23 53 04 01 63 45 76 08 64 27
08 45 93 15 22 60 21 75 46 91 98 77 27 85 42 28 88 61 08 84 69 62 03 42 73
07 08 55 18 40 45 44 75 13 90 24 94 96 61 02 57 55 66 83 15 73 42 37 11 61
01 85 89 95 66 51 10 19 34 88 15 84 97 19 75 12 76 39 43 78 64 63 91 08 25

72 84 71 14 35 19 11 58 49 26 50 11 17 17 76 86 31 57 20 18 95 60 78 46 75
88 78 28 16 84 13 52 53 94 53 75 45 69 30 96 73 89 65 70 31 99 17 43 48 76
45 17 75 65 57 28 40 19 72 12 25 12 74 75 67 60 40 60 81 19 24 62 01 61 16
96 76 28 12 54 22 01 11 94 25 71 96 16 16 88 68 64 36 74 45 19 59 50 88 92
43 31 67 72 30 24 02 94 08 63 38 32 36 66 02 69 36 38 25 39 48 03 45 15 22

50 44 66 44 21 66 06 58 05 62 68 15 54 35 02 42 35 48 96 32 14 52 41 52 48
22 66 22 15 86 26 63 75 41 99 58 42 36 72 24 58 37 52 18 51 03 37 18 39 11
96 24 40 14 51 23 22 30 88 57 95 67 47 29 83 94 69 40 06 07 18 16 36 78 86
31 73 91 61 19 60 20 72 93 48 98 57 07 23 89 65 95 39 69 58 56 80 30 19 44
78 60 73 99 84 43 89 94 36 45 56 69 47 07 41 90 22 91 07 12 78 35 34 08 72

84 37 90 61 56 70 10 23 98 05 85 11 34 76 60 76 48 45 34 60 01 64 18 39 96
36 67 10 08 23 98 93 35 08 86 99 29 76 29 81 33 34 91 58 93 63 14 52 32 52
07 28 59 07 48 89 64 58 89 75 83 85 62 27 89 30 14 78 56 27 86 63 59 80 02
10 15 83 87 60 79 24 31 66 56 21 48 24 06 93 91 98 94 05 49 01 47 59 38 00
55 19 68 97 65 03 73 52 16 56 00 53 55 90 27 33 42 29 38 87 22 13 88 83 34

53 81 29 13 39 35 01 20 71 34 62 33 74 74 14 53 73 19 09 03 56 54 29 56 93
51 86 32 68 92 33 98 74 66 99 40 14 71 82 58 45 94 19 38 81 14 44 99 81 07
35 91 70 29 13 80 03 54 07 27 96 94 78 94 66 50 95 52 74 33 13 80 55 62 54
37 71 67 95 13 20 02 44 95 94 64 85 04 05 72 01 32 90 76 14 53 89 74 60 41
93 66 13 83 27 92 79 64 64 72 28 54 96 53 84 48 14 52 98 94 56 07 93 89 30

02 96 08 45 65 13 05 00 41 84 93 07 54 72 59 21 45 57 09 77 19 48 56 27 44
49 83 43 48 35 82 88 33 69 96 72 36 04 19 76 47 45 15 18 60 82 11 08 95 97
84 60 71 62 46 40 80 81 30 37 34 39 23 05 38 25 15 35 71 30 88 12 57 21 77
18 17 30 88 71 44 91 14 88 47 89 23 30 63 15 56 34 20 47 89 99 82 93 24 98
79 69 10 61 78 71 32 76 95 62 87 00 22 58 40 92 54 01 75 25 43 11 71 99 31
```

94	26	13	54	74	86	63	68	42	96	65	90	97	21	74	11	82	14	20	56	83	57	36	93
09	08	92	32	04	67	93	08	29	61	63	84	06	25	62	38	39	81	28	06	03	29	92	30
09	77	63	55	18	44	49	48	15	76	77	74	02	97	51	80	95	75	57	31	34	10	50	29
36	54	14	47	70	76	94	90	83	52	33	10	16	24	73	74	53	81	79	37	24	86	38	31
06	11	09	96	54	45	42	23	55	16	92	20	14	10	42	67	37	23	02	58	88	87	23	01
39	25	84	80	58	92	26	80	43	81	32	69	57	02	87	18	00	72	74	68	95	22	17	33
35	07	90	98	47	18	79	23	05	96	35	89	77	32	39	38	87	59	36	13	60	79	36	84
79	42	16	72	23	80	50	70	13	16	32	08	25	24	28	95	56	20	97	09	62	98	77	40
30	21	30	49	69	97	18	47	03	80	70	99	99	63	65	72	68	82	84	20	89	03	43	31
60	98	67	39	35	94	26	59	58	82	49	20	09	16	27	77	71	93	23	57	73	05	28	59
47	03	82	24	58	06	95	13	09	61	51	57	04	02	87	35	92	23	35	07	59	27	68	53
74	62	51	83	47	62	30	18	52	85	09	77	79	77	39	55	37	93	41	92	29	84	27	95
25	47	47	05	23	78	59	05	71	16	93	25	05	06	28	21	25	87	19	99	31	17	23	88
21	99	21	81	69	22	93	26	38	46	61	99	26	67	65	64	32	90	09	84	16	24	76	57
47	75	44	07	35	99	28	09	69	88	05	20	09	30	27	05	04	32	77	87	98	59	28	43
69	72	57	55	39	51	85	13	44	08	88	47	91	04	34	47	76	67	24	33	56	35	27	22
09	19	92	69	15	44	27	18	33	82	45	65	20	38	55	70	96	06	22	49	72	50	86	76
80	70	10	90	90	86	61	05	77	56	34	56	79	06	10	83	02	02	07	65	96	96	48	68
06	29	98	86	98	47	07	26	87	22	28	52	36	75	27	76	38	38	29	92	94	93	89	39
02	23	92	74	63	49	79	09	54	49	44	17	31	51	65	07	68	68	57	98	98	87	00	71
81	59	86	16	90	66	38	27	18	08	70	47	45	18	55	94	24	59	72	27	53	88	56	12
03	12	37	52	65	11	31	73	84	64	18	45	06	84	06	72	22	29	48	86	95	09	72	96
62	23	87	56	51	12	35	19	64	24	68	90	86	17	02	33	07	31	03	48	88	12	96	94
03	03	47	21	70	09	78	94	81	29	85	69	27	24	38	63	29	16	26	89	57	85	47	57
10	92	65	23	78	63	93	05	98	40	44	62	67	59	68	87	57	98	31	00	43	38	59	43
75	70	86	16	90	75	77	56	18	08	57	47	70	34	35	33	59	27	53	56	88	75	38	51
15	97	37	52	65	15	42	72	84	64	48	70	18	38	41	49	29	84	95	72	09	90	46	20
12	39	87	56	51	12	60	31	64	24	61	83	68	75	19	65	31	17	88	96	12	46	21	71
12	90	47	21	70	12	22	09	81	29	36	76	85	00	09	92	16	24	57	94	85	36	18	29
18	41	65	23	78	10	91	51	98	40	18	07	44	51	77	98	98	59	43	64	38	71	03	58

Continued.

Table C-3. Random numbers—cont'd

53 40 02 95 35	26 77 46 37 61	93 21 95 97 69	04 61 85 21 15	02 87 98 10 47	22 67 27 33 13
44 76 17 17 76	29 80 40 56 65	43 96 20 86 92	31 06 93 74 69	89 18 83 08 90	85 80 62 78 13
09 66 79 82 22	13 20 66 08 61	69 60 47 21 06	17 98 85 32 53	08 15 71 58 56	61 43 50 80 92
42 26 18 06 42	56 75 44 18 68	64 12 97 78 34	21 03 86 47 82	04 89 94 21 10	68 79 96 87 66
72 84 05 53 92	41 82 52 09 66	07 99 97 73 13	56 91 88 45 80	49 79 22 66 08	90 33 72 15 99
00 57 12 31 96	85 72 91 77 37	34 11 27 10 59	33 87 72 73 79	20 85 59 72 88	49 12 79 38 47
41 99 59 51 11	47 82 36 53 27	18 20 37 65 71	73 14 87 96 96	21 43 97 68 02	64 83 44 30 24
86 99 52 10 83	04 32 74 84 47	04 99 83 81 74	99 77 08 07 23	14 01 50 49 84	92 11 61 06 49
79 90 57 96 44	66 99 43 46 39	52 45 28 92 17	19 43 62 94 53	68 72 99 29 27	85 41 40 38 57
79 37 02 46 80	08 90 53 47 19	35 18 71 59 32	87 96 40 52 10	86 73 52 31 83	44 16 15 21 74
68 36 22 92 34	34 63 30 31 84	56 48 00 58 27	26 43 16 09 65	87 08 08 89 42	16 25 14 14 32
47 63 07 06 68	72 95 82 91 83	27 13 06 76 55	72 00 06 65 39	63 61 52 85 29	40 58 53 47 25
22 32 90 88 35	57 73 13 18 70	09 93 41 17 10	39 65 10 90 07	93 74 85 84 72	12 19 40 47 43
00 08 47 07 48	59 76 54 95 07	24 55 41 14 24	27 98 89 77 16	95 51 08 46 23	89 68 65 07 62
20 58 03 77 77	13 73 00 58 48	86 34 74 97 19	67 50 20 47 29	17 69 40 06 19	88 70 39 26 17
35 37 28 56 33	82 89 78 24 53	61 18 45 04 23	53 45 23 25 45	11 89 87 59 66	50 77 27 54 10
55 40 14 11 42	43 73 45 16 21	85 37 89 76 71	77 60 21 76 33	29 74 80 73 56	14 02 31 96 97
31 13 11 50 40	80 44 63 74 40	53 79 09 62 82	57 33 34 16 02	01 39 61 19 45	49 54 58 87 11
51 68 30 81 90	46 99 98 11 06	83 49 39 16 13	68 01 74 19 43	95 82 65 85 65	81 00 50 53 69
51 97 79 69 60	15 05 35 53 71	45 90 84 17 74	93 07 97 33 70	80 15 31 23 79	06 52 28 32 84
00 87 20 40 73	38 48 55 44 95	19 65 51 17 63	60 98 76 53 02	35 94 91 65 20	01 53 11 40 99
83 64 69 23 96	26 67 03 10 06	90 97 67 95 52	61 99 38 05 87	14 51 51 09 71	82 43 39 36 63
63 81 22 72 53	61 26 36 13 79	70 38 11 70 52	97 46 03 70 40	97 33 80 29 53	77 37 03 40 22
22 07 40 51 97	70 43 67 85 88	99 20 52 45 01	22 50 29 53 41	35 41 32 75 20	45 15 34 96 32
55 83 98 39 86	04 18 68 57 54	00 46 49 80 41	61 47 63 30 45	33 67 44 63 25	12 26 25 76 98

```
47 47 25 78 26   09 15 12 14 04   98 82 04 31 54   23 36 54 50 71   23 96 53 27 10
89 11 62 76 94   62 09 65 71 39   56 05 36 36 83   18 20 27 85 64   88 61 50 41 28
46 87 50 97 84   07 70 67 24 05   98 30 03 30 80   48 97 18 19 59   02 57 42 21 34
28 39 43 34 42   43 55 39 07 44   96 58 70 28 53   08 54 11 82 82   23 23 77 81 61
59 01 63 01 52   17 51 90 53 14   09 55 80 74 90   88 26 20 86 16   54 13 18 15 61

29 70 25 08 56   77 75 32 80 84   54 66 62 31 75   97 32 13 91 44   64 64 21 76 91
48 85 99 19 30   73 59 39 74 01   40 53 68 56 53   85 59 28 30 37   06 08 79 97 00
25 34 61 69 67   68 73 18 43 08   00 16 69 91 78   77 27 80 20 75   94 34 18 46 36
02 67 29 76 46   66 71 47 56 43   96 89 40 62 93   94 42 79 95 65   50 60 99 98 88
91 12 33 51 55   82 01 86 34 92   51 56 81 97 47   17 24 03 02 05   21 87 59 37 04

30 97 01 88 79   83 83 81 95 29   94 16 45 76 72   09 55 78 21 94   41 34 06 57 63
23 47 11 85 14   43 79 92 38 12   07 70 70 23 09   71 45 92 41 34   90 53 23 54 78
36 99 42 03 50   35 40 48 24 59   15 70 33 47 54   25 59 36 14 53   43 15 62 50 87
12 22 70 65 61   06 71 64 68 48   04 07 69 25 66   52 11 53 59 88   77 10 92 29 47
33 16 01 83 81   79 94 06 41 50   31 37 88 79 95   53 67 04 28 65   41 59 87 65 56

75 77 44 69 06   84 67 61 09 77   29 93 87 26 44   48 34 78 43 73   67 86 45 57 02
01 51 25 60 14   76 16 79 24 46   28 64 93 12 68   60 90 92 62 48   17 13 14 54 31
96 71 61 28 59   54 54 36 70 24   23 76 52 22 67   99 58 36 97 28   36 43 16 50 28
48 47 13 63 92   20 43 78 24 83   75 54 47 63 67   38 52 53 63 02   50 66 62 29 63
12 62 01 88 44   55 14 76 67 44   46 71 45 57 86   72 38 04 96 76   51 26 58 65 45

61 73 88 34 49   95 67 36 53 30   22 35 39 13 74   51 50 85 45 77   70 63 36 65 39
94 58 25 58 08   63 16 96 93 79   86 84 94 51 76   23 51 94 18 29   04 16 98 71 73
89 24 17 71 09   48 54 72 48 97   91 13 95 57 79   86 08 71 65 72   11 20 56 68 72
87 72 18 33 53   51 43 05 97 26   46 95 61 31 77   01 70 20 37 89   76 99 26 60 75
47 84 00 56 45   48 14 37 87 06   29 93 75 38 48   14 39 15 30 81   29 82 60 88 37

17 56 06 74 97   46 03 56 39 02   29 88 95 17 89   49 30 46 71 83   72 80 02 08 68
99 47 99 83 18   41 19 98 62 10   43 78 02 84 01   50 01 85 52 70   67 61 98 23 14
72 78 53 96 41   91 39 74 42 19   66 34 08 41 07   28 41 99 27 25   44 21 96 08 49
16 73 80 12 56   62 00 23 24 09   96 10 95 68 39   29 42 62 61 63   43 08 06 37 78
58 74 79 15 91   77 34 67 73 44   31 15 60 84 56   56 23 83 96 76   68 17 34 21 37
```

Continued.

Table C-3. Random numbers—cont'd

```
29 43 67 38 69   47 94 06 72 40   90 43 81 88 94   83 76 59 97 41   89 29 74 85 91   33 43 85 90 55
09 28 67 88 59   10 14 54 77 24   35 80 31 07 30   19 59 77 77 60   65 43 62 54 46   18 13 40 90 53
34 06 29 39 09   25 63 18 63 13   89 69 96 10 05   76 61 96 72 76   87 65 60 96 96   08 37 25 65 09
04 36 70 54 51   62 19 66 48 27   95 98 82 05 39   16 81 47 73 83   08 42 53 72 86   51 00 24 77 48
87 49 80 86 85   97 75 09 84 79   01 46 00 24 28   94 43 55 09 44   13 78 51 66 19   51 79 73 63 86
83 52 62 97 39   05 89 18 08 26   61 68 57 98 10   11 63 78 62 88   50 66 57 86 83   78 68 52 99 28
07 83 80 37 52   31 11 94 31 88   16 05 25 65 99   68 64 99 06 96   63 28 32 65 52   57 96 93 25 30
55 51 03 44 85   03 47 06 55 86   96 14 60 63 00   84 61 95 65 07   04 55 22 64 47   26 26 70 69 02
07 14 42 22 13   61 11 19 58 30   94 82 59 21 27   26 61 24 72 80   23 80 27 60 53   17 60 50 02 35
76 47 10 00 07   20 31 98 24 01   50 90 46 47 12   23 65 37 87 83   25 47 12 56 65   34 70 48 09 71
58 56 80 95 28   26 56 40 33 31   78 78 72 21 73   54 76 55 12 05   47 46 72 59 00   87 39 21 04 30
30 91 21 01 37   36 34 07 45 60   13 50 60 61 73   20 36 85 49 83   57 41 72 75 51   96 83 47 03 32
83 29 38 31 07   31 19 17 77 10   69 05 18 88 99   86 95 78 03 38   91 90 27 36 93   23 66 74 35 06
64 34 84 76 61   62 09 81 58 39   36 62 77 32 12   85 90 78 60 96   13 08 77 75 51   95 56 63 78 47
87 05 90 17 11   68 79 22 80 53   37 77 55 27 49   23 18 01 41 73   52 55 44 46 30   89 62 17 19 93
29 87 56 16 16   69 57 45 45 58   68 79 66 80 99   86 48 48 15 70   62 98 67 44 80   99 03 27 79 74
25 31 35 29 36   86 92 44 67 47   53 13 12 30 57   66 27 41 20 66   24 78 32 33 05   93 55 27 95 21
58 06 35 56 27   95 36 84 93 70   37 57 12 21 94   99 45 19 76 81   19 10 23 63 19   39 86 51 07 86
84 95 09 63 03   44 59 11 82 93   31 44 11 60 82   07 68 10 27 90   94 70 13 71 29   79 57 26 21 33
86 12 43 38 78   84 14 24 75 85   71 59 08 10 96   36 27 35 50 30   91 49 67 54 56   11 77 35 02 49
50 45 12 78 86   95 93 62 70 81   26 60 99 92 88   37 23 19 47 56   67 92 95 50 23   28 55 96 84 90
60 57 74 94 72   48 87 20 16 56   35 10 55 35 57   34 65 54 02 10   48 05 07 06 27   94 33 29 48 21
00 09 49 49 04   46 81 42 08 39   03 39 64 36 17   92 30 07 29 48   57 12 76 44 19   15 62 00 51 69
25 09 14 81 95   45 40 31 24 38   71 66 57 12 91   09 72 73 16 59   10 07 30 75 03   52 02 45 97 74
```

```
13 52 28 27 75   46 90 16 18 17   36 87 24 33 56   97 59 47 96 97   80 69 40 83 89
31 04 85 42 92   83 81 13 37 42   59 79 81 50 97   07 96 69 41 93   68 05 96 20 73
96 36 43 59 34   61 31 02 63 35   24 46 04 33 40   42 36 74 24 40   21 76 07 89 10
33 94 94 63 71   37 63 77 41 26   85 36 80 78 17   98 25 16 06 06   37 78 27 50 91
92 25 00 63 61   15 33 39 10 98   17 21 67 46 39   89 03 26 81 97   88 66 44 45 03

43 67 99 15 32   60 87 88 16 56   55 61 79 14 90   84 97 59 99 65   63 91 58 41 89
29 43 20 49 68   07 69 33 85 31   17 72 66 22 60   41 32 21 91 16   26 97 00 43 13
56 35 19 93 50   70 09 03 12 78   25 18 99 27 35   32 26 89 03 62   72 51 00 71 71
67 39 32 20 92   29 37 99 81 98   16 75 05 11 37   38 40 73 27 92   41 00 15 28 19
79 95 40 68 21   09 01 39 66 95   37 36 14 84 00   04 69 94 51 45   30 92 30 38 56

58 67 20 81 13   77 05 63 35 03   26 75 05 08 12   48 28 06 81 00   11 89 52 27 39
03 54 01 76 25   36 04 78 93 72   93 99 29 60 60   07 24 42 06 05   01 58 28 13 73
66 20 68 79 83   91 95 10 81 70   89 87 71 09 60   89 55 46 68 12   57 51 84 60 81
05 08 87 58 61   23 48 76 79 85   41 37 72 85 67   61 69 26 79 07   85 07 98 62 05
65 37 60 84 48   36 03 34 25 32   63 97 80 95 62   56 23 16 16 52   18 29 16 97 62

59 61 66 28 07   38 91 80 64 08   72 73 74 79 48   21 58 92 01 16   08 21 63 13 31
96 65 95 13 46   69 01 86 96 97   88 54 31 09 88   47 34 05 84 89   19 34 35 38 97
59 16 31 36 42   97 94 39 66 80   36 60 10 75 12   39 44 98 99 51   82 33 78 11 32
30 06 69 18 96   95 37 04 02 26   18 89 84 73 61   23 39 60 12 08   05 37 13 99 81
05 44 71 10 66   59 55 28 30 03   18 00 30 06 48   52 26 47 99 69   05 03 00 74 45

59 45 90 77 88   36 01 96 59 98   55 96 14 42 71   50 79 28 91 88   01 69 13 84 11
56 65 36 98 67   44 59 08 72 64   41 85 23 64 85   51 08 27 45 59   22 87 12 66 14
63 35 06 39 95   11 58 50 02 98   58 02 49 69 48   37 30 17 27 84   82 87 67 25 40
84 69 33 54 90   08 60 63 66 76   11 74 46 83 14   07 41 53 45 65   43 49 97 48 44
72 69 95 30 22   06 74 44 28 97   73 91 21 11 09   84 83 01 28 48   57 06 54 94 41

75 92 63 19 47   05 66 54 58 53   91 29 62 52 54   45 83 31 18 93   84 58 15 12 07
23 76 96 87 73   85 64 39 96 14   57 27 45 58 50   83 96 32 26 18   52 43 90 27 64
41 83 21 63 69   74 04 52 22 32   94 10 34 69 35   88 40 63 62 45   03 41 86 71 80
57 92 90 56 33   42 38 12 32 24   79 14 22 58 38   27 28 59 22 26   92 09 08 06 27
03 27 52 61 58   49 92 01 28 30   48 13 19 22 74   30 03 74 26 33   54 20 97 68 54
```

Continued.

Table C-3. Random numbers—cont'd

02	92	65	68	99	05	53	15	26	70	04	69	22	64	07	04	73	25	74	82	78	35	22	21	88
83	52	57	78	62	98	61	70	48	22	68	50	64	55	75	42	70	32	09	60	58	70	61	43	97
82	82	76	31	33	85	13	41	38	10	16	47	61	43	77	83	27	19	70	41	34	78	77	60	25
38	61	34	09	49	04	41	66	09	76	20	50	73	40	95	24	77	95	73	20	47	42	80	61	03
01	01	11	88	38	03	10	16	82	24	39	58	20	12	39	82	77	02	18	88	33	11	49	15	16
21	66	14	38	28	54	08	18	07	04	92	17	63	36	75	33	14	11	11	78	97	30	53	62	38
32	29	30	69	59	68	50	33	31	47	15	64	88	75	27	04	51	41	61	96	86	62	93	66	71
04	59	21	65	47	39	90	89	86	77	46	86	86	88	86	50	09	13	24	91	54	80	67	78	66
38	64	50	07	36	56	50	45	94	25	48	28	48	30	51	60	73	73	03	87	68	47	37	10	84
48	33	50	83	53	59	77	64	59	90	58	92	62	50	18	93	09	45	89	06	13	26	98	86	29
25	19	64	82	84	62	74	29	92	24	61	03	91	22	48	64	94	63	15	07	66	85	12	00	27
23	02	41	46	04	44	31	52	43	07	44	06	03	09	34	19	83	94	62	94	48	28	01	51	92
55	85	66	96	28	28	30	62	58	83	65	68	62	42	45	13	08	60	46	28	95	68	45	52	43
68	45	19	69	59	35	14	82	56	80	22	06	52	26	39	59	78	98	76	14	36	09	03	01	86
69	31	46	29	85	18	88	26	95	54	01	02	14	03	05	48	00	26	43	85	33	93	81	45	95
37	31	61	28	98	94	61	47	03	10	67	80	84	41	26	88	84	59	69	14	77	32	82	81	89
66	42	19	24	94	13	13	38	69	96	76	69	76	24	13	43	83	10	13	24	18	32	84	85	04
33	65	78	12	35	91	59	11	38	44	23	31	48	75	74	05	30	08	46	32	90	04	93	56	16
76	32	06	19	35	22	95	30	19	29	57	74	43	20	90	20	25	36	70	69	38	32	11	01	01
43	33	42	02	59	20	39	84	95	61	58	22	04	02	99	99	78	78	83	82	43	67	16	38	95
28	31	93	43	94	87	73	19	38	47	54	36	90	98	10	83	43	32	26	26	22	00	90	59	22
97	19	21	63	34	69	33	17	03	02	11	15	50	46	08	42	69	60	17	42	14	68	61	14	48
82	80	37	14	20	56	39	59	89	63	33	90	38	44	50	78	22	87	10	88	06	58	87	39	67
03	68	03	13	60	64	13	09	37	11	86	02	57	41	99	31	66	60	65	64	03	03	02	58	97
65	16	58	11	01	98	78	80	63	23	07	37	66	20	56	20	96	06	79	80	33	39	40	49	42
24	65	58	57	04	18	62	85	28	24	26	45	17	82	76	39	65	01	73	91	50	37	49	38	73
02	72	64	07	75	85	66	48	38	73	75	10	96	59	31	48	78	58	08	88	72	08	54	57	17
79	16	78	63	99	43	61	00	66	42	76	26	71	14	33	33	86	76	71	66	37	85	05	56	07
04	75	14	93	39	68	52	16	83	34	64	09	44	62	58	48	32	72	26	95	32	67	35	49	71
40	64	64	57	60	97	00	12	91	33	22	14	73	01	11	83	97	68	95	65	67	77	80	98	87

32	07	26	39	07	41	65	06	66	08	41	82	49	13	66	50	80	78	42	30	30	25	29	44	78	11	85	68	33	32
02	47	78	13	00	80	07	88	92	51	83	12	73	28	17	38	40	77	15	40	59	24	64	47	58	21	80	85	92	40
73	18	13	35	77	61	08	14	19	55	25	96	14	76	48	54	56	06	00	95	22	90	61	18	70	22	20	27	34	40
85	45	71	75	84	61	99	82	51	49	97	96	92	19	33	10	24	19	54	62	05	44	10	13	76	61	25	18	63	59
86	96	03	53	88	81	91	57	07	15	35	60	09	73	01	55	43	83	77	60	21	68	55	66	53	31	94	39	05	63
33	98	84	43	45	00	45	79	69	37	73	06	19	66	59	45	06	92	30	37	35	54	14	14	06	75	39	77	46	28
89	84	79	83	19	54	69	39	35	40	49	54	44	02	82	35	24	42	07	71	52	91	17	81	65	43	11	60	73	31
03	04	04	36	71	88	48	71	08	38	51	78	68	95	82	13	26	48	43	80	96	32	18	43	89	61	55	30	41	62
41	73	29	49	10	68	36	50	93	71	72	42	61	79	36	40	36	84	65	79	79	48	17	95	59	32	48	07	49	10
02	60	88	41	10	68	92	97	57	44	70	56	80	37	35	43	78	98	84	23	17	33	82	91	83	22	49	39	52	47
96	20	07	45	25	08	26	29	19	37	09	64	31	85	20	43	68	52	29	82	64	03	94	29	05	73	87	11	50	93
55	94	03	12	89	49	04	67	04	29	43	40	92	49	58	39	76	19	95	18	43	64	64	24	00	67	54	52	57	37
53	60	84	41	22	05	02	74	57	12	59	58	02	50	15	27	98	92	14	54	59	58	98	04	92	11	70	14	61	58
17	56	25	66	12	41	30	40	11	89	27	40	39	28	23	48	70	34	67	50	85	90	54	55	48	10	26	04	86	06
19	35	74	49	86	58	69	52	27	34	91	25	34	67	76	73	27	16	53	18	90	69	32	52	72	38	64	81	79	38
57	94	95	09	85	70	63	22	37	80	29	83	63	85	68	88	26	48	42	14	64	38	23	08	77	54	98	82	14	17
69	46	27	46	89	64	93	61	22	22	98	08	12	36	73	06	39	18	95	85	98	20	73	64	44	51	82	15	70	53
48	22	63	83	00	64	81	72	34	33	33	34	07	73	93	35	55	17	37	36	08	79	12	64	51	67	25	91	40	33
52	88	51	55	98	12	12	35	96	85	83	82	42	02	38	58	93	42	62	54	03	26	28	31	46	53	28	21	77	37
01	96	91	98	01	65	09	99	89	89	81	68	62	61	61	80	74	60	59	49	37	53	95	84	21	12	16	64	12	44
26	10	97	91	78	78	10	60	76	06	09	97	28	61	23	88	06	97	51	23	96	47	42	02	73	49	34	81	04	63
34	87	18	18	25	97	93	77	52	03	06	06	20	75	67	70	44	96	06	78	21	17	67	22	64	70	16	71	55	54
07	03	48	19	52	80	92	41	46	61	53	92	24	74	74	12	36	96	70	07	76	55	64	70	61	51	36	37	57	95
27	40	98	64	54	86	72	21	05	90	88	05	94	89	19	64	49	82	10	00	37	57	74	04	74	73	18	17	95	99
06	62	00	50	38	46	90	66	87	46	11	11	33	24	15	05	57	77	24	50	44	90	50	44	32	75	76	00	54	69

Continued.

Table C-4.* Areas of the normal curve in terms of x/σ

(1) z Standard score $\left(\frac{x}{\sigma}\right)$	(2) A Area from mean to $\frac{x}{\sigma}$	(3) B Area in larger portion	(4) C Area in smaller portion	(1) z Standard score $\left(\frac{x}{\sigma}\right)$	(2) A Area from mean to $\frac{x}{\sigma}$	(3) B Area in larger portion	(4) C Area in smaller portion
0.00	.0000	.5000	.5000	0.45	.1736	.6736	.3264
0.01	.0040	.5040	.4960	0.46	.1772	.6772	.3228
0.02	.0080	.5080	.4920	0.47	.1808	.6808	.3192
0.03	.0120	.5120	.4880	0.48	.1844	.6844	.3156
0.04	.0160	.5160	.4840	0.49	.1879	.6879	.3121
0.05	.0199	.5199	.4801	0.50	.1915	.6915	.3085
0.06	.0239	.5239	.4761	0.51	.1950	.6950	.3050
0.07	.0279	.5279	.4721	0.52	.1985	.6985	.3015
0.08	.0319	.5319	.4681	0.53	.2019	.7019	.2981
0.09	.0359	.5359	.4641	0.54	.2054	.7054	.2946
0.10	.0398	.5398	.4602	0.55	.2088	.7088	.2912
0.11	.0438	.5438	.4562	0.56	.2123	.7123	.2877
0.12	.0478	.5478	.4522	0.57	.2157	.7157	.2843
0.13	.0517	.5517	.4483	0.58	.2190	.7190	.2810
0.14	.0557	.5557	.4443	0.59	.2224	.7224	.2776
0.15	.0596	.5596	.4404	0.60	.2257	.7257	.2743
0.16	.0636	.5636	.4364	0.61	.2291	.7291	.2709
0.17	.0675	.5675	.4325	0.62	.2324	.7324	.2676
0.18	.0714	.5714	.4286	0.63	.2357	.7357	.2643
0.19	.0753	.5753	.4247	0.64	.2389	.7389	.2611
0.20	.0793	.5793	.4207	0.65	.2422	.7422	.2578
0.21	.0832	.5832	.4168	0.66	.2454	.7454	.2546
0.22	.0871	.5871	.4129	0.67	.2486	.7486	.2514
0.23	.0910	.5910	.4090	0.68	.2517	.7517	.2483
0.24	.0948	.5948	.4052	0.69	.2549	.7549	.2451
0.25	.0987	.5987	.4013	0.70	.2580	.7580	.2420
0.26	.1026	.6026	.3974	0.71	.2611	.7611	.2389
0.27	.1064	.6064	.3936	0.72	.2642	.7642	.2358
0.28	.1103	.6103	.3897	0.73	.2673	.7673	.2327
0.29	.1141	.6141	.3859	0.74	.2704	.7704	.2296
0.30	.1179	.6179	.3821	0.75	.2734	.7734	.2266
0.31	.1217	.6217	.3783	0.76	.2764	.7764	.2236
0.32	.1255	.6255	.3745	0.77	.2794	.7794	.2206
0.33	.1293	.6293	.3707	0.78	.2823	.7823	.2177
0.34	.1331	.6331	.3669	0.79	.2852	.7852	.2148
0.35	.1368	.6368	.3632	0.80	.2881	.7881	.2119
0.36	.1406	.6406	.3594	0.81	.2910	.7910	.2090
0.37	.1443	.6443	.3557	0.82	.2939	.7939	.2061
0.38	.1480	.6480	.3520	0.83	.2967	.7967	.2033
0.39	.1517	.6517	.3483	0.84	.2995	.7995	.2005
0.40	.1554	.6554	.3446	0.85	.3023	.8023	.1977
0.41	.1591	.6591	.3409	0.86	.3051	.8051	.1949
0.42	.1628	.6628	.3372	0.87	.3078	.8078	.1922
0.43	.1664	.6664	.3336	0.88	.3106	.8106	.1894
0.44	.1700	.6700	.3300	0.89	.3133	.8133	.1867

*From Edwards, Allen L.: Statistical analysis, New York, 1958, Holt, Rinehart & Winston; by permission of the author and publishers.

Table C-4. Areas of the normal curve in terms of x/σ—cont'd

(1) z Standard score $\left(\frac{x}{\sigma}\right)$	(2) A Area from mean to $\frac{x}{\sigma}$	(3) B Area in larger portion	(4) C Area in smaller portion	(1) z Standard score $\left(\frac{x}{\sigma}\right)$	(2) A Area from mean to $\frac{x}{\sigma}$	(3) B Area in larger portion	(4) C Area in smaller portion
0.90	.3159	.8159	.1841	1.35	.4115	.9115	.0885
0.91	.3186	.8186	.1814	1.36	.4131	.9131	.0869
0.92	.3212	.8212	.1788	1.37	.4147	.9147	.0853
0.93	.3238	.8238	.1762	1.38	.4162	.9162	.0838
0.94	.3264	.8264	.1736	1.39	.4177	.9177	.0823
0.95	.3289	.8289	.1711	1.40	.4192	.9192	.0808
0.96	.3315	.8315	.1685	1.41	.4207	.9207	.0793
0.97	.3340	.8340	.1660	1.42	.4222	.9222	.0778
0.98	.3365	.8365	.1635	1.43	.4236	.9236	.0764
0.99	.3389	.8389	.1611	1.44	.4251	.9251	.0749
1.00	.3413	.8413	.1587	1.45	.4265	.9265	.0735
1.01	.3438	.8438	.1562	1.46	.4279	.9279	.0721
1.02	.3461	.8461	.1539	1.47	.4292	.9292	.0708
1.03	.3485	.8485	.1515	1.48	.4306	.9306	.0694
1.04	.3508	.8508	.1492	1.49	.4319	.9319	.0681
1.05	.3531	.8531	.1469	1.50	.4332	.9332	.0668
1.06	.3554	.8554	.1446	1.51	.4345	.9345	.0655
1.07	.3577	.8577	.1423	1.52	.4357	.9357	.0643
1.08	.3599	.8599	.1401	1.53	.4370	.9370	.0630
1.09	.3621	.8621	.1379	1.54	.4382	.9382	.0618
1.10	.3643	.8643	.1357	1.55	.4394	.9394	.0606
1.11	.3665	.8665	.1335	1.56	.4406	.9406	.0594
1.12	.3686	.8686	.1314	1.57	.4418	.9418	.0582
1.13	.3708	.8708	.1292	1.58	.4429	.9429	.0571
1.14	.3729	.8729	.1271	1.59	.4441	.9441	.0559
1.15	.3749	.8749	.1251	1.60	.4452	.9452	.0548
1.16	.3770	.8770	.1230	1.61	.4463	.9463	.0537
1.17	.3790	.8790	.1210	1.62	.4474	.9474	.0526
1.18	.3810	.8810	.1190	1.63	.4484	.9484	.0516
1.19	.3830	.8830	.1170	1.64	.4495	.9495	.0505
1.20	.3849	.8849	.1151	1.65	.4505	.9505	.0495
1.21	.3869	.8869	.1131	1.66	.4515	.9515	.0485
1.22	.3888	.8888	.1112	1.67	.4525	.9525	.0475
1.23	.3907	.8907	.1093	1.68	.4535	.9535	.0465
1.24	.3925	.8925	.1075	1.69	.4545	.9545	.0455
1.25	.3944	.8944	.1056	1.70	.4554	.9554	.0446
1.26	.3962	.8962	.1038	1.71	.4564	.9564	.0436
1.27	.3980	.8980	.1020	1.72	.4573	.9573	.0427
1.28	.3997	.8997	.1003	1.73	.4582	.9582	.0418
1.29	.4015	.9015	.0985	1.74	.4591	.9591	.0409
1.30	.4032	.9032	.0968	1.75	.4599	.9599	.0401
1.31	.4049	.9049	.0951	1.76	.4608	.9608	.0392
1.32	.4066	.9066	.0934	1.77	.4616	.9616	.0384
1.33	.4082	.9082	.0918	1.78	.4625	.9625	.0375
1.34	.4099	.9099	.0901	1.79	.4633	.9633	.0367

Continued.

Table C-4. Areas of the normal curve in terms of x/σ—cont'd

(1) z Standard score $\left(\frac{x}{\sigma}\right)$	(2) A Area from mean to $\frac{x}{\sigma}$	(3) B Area in larger portion	(4) C Area in smaller portion	(1) z Standard score $\left(\frac{x}{\sigma}\right)$	(2) A Area from mean to $\frac{x}{\sigma}$	(3) B Area in larger portion	(4) C Area in smaller portion
1.80	.4641	.9641	.0359	2.25	.4878	.9878	.0122
1.81	.4649	.9649	.0351	2.26	.4881	.9881	.0119
1.82	.4656	.9656	.0344	2.27	.4884	.9884	.0116
1.83	.4664	.9664	.0336	2.28	.4887	.9887	.0113
1.84	.4671	.9671	.0329	2.29	.4890	.9890	.0110
1.85	.4678	.9678	.0322	2.30	.4893	.9893	.0107
1.86	.4686	.9686	.0314	2.31	.4896	.9896	.0104
1.87	.4693	.9693	.0307	2.32	.4898	.9898	.0102
1.88	.4699	.9699	.0301	2.33	.4901	.9901	.0099
1.89	.4706	.9706	.0294	2.34	.4904	.9904	.0096
1.90	.4713	.9713	.0287	2.35	.4906	.9906	.0094
1.91	.4719	.9719	.0281	2.36	.4909	.9909	.0091
1.92	.4726	.9726	.0274	2.37	.4911	.9911	.0089
1.93	.4732	.9732	.0268	2.38	.4913	.9913	.0087
1.94	.4738	.9738	.0262	2.39	.4916	.9916	.0084
1.95	.4744	.9744	.0256	2.40	.4918	.9918	.0082
1.96	.4750	.9750	.0250	2.41	.4920	.9920	.0080
1.97	.4756	.9756	.0244	2.42	.4922	.9922	.0078
1.98	.4761	.9761	.0239	2.43	.4925	.9925	.0075
1.99	.4767	.9767	.0233	2.44	.4927	.9927	.0073
2.00	.4772	.9772	.0228	2.45	.4929	.9929	.0071
2.01	.4778	.9778	.0222	2.46	.4931	.9931	.0069
2.02	.4783	.9783	.0217	2.47	.4932	.9932	.0068
2.03	.4788	.9788	.0212	2.48	.4934	.9934	.0066
2.04	.4793	.9793	.0207	2.49	.4936	.9936	.0064
2.05	.4798	.9798	.0202	2.50	.4938	.9938	.0062
2.06	.4803	.9803	.0197	2.51	.4940	.9940	.0060
2.07	.4808	.9808	.0192	2.52	.4941	.9941	.0059
2.08	.4812	.9812	.0188	2.53	.4943	.9943	.0057
2.09	.4817	.9817	.0183	2.54	.4945	.9945	.0055
2.10	.4821	.9821	.0179	2.55	.4946	.9946	.0054
2.11	.4826	.9826	.0174	2.56	.4948	.9948	.0052
2.12	.4830	.9830	.0170	2.57	.4949	.9949	.0051
2.13	.4834	.9834	.0166	2.58	.4951	.9951	.0049
2.14	.4838	.9838	.0162	2.59	.4952	.9952	.0048
2.15	.4832	.9842	.0158	2.60	.4953	.9953	.0047
2.16	.4846	.9846	.0154	2.61	.4955	.9955	.0045
2.17	.4850	.9850	.0150	2.62	.4956	.9956	.0044
2.18	.4854	.9854	.0146	2.63	.4957	.9957	.0043
2.19	.4857	.9857	.0143	2.64	.4959	.9959	.0041
2.20	.4861	.9861	.0139	2.65	.4960	.9960	.0040
2.21	.4864	.9864	.0136	2.66	.4961	.9961	.0039
2.22	.4868	.9868	.0132	2.67	.4962	.9962	.0038
2.23	.4871	.9871	.0129	2.68	.4963	.9963	.0037
2.24	.4875	.9875	.0125	2.69	.4964	.9964	.0036

Table C-4. Areas of the normal curve in terms of x/σ—cont'd

(1) z Standard score $\left(\frac{x}{\sigma}\right)$	(2) A Area from mean to $\frac{x}{\sigma}$	(3) B Area in larger portion	(4) C Area in smaller portion	(1) z Standard score $\left(\frac{x}{\sigma}\right)$	(2) A Area from mean to $\frac{x}{\sigma}$	(3) B Area in larger portion	(4) C Area in smaller portion
2.70	.4965	.9965	.0035	3.00	.4987	.9987	.0013
2.71	.4966	.9966	.0034	3.01	.4987	.9987	.0013
2.72	.4967	.9967	.0033	3.02	.4987	.9987	.0013
2.73	.4968	.9968	.0032	3.03	.4988	.9988	.0012
2.74	.4969	.9969	.0031	3.04	.4988	.9988	.0012
2.75	.4970	.9970	.0030	3.05	.4989	.9989	.0011
2.76	.4971	.9971	.0029	3.06	.4989	.9989	.0011
2.77	.4972	.9972	.0028	3.07	.4989	.9989	.0011
2.78	.4973	.9973	.0027	3.08	.4990	.9990	.0010
2.79	.4974	.9974	.0026	3.09	.4990	.9990	.0010
2.80	.4974	.9974	.0026	3.10	.4990	.9990	.0010
2.81	.4975	.9975	.0025	3.11	.4991	.9991	.0009
2.82	.4976	.9976	.0024	3.12	.4991	.9991	.0009
2.83	.4977	.9977	.0023	3.13	.4991	.9991	.0009
2.84	.4977	.9977	.0023	3.14	.4992	.9992	.0008
2.85	.4978	.9978	.0022	3.15	.4992	.9992	.0008
2.86	.4979	.9979	.0021	3.16	.4992	.9992	.0008
2.87	.4979	.9979	.0021	3.17	.4992	.9992	.0008
2.88	.4980	.9980	.0020	3.18	.4993	.9993	.0007
2.89	.4981	.9981	.0019	3.19	.4993	.9993	.0007
2.90	.4981	.9981	.0019	3.20	.4993	.9993	.0007
2.91	.4982	.9982	.0018	3.21	.4993	.9993	.0007
2.92	.4982	.9982	.0018	3.22	.4994	.9994	.0006
2.93	.4983	.9983	.0017	3.23	.4994	.9994	.0006
2.94	.4984	.9984	.0016	3.24	.4994	.9994	.0006
2.95	.4984	.9984	.0016	3.30	.4995	.9995	.0005
2.96	.4985	.9985	.0015	3.40	.4997	.9997	.0003
2.97	.4985	.9985	.0015	3.50	.4998	.9998	.0002
2.98	.4986	.9986	.0014	3.60	.4998	.9998	.0002
2.99	.4986	.9986	.0014	3.70	.4999	.9999	.0001

Table C-5. Values of the correlation coefficient for different levels of significance*

n	.1	.05	.02	.01	.001
1	.98769	.99692	.999507	.999877	.9999988
2	.90000	.95000	.98000	.990000	.99900
3	.8054	.8783	.93433	.95873	.99116
4	.7293	.8114	.8822	.91720	.97406
5	.6694	.7545	.8329	.8745	.95074
6	.6215	.7067	.7887	.8343	.92493
7	.5822	.6664	.7498	.7977	.8982
8	.5494	.6319	.7155	.7646	.8721
9	.5214	.6021	.6851	.7348	.8471
10	.4973	.5760	.6581	.7079	.8233
11	.4762	.5529	.6339	.6835	.8010
12	.4575	.5324	.6120	.6614	.7800
13	.4409	.5139	.5923	.6411	.7603
14	.4259	.4973	.5742	.6226	.7420
15	.4124	.4821	.5577	.6055	.7246

n	.1	.05	.02	.01	.001
16	.4000	.4683	.5425	.5897	.7084
17	.3887	.4555	.5285	.5751	.6932
18	.3783	.4438	.5155	.5614	.6787
19	.3687	.4329	.5034	.5487	.6652
20	.3598	.4227	.4921	.5368	.6524
25	.3233	.3809	.4451	.4869	.5974
30	.2960	.3494	.4093	.4487	.5541
35	.2746	.3246	.3810	.4182	.5189
40	.2573	.3044	.3578	.3932	.4896
45	.2428	.2875	.3384	.3721	.4648
50	.2306	.2732	.3218	.3541	.4433
60	.2108	.2500	.2948	.3248	.4078
70	.1954	.2319	.2737	.3017	.3799
80	.1829	.2172	.2565	.2830	.3568
90	.1726	.2050	.2422	.2673	.3375
100	.1638	.1946	.2301	.2540	.3211

*From Fisher, Sir Ronald A., and Yates, Frank: Statistical tables for biological, agricultural, and medical research, ed. 6, Edinburgh, 1963, Oliver & Boyd Ltd.; by permission of the authors and publishers.

Table C-6. Percentage points (q) of the studentized range*

alpha = .10

n = total number of means compared   v = d.f. of denominator of prior F test

v	2	3	4	5	6	7	8	9	10	11	12	13	14	15	16	17	18	19	20
1	8.93	13.44	16.36	18.49	20.15	21.51	22.64	23.62	24.48	25.24	25.92	26.54	27.10	27.62	28.10	28.54	28.96	29.35	29.71
2	4.13	5.73	6.77	7.54	8.14	8.63	9.05	9.41	9.72	10.01	10.26	10.49	10.70	10.89	11.07	11.24	11.39	11.54	11.68
3	3.33	4.47	5.20	5.74	6.16	6.51	6.81	7.06	7.29	7.49	7.67	7.83	7.98	8.12	8.25	8.37	8.48	8.58	8.68
4	3.01	3.98	4.59	5.03	5.39	5.68	5.93	6.14	6.33	6.49	6.65	6.78	6.91	7.02	7.13	7.23	7.33	7.41	7.50
5	2.85	3.72	4.26	4.66	4.98	5.24	5.46	5.65	5.82	5.97	6.10	6.22	6.34	6.44	6.54	6.63	6.71	6.79	6.86
6	2.75	3.56	4.07	4.44	4.73	4.97	5.17	5.34	5.50	5.64	5.76	5.87	5.98	6.07	6.16	6.25	6.32	6.40	6.47
7	2.68	3.45	3.93	4.28	4.55	4.78	4.97	5.14	5.28	5.41	5.53	5.64	5.74	5.83	5.91	5.99	6.06	6.13	6.19
8	2.63	3.37	3.83	4.17	4.43	4.65	4.83	4.99	5.13	5.25	5.36	5.46	5.56	5.64	5.72	5.80	5.87	5.93	6.00
9	2.59	3.32	3.76	4.08	4.34	4.54	4.72	4.87	5.01	5.13	5.23	5.33	5.42	5.51	5.58	5.66	5.72	5.79	5.85
10	2.56	3.27	3.70	4.02	4.26	4.47	4.64	4.78	4.91	5.03	5.13	5.23	5.32	5.40	5.47	5.54	5.61	5.67	5.73
11	2.54	3.23	3.66	3.96	4.20	4.40	4.57	4.71	4.84	4.95	5.05	5.15	5.23	5.31	5.38	5.45	5.51	5.57	5.63
12	2.52	3.20	3.62	3.92	4.16	4.35	4.51	4.65	4.78	4.89	4.99	5.08	5.16	5.24	5.31	5.37	5.44	5.49	5.55
13	2.50	3.18	3.59	3.88	4.12	4.30	4.46	4.60	4.72	4.83	4.93	5.02	5.10	5.18	5.25	5.31	5.37	5.43	5.48
14	2.49	3.16	3.56	3.85	4.08	4.27	4.42	4.56	4.68	4.79	4.88	4.97	5.05	5.12	5.19	5.26	5.32	5.37	5.43
15	2.48	3.14	3.54	3.83	4.05	4.23	4.39	4.52	4.64	4.75	4.84	4.93	5.01	5.08	5.15	5.21	5.27	5.32	5.38
16	2.47	3.12	3.52	3.80	4.03	4.21	4.36	4.49	4.61	4.71	4.81	4.89	4.97	5.04	5.11	5.17	5.23	5.28	5.33
17	2.46	3.11	3.50	3.78	4.00	4.18	4.33	4.46	4.58	4.68	4.77	4.86	4.93	5.01	5.07	5.13	5.19	5.24	5.30
18	2.45	3.10	3.49	3.77	3.98	4.16	4.31	4.44	4.55	4.65	4.75	4.83	4.90	4.98	5.04	5.10	5.16	5.21	5.26
19	2.45	3.09	3.47	3.75	3.97	4.14	4.29	4.42	4.53	4.63	4.72	4.80	4.88	4.95	5.01	5.07	5.13	5.18	5.23
20	2.44	3.08	3.46	3.74	3.95	4.12	4.27	4.40	4.51	4.61	4.70	4.78	4.85	4.92	4.99	5.05	5.10	5.16	5.20
24	2.42	3.05	3.42	3.69	3.90	4.07	4.21	4.34	4.44	4.54	4.63	4.71	4.78	4.85	4.91	4.97	5.02	5.07	5.12
30	2.40	3.02	3.39	3.65	3.85	4.02	4.16	4.28	4.38	4.47	4.56	4.64	4.71	4.77	4.83	4.89	4.94	4.99	5.03
40	2.38	2.99	3.35	3.60	3.80	3.96	4.10	4.21	4.32	4.41	4.49	4.56	4.63	4.69	4.75	4.81	4.86	4.90	4.95
60	2.36	2.96	3.31	3.56	3.75	3.91	4.04	4.16	4.25	4.34	4.42	4.49	4.56	4.62	4.67	4.73	4.78	4.82	4.86
120	2.34	2.93	3.28	3.52	3.71	3.86	3.99	4.10	4.19	4.28	4.35	4.42	4.48	4.54	4.60	4.65	4.69	4.74	4.78
∞	2.33	2.90	3.24	3.48	3.66	3.81	3.93	4.04	4.13	4.21	4.28	4.35	4.41	4.47	4.52	4.57	4.61	4.65	4.69

*From Pearson, E. S., and Hartley, H. O., editors: Biometrika tables for statisticians, ed. 3, Cambridge, 1966, Cambridge University Press, vol. 1.

Continued.

Table C-6. Percentage points (q) of the studentized range—cont'd

alpha = .05

v \ n	2	3	4	5	6	7	8	9	10	11	12	13	14	15	16	17	18	19	20
1	17.97	26.98	32.82	37.08	40.41	43.12	45.40	47.36	49.07	50.59	51.96	53.20	54.33	55.36	56.32	57.22	58.04	58.83	59.56
2	6.08	8.33	9.80	10.88	11.74	12.44	13.03	13.54	13.99	14.39	14.75	15.08	15.38	15.65	15.91	16.14	16.37	16.57	16.77
3	4.50	5.91	6.82	7.50	8.04	8.48	8.85	9.18	9.46	9.72	9.95	10.15	10.35	10.52	10.69	10.84	10.98	11.11	11.24
4	3.93	5.04	5.76	6.29	6.71	7.05	7.35	7.60	7.83	8.03	8.21	8.37	8.52	8.66	8.79	8.91	9.03	9.13	9.23
5	3.64	4.60	5.22	5.67	6.03	6.33	6.58	6.80	6.99	7.17	7.32	7.47	7.60	7.72	7.83	7.93	8.03	8.12	8.21
6	3.46	4.34	4.90	5.30	5.63	5.90	6.12	6.32	6.49	6.65	6.79	6.92	7.03	7.14	7.24	7.34	7.43	7.51	7.59
7	3.34	4.16	4.68	5.06	5.36	5.61	5.82	6.00	6.16	6.30	6.43	6.55	6.66	6.76	6.85	6.94	7.02	7.10	7.17
8	3.26	4.04	4.53	4.89	5.17	5.40	5.60	5.77	5.92	6.05	6.18	6.29	6.39	6.48	6.57	6.65	6.73	6.80	6.87
9	3.20	3.95	4.41	4.76	5.02	5.24	5.43	5.59	5.74	5.87	5.98	6.09	6.19	6.28	6.36	6.44	6.51	6.58	6.64
10	3.15	3.88	4.33	4.65	4.91	5.12	5.30	5.46	5.60	5.72	5.83	5.93	6.03	6.11	6.19	6.27	6.34	6.40	6.47
11	3.11	3.82	4.26	4.57	4.82	5.03	5.20	5.35	5.49	5.61	5.71	5.81	5.90	5.98	6.06	6.13	6.20	6.27	6.33
12	3.08	3.77	4.20	4.51	4.75	4.95	5.12	5.27	5.39	5.51	5.61	5.71	5.80	5.88	5.95	6.02	6.09	6.15	6.21
13	3.06	3.73	4.15	4.45	4.69	4.88	5.05	5.19	5.32	5.43	5.53	5.63	5.71	5.79	5.86	5.93	5.99	6.05	6.11
14	3.03	3.70	4.11	4.41	4.64	4.83	4.99	5.13	5.25	5.36	5.46	5.55	5.64	5.71	5.79	5.85	5.91	5.97	6.03
15	3.01	3.67	4.08	4.37	4.59	4.78	4.94	5.08	5.20	5.31	5.40	5.49	5.57	5.65	5.72	5.78	5.85	5.90	5.96
16	3.00	3.65	4.05	4.33	4.56	4.74	4.90	5.03	5.15	5.26	5.35	5.44	5.52	5.59	5.66	5.73	5.79	5.84	5.90
17	2.98	3.63	4.02	4.30	4.52	4.70	4.86	4.99	5.11	5.21	5.31	5.39	5.47	5.54	5.61	5.67	5.73	5.79	5.84
18	2.97	3.61	4.00	4.28	4.49	4.67	4.82	4.96	5.07	5.17	5.27	5.35	5.43	5.50	5.57	5.63	5.69	5.74	5.79
19	2.96	3.59	3.98	4.25	4.47	4.65	4.79	4.92	5.04	5.14	5.23	5.31	5.39	5.46	5.53	5.59	5.65	5.70	5.75
20	2.95	3.58	3.96	4.23	4.45	4.62	4.77	4.90	5.01	5.11	5.20	5.28	5.36	5.43	5.49	5.55	5.61	5.66	5.71
24	2.92	3.53	3.90	4.17	4.37	4.54	4.68	4.81	4.92	5.01	5.10	5.18	5.25	5.32	5.38	5.44	5.49	5.55	5.59
30	2.89	3.49	3.85	4.10	4.30	4.46	4.60	4.72	4.82	4.92	5.00	5.08	5.15	5.21	5.27	5.33	5.38	5.43	5.47
40	2.86	3.44	3.79	4.04	4.23	4.39	4.52	4.63	4.73	4.82	4.90	4.98	5.04	5.11	5.16	5.22	5.27	5.31	5.36
60	2.83	3.40	3.74	3.98	4.16	4.31	4.44	4.55	4.65	4.73	4.81	4.88	4.94	5.00	5.06	5.11	5.15	5.20	5.24
120	2.80	3.36	3.68	3.92	4.10	4.24	4.36	4.47	4.56	4.64	4.71	4.78	4.84	4.90	4.95	5.00	5.04	5.09	5.13
∞	2.77	3.31	3.63	3.86	4.03	4.17	4.29	4.39	4.47	4.55	4.62	4.68	4.74	4.80	4.85	4.89	4.93	4.97	5.01

alpha = .01

ν \ n	2	3	4	5	6	7	8	9	10	11	12	13	14	15	16	17	18	19	20
1	90.03	135.0	164.3	185.6	202.2	215.8	227.2	237.0	245.6	253.2	260.0	266.2	271.8	277.0	281.8	286.3	290.4	294.3	298.0
2	14.04	19.02	22.29	24.72	26.63	28.20	29.53	30.68	31.69	32.59	33.40	34.13	34.81	35.43	36.00	36.53	37.03	37.50	37.95
3	8.26	10.62	12.17	13.33	14.24	15.00	15.64	16.20	16.69	17.13	17.53	17.89	18.22	18.52	18.81	19.07	19.32	19.55	19.77
4	6.51	8.12	9.17	9.96	10.58	11.10	11.55	11.93	12.27	12.57	12.84	13.09	13.32	13.53	13.73	13.91	14.08	14.24	14.40
5	5.70	6.98	7.80	8.42	8.91	9.32	9.67	9.97	10.24	10.48	10.70	10.89	11.08	11.24	11.40	11.55	11.68	11.81	11.93
6	5.24	6.33	7.03	7.56	7.97	8.32	8.61	8.87	9.10	9.30	9.48	9.65	9.81	9.95	10.08	10.21	10.32	10.43	10.54
7	4.95	5.92	6.54	7.01	7.37	7.68	7.94	8.17	8.37	8.55	8.71	8.86	9.00	9.12	9.24	9.35	9.46	9.55	9.65
8	4.75	5.64	6.20	6.62	6.96	7.24	7.47	7.68	7.86	8.03	8.18	8.31	8.44	8.55	8.66	8.76	8.85	8.94	9.03
9	4.60	5.43	5.96	6.35	6.66	6.91	7.13	7.33	7.49	7.65	7.78	7.91	8.03	8.13	8.23	8.33	8.41	8.49	8.57
10	4.48	5.27	5.77	6.14	6.43	6.67	6.87	7.05	7.21	7.36	7.49	7.60	7.71	7.81	7.91	7.99	8.08	8.15	8.23
11	4.39	5.15	5.62	5.97	6.25	6.48	6.67	6.84	6.99	7.13	7.25	7.36	7.46	7.56	7.65	7.73	7.81	7.88	7.95
12	4.32	5.05	5.50	5.84	6.10	6.32	6.51	6.67	6.81	6.94	7.06	7.17	7.26	7.36	7.44	7.52	7.59	7.66	7.73
13	4.26	4.96	5.40	5.73	5.98	6.19	6.37	6.53	6.67	6.79	6.90	7.01	7.10	7.19	7.27	7.35	7.42	7.48	7.55
14	4.21	4.89	5.32	5.63	5.88	6.08	6.26	6.41	6.54	6.66	6.77	6.87	6.96	7.05	7.13	7.20	7.27	7.33	7.39
15	4.17	4.84	5.25	5.56	5.80	5.99	6.16	6.31	6.44	6.55	6.66	6.76	6.84	6.93	7.00	7.07	7.14	7.20	7.26
16	4.13	4.79	5.19	5.49	5.72	5.92	6.08	6.22	6.35	6.46	6.56	6.66	6.74	6.82	6.90	6.97	7.03	7.09	7.15
17	4.10	4.74	5.14	5.43	5.66	5.85	6.01	6.15	6.27	6.38	6.48	6.57	6.66	6.73	6.81	6.87	6.94	7.00	7.05
18	4.07	4.70	5.09	5.38	5.60	5.79	5.94	6.08	6.20	6.31	6.41	6.50	6.58	6.65	6.73	6.79	6.85	6.91	6.97
19	4.05	4.67	5.05	5.33	5.55	5.73	5.89	6.02	6.14	6.25	6.34	6.43	6.51	6.58	6.65	6.72	6.78	6.84	6.89
20	4.02	4.64	5.02	5.29	5.51	5.69	5.84	5.97	6.09	6.19	6.28	6.37	6.45	6.52	6.59	6.65	6.71	6.77	6.82
24	3.96	4.55	4.91	5.17	5.37	5.54	5.69	5.81	5.92	6.02	6.11	6.19	6.26	6.33	6.39	6.45	6.51	6.56	6.61
30	3.89	4.45	4.80	5.05	5.24	5.40	5.54	5.65	5.76	5.85	5.93	6.01	6.08	6.14	6.20	6.26	6.31	6.36	6.41
40	3.82	4.37	4.70	4.93	5.11	5.26	5.39	5.50	5.60	5.69	5.76	5.83	5.90	5.96	6.02	6.07	6.12	6.16	6.21
60	3.76	4.28	4.59	4.82	4.99	5.13	5.25	5.36	5.45	5.53	5.60	5.67	5.73	5.78	5.84	5.89	5.93	5.97	6.01
120	3.70	4.20	4.50	4.71	4.87	5.01	5.12	5.21	5.30	5.37	5.44	5.50	5.56	5.61	5.66	5.71	5.75	5.79	5.83
∞	3.64	4.12	4.40	4.60	4.76	4.88	4.99	5.08	5.16	5.23	5.29	5.35	5.40	5.45	5.49	5.54	5.57	5.61	5.65

Totally Meler.

Table C-7. Percentage points of the χ^2 distribution*

d.f. \ alpha	0.995	0.990	0.975	0.950	0.900	0.750	0.500
1	392704.10^{-10}	157088.10^{-9}	980069.10^{-9}	393214.10^{-8}	0.0157908	0.1015308	0.454936
2	0.0100251	0.0201007	0.0506356	0.102587	0.210721	0.575364	1.38629
3	0.0717218	0.114832	0.215795	0.351846	0.584374	1.212534	2.36597
4	0.206989	0.297109	0.484419	0.710723	1.063623	1.92256	3.35669
5	0.411742	0.554298	0.831212	1.145476	1.61031	2.67460	4.35146
6	0.675727	0.872090	1.23734	1.63538	2.20413	3.45460	5.34812
7	0.989256	1.239043	1.68987	2.16735	2.83311	4.25485	6.34581
8	1.34441	1.64650	2.17973	2.73264	3.48954	5.07064	7.34412
9	1.73493	2.08790	2.70039	3.32511	4.16816	5.89883	8.34283
10	2.15586	2.55821	3.24697	3.94030	4.86518	6.73720	9.34182
11	2.60322	3.05348	3.81575	4.57481	5.57778	7.58414	10.3410
12	3.07382	3.57057	4.40379	5.22603	6.30380	8.43842	11.3403
13	3.56503	4.10692	5.00875	5.89186	7.04150	9.29907	12.3398
14	4.07467	4.66043	5.62873	6.57063	7.78953	10.1653	13.3393
15	4.60092	5.22935	6.26214	7.26094	8.54676	11.0365	14.3389
16	5.14221	5.81221	6.90766	7.96165	9.31224	11.9122	15.3385
17	5.69722	6.40776	7.56419	8.67176	10.0852	12.7919	16.3382
18	6.26480	7.01491	8.23075	9.39046	10.8649	13.6753	17.3379
19	6.84397	7.63273	8.90652	10.1170	11.6509	14.5620	18.3377
20	7.43384	8.26040	9.59078	10.8508	12.4426	15.4518	19.3374
21	8.03365	8.89720	10.28293	11.5913	13.2396	16.3444	20.3372
22	8.64272	9.54249	10.9823	12.3380	14.0415	17.2396	21.3370
23	9.26043	10.19567	11.6886	13.0905	14.8480	18.1373	22.3369
24	9.88623	10.8564	12.4012	13.8484	15.6587	19.0373	23.3367

n	.250	.100	.05	.025	.01	.005	.001
25	10.5197	11.5240	13.1197	14.6114	16.4734	19.9393	24.3366
26	11.1602	12.1981	13.8439	15.3792	17.2919	20.8434	25.3365
27	11.8076	12.8785	14.5734	16.1514	18.1139	21.7494	26.3363
28	12.4613	13.5647	15.3079	16.9279	18.9392	22.6572	27.3362
29	13.1211	14.2565	16.0471	17.7084	19.7677	23.5666	28.3361
30	13.7867	14.9535	16.7908	18.4927	20.5992	24.4776	29.3360
40	20.7065	22.1643	24.4330	26.5093	29.0505	33.6603	39.3353
50	27.9907	29.7067	32.3574	34.7643	37.6886	42.9421	49.3349
60	35.5345	37.4849	40.4817	43.1880	46.4589	52.2938	59.3347
70	43.2752	45.4417	48.7576	51.7393	55.3289	61.6983	69.3345
80	51.1719	53.5401	57.1532	60.3915	64.2778	71.1445	79.3343
90	59.1963	61.7541	65.6466	69.1260	73.2911	80.6247	89.3342
100	67.3276	70.0649	74.2219	77.9295	82.3581	90.1332	99.3341
Q	−2.6758	−2.3263	−1.9600	−1.6449	−1.2816	−0.6745	−0.0000
1	1.32330	2.70554	3.84146	5.02389	6.63490	7.87944	10.828
2	2.77259	4.60517	5.99146	7.37776	9.21034	10.5966	13.816
3	4.10834	6.25139	7.81473	9.34840	11.3449	12.8382	16.266
4	5.38527	7.77944	9.48773	11.1433	13.2767	14.8603	18.467
5	6.62568	9.23636	11.0705	12.8325	15.0863	16.7496	20.515
6	7.84080	10.6446	12.5916	14.4494	16.8119	18.5476	22.458
7	9.03715	12.0170	14.0671	16.0128	18.4753	20.2777	24.322
8	10.2189	13.3616	15.5073	17.5345	20.0902	21.9550	26.125
9	11.3888	14.6837	16.9190	19.0228	21.6660	23.5894	27.877
10	12.5489	15.9872	18.3070	20.4832	23.2093	25.1882	29.588
11	13.7007	17.2750	19.6751	21.9200	24.7250	26.7568	31.264
12	14.8454	18.5493	21.0261	23.3367	26.2170	28.2995	32.909
13	15.9839	19.8119	22.3620	24.7356	27.6882	29.8195	34.528
14	17.1169	21.0641	23.6848	26.1189	29.1412	31.3194	36.123

*From Pearson, E. S., and Hartley, H. O., editors: Biometrika tables for statisticians, ed. 3, Cambridge, 1966, Cambridge University Press, vol 1. *Continued.*

Table C-7. Percentage points of the χ^2 distribution—cont'd

d.f. \ alpha	0.250	0.100	0.050	0.025	0.010	0.005	0.001
15	18.2451	22.3071	24.9958	27.4884	30.5779	32.8013	37.697
16	19.3689	23.5418	26.2962	28.8454	31.9999	34.2672	39.252
17	20.4887	24.7690	27.5871	30.1910	33.4087	35.7185	40.790
18	21.6049	25.9894	28.8693	31.5264	34.8053	37.1565	42.312
19	22.7178	27.2036	30.1435	32.8523	36.1909	38.5823	43.820
20	23.8277	28.4120	31.4104	34.1696	37.5662	39.9968	45.315
21	24.9348	29.6151	32.6706	35.4789	38.9322	41.4011	46.797
22	26.0393	30.8133	33.9244	36.7807	40.2894	42.7957	48.268
23	27.1413	32.0069	35.1725	38.0756	41.6384	44.1813	49.728
24	28.2412	33.1962	36.4150	39.3641	42.9798	44.5585	51.179
25	29.3389	34.3816	37.6525	40.6465	44.3141	46.9279	52.618
26	30.4346	35.5632	38.8851	41.9232	45.6417	48.2899	54.052
27	31.5284	36.7412	40.1133	43.1945	46.9629	49.6449	55.476
28	32.6205	37.9159	41.3371	44.4608	48.2782	50.9934	56.892
29	33.7109	39.0875	42.5570	45.7223	49.5879	52.3356	58.301
30	34.7997	40.2560	43.7730	46.9792	50.8922	53.6720	59.703
40	45.6160	51.8051	55.7585	59.3417	63.6907	66.7660	73.402
50	56.3336	63.1671	67.5048	71.4202	76.1539	79.4900	86.661
60	66.9815	74.3970	79.0819	83.2977	88.3794	91.9517	99.607
70	77.5767	85.5270	90.5312	95.0232	100.425	104.215	112.317
80	88.1303	96.5782	101.879	106.629	112.329	116.321	124.839
90	98.6499	107.565	113.145	118.136	124.116	128.299	137.208
100	109.141	118.498	124.342	129.561	135.807	140.169	149.449
X	+0.6745	+1.2816	+1.6449	+1.9600	+2.3263	+2.5758	+3.0902

Table C-8. Percentage points of the t distribution*

d.f.	alpha = 0.4 alpha = 0.8	0.25 0.5	0.1 0.2	0.05 0.1	0.025 0.05	0.01 0.02	0.005 0.01	0.0025 0.005	0.001 0.002	0.0005 0.001
1	0.325	1.000	3.078	6.314	12.706	31.821	63.657	127.32	318.31	636.62
2	.289	0.816	1.886	2.920	4.303	6.965	9.925	14.089	22.327	31.598
3	.277	.765	1.638	2.353	3.182	4.541	5.841	7.453	10.214	12.924
4	.271	.741	1.533	2.132	2.776	3.747	4.604	5.598	7.173	8.610
5	0.267	0.727	1.476	2.015	2.571	3.365	4.032	4.773	5.893	6.869
6	.265	.718	1.440	1.943	2.447	3.143	3.707	4.317	5.208	5.959
7	.263	.711	1.415	1.895	2.365	2.998	3.499	4.029	4.785	5.408
8	.262	.706	1.397	1.860	2.306	2.896	3.355	3.833	4.501	5.041
9	.261	.703	1.383	1.833	2.262	2.821	3.250	3.690	4.297	4.781
10	0.260	0.700	1.372	1.812	2.228	2.764	3.169	3.581	4.144	4.587
11	.260	.697	1.363	1.796	2.201	2.718	3.106	3.497	4.025	4.437
12	.259	.695	1.356	1.782	2.179	2.681	3.055	3.428	3.930	4.318
13	.259	.694	1.350	1.771	2.160	2.650	3.012	3.372	3.852	4.221
14	.258	.692	1.345	1.761	2.145	2.624	2.977	3.326	3.787	4.140
15	0.258	0.691	1.341	1.753	2.131	2.602	2.947	3.286	3.733	4.073
16	.258	.690	1.337	1.746	2.120	2.583	2.921	3.252	3.686	4.015
17	.257	.689	1.333	1.740	2.110	2.567	2.898	3.222	3.646	3.965
18	.257	.688	1.330	1.734	2.101	2.552	2.878	3.197	3.610	3.922
19	.257	.688	1.328	1.729	2.093	2.539	2.861	3.174	3.579	3.883
20	0.257	0.687	1.325	1.725	2.086	2.528	2.845	3.153	3.552	3.850
21	.257	.686	1.323	1.721	2.080	2.518	2.831	3.135	3.527	3.819
22	.256	.686	1.321	1.717	2.074	2.508	2.819	3.119	3.505	3.792
23	.256	.685	1.319	1.714	2.069	2.500	2.807	3.104	3.485	3.767
24	.256	.685	1.318	1.711	2.064	2.492	2.797	3.091	3.467	3.745
25	0.256	0.684	1.316	1.708	2.060	2.485	2.787	3.078	3.450	3.725
26	.256	.684	1.315	1.706	2.056	2.470	2.779	3.067	3.435	3.707
27	.256	.684	1.314	1.703	2.052	2.473	2.771	3.057	3.421	3.690
28	.256	.683	1.313	1.701	2.048	2.467	2.763	3.047	3.408	3.674
29	.256	.683	1.311	1.699	2.045	2.462	2.756	3.038	3.396	3.659
30	0.256	0.683	1.310	1.697	2.042	2.457	2.750	3.030	3.385	3.646
40	.255	.681	1.303	1.684	2.021	2.423	2.704	2.971	3.307	3.551
60	.254	.679	1.296	1.671	2.000	2.390	2.660	2.915	3.232	3.460
120	.254	.677	1.289	1.658	1.980	2.358	2.617	2.860	3.160	3.373
∞	.253	.674	1.282	1.645	1.960	2.326	2.576	2.807	3.090	3.291

Alpha $= 1 - P(t/d.f.)$ is the upper-tail area of the distribution for d.f. degrees of freedom, appropriate for use in a single-tail test. For a two-tail test, ½ alpha must be used.

*From Pearson, E. S., and Hartley, H. O., editors: Biometrika tables for statisticians, ed. 3, Cambridge University Press, vol. 1.

Table C-9. The F distribution

alpha = .05

v_1 = d.f. of numerator v_2 = d.f. of denominator

v_1 / v_2	1	2	3	4	5	6	7	8	9	10
1	161.4	199.5	215.7	224.6	230.2	234.0	236.8	238.9	240.5	241.9
2	18.51	19.00	19.16	19.25	19.30	19.33	19.35	19.37	19.38	19.40
3	10.13	9.55	9.28	9.12	9.01	8.94	8.89	8.85	8.81	8.79
4	7.71	6.94	6.59	6.39	6.26	6.16	6.09	6.04	6.00	5.96
5	6.61	5.79	5.41	5.19	5.05	4.95	4.88	4.82	4.77	4.74
6	5.99	5.14	4.76	4.53	4.39	4.28	4.21	4.15	4.10	4.06
7	5.59	4.74	4.35	4.12	3.97	3.87	3.79	3.73	3.68	3.64
8	5.32	4.46	4.07	3.84	3.69	3.58	3.50	3.44	3.39	3.35
9	5.12	4.26	3.86	3.63	3.48	3.37	3.29	3.23	3.18	3.14
10	4.96	4.10	3.71	3.48	3.33	3.22	3.14	3.07	3.02	2.98
11	4.84	3.98	3.59	3.36	3.20	3.09	3.01	2.95	2.90	2.85
12	4.75	3.89	3.49	3.26	3.11	3.00	2.91	2.85	2.80	2.75
13	4.67	3.81	3.41	3.18	3.03	2.92	2.83	2.77	2.71	2.67
14	4.60	3.74	3.34	3.11	2.96	2.85	2.76	2.70	2.65	2.60
15	4.54	3.68	3.29	3.06	2.90	2.79	2.71	2.64	2.59	2.54
16	4.49	3.63	3.24	3.01	2.85	2.74	2.66	2.59	2.54	2.49
17	4.45	3.59	3.20	2.96	2.81	2.70	2.61	2.55	2.49	2.45
18	4.41	3.55	3.16	2.93	2.77	2.66	2.58	2.51	2.46	2.41
19	4.38	3.52	3.13	2.90	2.74	2.63	2.54	2.48	2.42	2.38
20	4.35	3.49	3.10	2.87	2.71	2.60	2.51	2.45	2.39	2.35
21	4.32	3.47	3.07	2.84	2.68	2.57	2.49	2.42	2.37	2.32
22	4.30	3.44	3.05	2.82	2.66	2.55	2.46	2.40	2.34	2.30
23	4.28	3.42	3.03	2.80	2.64	2.53	2.44	2.37	2.32	2.27
24	4.26	3.40	3.01	2.78	2.62	2.51	2.42	2.36	2.30	2.25
25	4.24	3.39	2.99	2.76	2.60	2.49	2.40	2.34	2.28	2.24
26	4.23	3.37	2.98	2.74	2.59	2.47	2.39	2.32	2.27	2.22
27	4.21	3.35	2.96	2.73	2.57	2.46	2.37	2.31	2.25	2.20
28	4.20	3.34	2.95	2.71	2.56	2.45	2.36	2.29	2.24	2.19
29	4.18	3.33	2.93	2.70	2.55	2.43	2.35	2.28	2.22	2.18
30	4.17	3.32	2.92	2.69	2.53	2.42	2.33	2.27	2.21	2.16
40	4.08	3.23	2.84	2.61	2.45	2.34	2.25	2.18	2.12	2.08
60	4.00	3.15	2.76	2.53	2.37	2.25	2.17	2.10	2.04	1.99
120	3.92	3.07	2.68	2.45	2.29	2.17	2.09	2.02	1.96	1.91
∞	3.84	3.00	2.60	2.37	2.21	2.10	2.01	1.94	1.88	1.83

*From Pearson, E. S., and Hartley, H. O., editors: Biometrika tables for statisticians, ed. 3,

v_1	12	15	20	24	30	40	60	120	∞
v_2									
1	243.9	245.9	248.0	249.1	250.1	251.1	252.2	253.3	254.3
2	19.41	19.43	19.45	19.45	19.46	19.47	19.48	19.49	19.50
3	8.74	8.70	8.66	8.64	8.62	8.59	8.57	8.55	8.53
4	5.91	5.86	5.80	5.77	5.75	5.72	5.69	5.66	5.63
5	4.68	4.62	4.56	4.53	4.50	4.46	4.43	4.40	4.36
6	4.00	3.94	3.87	3.84	3.81	3.77	3.74	3.70	3.67
7	3.57	3.51	3.44	3.41	3.38	3.34	3.30	3.27	3.23
8	3.28	3.22	3.15	3.12	3.08	3.04	3.01	2.97	2.93
9	3.07	3.01	2.94	2.90	2.86	2.83	2.79	2.75	2.71
10	2.91	2.85	2.77	2.74	2.70	2.66	2.62	2.58	2.54
11	2.79	2.72	2.65	2.61	2.57	2.53	2.49	2.45	2.40
12	2.69	2.62	2.54	2.51	2.47	2.43	2.38	2.34	2.30
13	2.60	2.53	2.46	2.42	2.38	2.34	2.30	2.25	2.21
14	2.53	2.46	2.39	2.35	2.31	2.27	2.22	2.18	2.13
15	2.48	2.40	2.33	2.29	2.25	2.20	2.16	2.11	2.07
16	2.42	2.35	2.28	2.24	2.19	2.15	2.11	2.06	2.01
17	2.38	2.31	2.23	2.19	2.15	2.10	2.06	2.01	1.96
18	2.34	2.27	2.19	2.15	2.11	2.06	2.02	1.97	1.92
19	2.31	2.23	2.16	2.11	2.07	2.03	1.98	1.93	1.88
20	2.28	2.20	2.12	2.08	2.04	1.99	1.95	1.90	1.84
21	2.25	2.18	2.10	2.05	2.01	1.96	1.92	1.87	1.81
22	2.23	2.15	2.07	2.03	1.98	1.94	1.89	1.84	1.78
23	2.20	2.13	2.05	2.01	1.96	1.91	1.86	1.81	1.76
24	2.18	2.11	2.03	1.98	1.94	1.89	1.84	1.79	1.73
25	2.16	2.09	2.01	1.96	1.92	1.87	1.82	1.77	1.71
26	2.15	2.07	1.99	1.95	1.90	1.85	1.80	1.75	1.69
27	2.13	2.06	1.97	1.93	1.88	1.84	1.79	1.73	1.67
28	2.12	2.04	1.96	1.91	1.87	1.82	1.77	1.71	1.65
29	2.10	2.03	1.94	1.90	1.85	1.81	1.75	1.70	1.64
30	2.09	2.01	1.93	1.89	1.84	1.79	1.74	1.68	1.62
40	2.00	1.92	1.84	1.79	1.74	1.69	1.64	1.58	1.51
60	1.92	1.84	1.75	1.70	1.65	1.59	1.53	1.47	1.39
120	1.83	1.75	1.66	1.61	1.55	1.50	1.43	1.35	1.25
∞	1.75	1.67	1.57	1.52	1.46	1.39	1.32	1.22	1.00

Cambridge, 1966, Cambridge University Press, vol 1. *Continued.*

Table C-9. The F distribution—cont'd

alpha = .01

v_2 \ v_1	1	2	3	4	5	6	7	8	9	10
1	4052	4999.5	5403	5625	5764	5859	5928	5981	6022	6056
2	98.50	99.00	99.17	99.25	99.30	99.33	99.36	99.37	99.39	99.40
3	34.12	30.82	29.46	28.71	28.24	27.91	27.67	27.49	27.35	27.23
4	21.20	18.00	16.69	15.98	15.52	15.21	14.98	14.80	14.66	14.55
5	16.26	13.27	12.06	11.39	10.97	10.67	10.46	10.29	10.16	10.05
6	13.75	10.92	9.78	9.15	8.75	8.47	8.26	8.10	7.98	7.87
7	12.25	9.55	8.45	7.85	7.46	7.19	6.99	6.84	6.72	6.62
8	11.26	8.65	7.59	7.01	6.63	6.37	6.18	6.03	5.91	5.81
9	10.56	8.02	6.99	6.42	6.06	5.80	5.61	5.47	5.35	5.26
10	10.04	7.56	6.55	5.99	5.64	5.39	5.20	5.06	4.94	4.85
11	9.65	7.21	6.22	5.67	5.32	5.07	4.89	4.74	4.63	4.54
12	9.33	6.93	5.95	5.41	5.06	4.82	4.64	4.50	4.39	4.30
13	9.07	6.70	5.74	5.21	4.86	4.62	4.44	4.30	4.19	4.10
14	8.86	6.51	5.56	5.04	4.69	4.46	4.28	4.14	4.03	3.94
15	8.68	6.36	5.42	4.89	4.56	4.32	4.14	4.00	3.89	3.80
16	8.53	6.23	5.29	4.77	4.44	4.20	4.03	3.89	3.78	3.69
17	8.40	6.11	5.18	4.67	4.34	4.10	3.93	3.79	3.68	3.59
18	8.29	6.01	5.09	4.58	4.25	4.01	3.84	3.71	3.60	3.51
19	8.18	5.93	5.01	4.50	4.17	3.94	3.77	3.63	3.52	3.43
20	8.10	5.85	4.94	4.43	4.10	3.87	3.70	3.56	3.46	3.37
21	8.02	5.78	4.87	4.37	4.04	3.81	3.64	3.51	3.40	3.31
22	7.95	5.72	4.82	4.31	3.99	3.76	3.59	3.45	3.35	3.26
23	7.88	5.66	4.76	4.26	3.94	3.71	3.54	3.41	3.30	3.21
24	7.82	5.61	4.72	4.22	3.90	3.67	3.50	3.36	3.26	3.17
25	7.77	5.57	4.68	4.18	3.85	3.63	3.46	3.32	3.22	3.13
26	7.72	5.53	4.64	4.14	3.82	3.59	3.42	3.29	3.18	3.09
27	7.68	5.49	4.60	4.11	3.78	3.56	3.39	3.26	3.15	3.06
28	7.64	5.45	4.57	4.07	3.75	3.53	3.36	3.23	3.12	3.03
29	7.60	5.42	4.54	4.04	3.73	3.50	3.33	3.20	3.09	3.00
30	7.56	5.39	4.51	4.02	3.70	3.47	3.30	3.17	3.07	2.98
40	7.31	5.18	4.31	3.83	3.51	3.29	3.12	2.99	2.89	2.80
60	7.08	4.98	4.13	3.65	3.34	3.12	2.95	2.82	2.72	2.63
120	6.85	4.79	3.95	3.48	3.17	2.96	2.79	2.66	2.56	2.47
∞	6.63	4.61	3.78	3.32	3.02	2.80	2.64	2.51	2.41	2.32

v_1 v_2	12	15	20	24	30	40	60	120	∞
1	6106	6157	6209	6235	6261	6287	6313	6339	6366
2	99.42	99.43	99.45	99.46	99.47	99.47	99.48	99.49	99.50
3	27.05	26.87	26.69	26.60	26.50	26.41	26.32	26.22	26.13
4	14.37	14.20	14.02	13.93	13.84	13.75	13.65	13.56	13.46
5	9.89	9.72	9.55	9.47	9.38	9.29	9.20	9.11	9.02
6	7.72	7.56	7.40	7.31	7.23	7.14	7.06	6.97	6.88
7	6.47	6.31	6.16	6.07	5.99	5.91	5.82	5.74	5.65
8	5.67	5.52	5.36	5.28	5.20	5.12	5.03	4.95	4.86
9	5.11	4.96	4.81	4.73	4.65	4.57	4.48	4.40	4.31
10	4.71	4.56	4.41	4.33	4.25	4.17	4.08	4.00	3.91
11	4.40	4.25	4.10	4.02	3.94	3.86	3.78	3.69	3.60
12	4.16	4.01	3.86	3.78	3.70	3.62	3.54	3.45	3.36
13	3.96	3.82	3.66	3.59	3.51	3.43	3.34	3.25	3.17
14	3.80	3.66	3.51	3.43	3.35	3.27	3.18	3.09	3.00
15	3.67	3.52	3.37	3.29	3.21	3.13	3.05	2.96	2.87
16	3.55	3.41	3.26	3.18	3.10	3.02	2.93	2.84	2.75
17	3.46	3.31	3.16	3.08	3.00	2.92	2.83	2.75	2.65
18	3.37	3.23	3.08	3.00	2.92	2.84	2.75	2.66	2.57
19	3.30	3.15	3.00	2.92	2.84	2.76	2.67	2.58	2.49
20	3.23	3.09	2.94	2.86	2.78	2.69	2.61	2.52	2.42
21	3.17	3.03	2.88	2.80	2.72	2.64	2.55	2.46	2.36
22	3.12	2.98	2.83	2.75	2.67	2.58	2.50	2.40	2.31
23	3.07	2.93	2.78	2.70	2.62	2.54	2.45	2.35	2.26
24	3.03	2.89	2.74	2.66	2.58	2.49	2.40	2.31	2.21
25	2.99	2.85	2.70	2.62	2.54	2.45	2.36	2.27	2.17
26	2.96	2.81	2.66	2.58	2.50	2.42	2.33	2.23	2.13
27	2.93	2.78	2.63	2.55	2.47	2.38	2.29	2.20	2.10
28	2.90	2.75	2.60	2.52	2.44	2.35	2.26	2.17	2.06
29	2.87	2.73	2.57	2.49	2.41	2.33	2.23	2.14	2.03
30	2.84	2.70	2.55	2.47	2.39	2.30	2.21	2.11	2.01
40	2.66	2.52	2.37	2.29	2.20	2.11	2.02	1.92	1.80
60	2.50	2.35	2.20	2.12	2.03	1.94	1.84	1.73	1.60
120	2.34	2.19	2.03	1.95	1.86	1.76	1.66	1.53	1.38
∞	2.18	2.04	1.88	1.79	1.70	1.59	1.47	1.32	1.00

Index

A

Analysis
  factor, 170-171
  of variance; *see* Variance
Assignment, random, 54
Attitudes, tests of, 187
Average deviation, 24-26

B

Beta weights, Doolittle method for, 161, 162
Binomial test, 175
Biserial coefficient, 87-89
Body mechanics, tests of, 186-187

C

Category scale, 7-8
Central tendency measures, 17-22
  importance of, 17-21
Chi square, 80-85, 177, 179
  cases
    expected, 80
    observed, 80
  contingency tables, 82-83
  correction for continuity, 83-84
  frequencies
    expected, 80
    observed, 80
Cochran Q test, 179
Coefficient
  biserial, 87-89
    point, 87-89
  contingency; 87
  correlation
    partial, 167-169
    partial, computation of, 168-169
    partial, purpose of, 167
    values for different levels of significance, 222
  Kendall, 176, 177
  multiple determination, 164
  Pearson, 176
  phi, 86-87
  rank-order, 90-91

Coefficient—cont'd
  regression, partial, estimated, 161
  Spearman, 176
    Rho, 90
  tetrachoric, 86
Collection of data, 7-14
Contingency
  coefficient, 87
  tables, 82-83
Continuity, correction for, 83-84
Continuous scores, 7
Control groups, 52
Correction for continuity, 83-84
Correlation
  coefficient, values for different levels of significance, 222
  linear, simple, 59-72
    r; *see* r
  meaning of, 59
  multiple, 164-167
    assumptions of, 160
    purpose of, 164
    R, interpretation of, 165
    R, significance of difference between multiple R's, 167
    R, significance test for multiple R, 165-166
    R^2, computation of, 164
    R^2, correction for small samples, 164-165
    R^2, interpretation of, 165
    relative contribution of independent variables to variance of dependent variable, 166-167
  partial, coefficients, 167-169
    computation of, 168-169
    purpose of, 167
  ratio, 89
  representing, 59-63
Covariance analysis, 146-157
  completely randomized model, 146-157
    analytical procedure, 148-150
    analytical procedure, example, 151-157
    assumptions of test, 148

Covariance analysis—cont'd
  completely randomized model—cont'd
    example, 151-157
    layout of data, 146-147
    purpose, 146
    summary of results, 150
    summary of results, example, 155
Curve, normal
  areas of, tables of, 218-221
  measures that fit, 15-16

D

Data
  collection of, 7-14
  layout
    covariance analysis, 146-147
    variance analysis, one-way, 104
    variance analysis, one-way, fixed effects,
      randomized blocks model, 114
    variance analysis, repeated observations
      on same subjects—single-factor model,
      134
    variance analysis, repeated observations
      on same subjects—two-factor model,
      136, 137
    variance analysis, two-way, fixed effects,
      completely randomized model, 124-125
  presentation of, 7-14
    graphic, 11-14
  relationship of data to problem, 43-44
Deciles, 33
Decimals, 190
Dependent variable and multiple correlation,
  166-167
Descriptive research, 36-37
Designs
  factorial, 180
  group; *see* Group designs
  research; *see* Research design
Determination coefficient, multiple, 164
Deviation, 192
  average, 24-26
  standard, 26-28
Difference, significance of, between multiple
  R's, 167
Discrete scores, 7
Distributions
  frequency, 8-11
    choosing step interval for, 9-11
  normal, 15-17
    characteristics of, 16-17
    importance of, 15
    position of mean, median, and mode in, 21-22
Doolittle method for beta weights, 161, 162

E

Equations, 193-196
  multiple regression prediction, 159-164
    computational methods, 161-163
    form of, 160
    interpretation of, 163-164

Error
  standard
    of estimate, 77-78
    of mean, 30-31
  statistical
    type I, 48
    type II, 48
    types of, 48
Estimate, standard error of, 77-78
Estimated partial regression coefficients, 161
Experimental research, 40-42

F

F
  distribution, tables of, 230-233
  test, 117
Factor analysis, 170-171
Factorial designs, 180
Feasibility of tests, 184
Fisher test, 177
Fitness, tests of, 186
Fractions, 189-190
  divided, 189
  multiplied, 189
Frequency(ies)
  distributions, 8-11
    choosing step interval for, 9-11
  expected, and chi square, 80
  observed, and chi square, 80
Friedman variance analysis, 176, 179

G

Graphs, 11-14
Group designs
  r-, where $r > 2$, 179-180
    factorial designs—more than one indepen-
      dent variable manipulated interaction
      effects of interest, 180
    one variable manipulated, one observa-
      tion per subject, 179
    one variable manipulated, one pair of
      observations per subject in each of *r*
      treatments or groups, 179
  single, 174-177
    $r > 2$ variables, one observation on each
      variable for each subject, 176-177
    single variable, one observation per sub-
      ject, 174-175
    single variable, $r > 2$ treatments or ob-
      servations per subject, 175-176
    single variable, two observations per sub-
      ject, pretest and posttest experiments,
      175
    two variables, one pair of observations per
      subject, 176
  two-, 177-178
    single variable, one observation per sub-
      ject, 177-178
    single variable, two observations per sub-
      ject, pretest and posttest experiments,
      178

Group designs—cont'd
  single—cont'd
    two correlated variables, one pair of
      observations per subject, 178

H

Hypothesis
  alternative, selection of, 48-50
  scientific, 45-46, 50
    answering question of, 51-55
  statistical, 45, 46-47, 50
  test, 50
    selection of, 48-50
  testable, 51
  testing, 45-50
    nonexperimental, 39-40
    probabilities of false conclusions, 47
    relative consequences of false conclusions,
      47
    summary of, 50

I

Independent variables and multiple correlation, 166-167
Investigation, descriptive, 36-37

K

Kendall coefficient, 176, 177
Knowledge, tests of, 184-185
Kolmogorov-Smirnov test, 175, 177
Kruskal-Wallis variance analysis, 179

L

Linear correlation, 59-72
  r; see r
Linear regression, 73-79
  standard error of estimate, 77-78

M

Mann-Whitney U test, 177
Mathematics skills, review of, 188-196
  order of operations, 193
McNemar test, 175, 178
Mean(s), 17-19
  position in distributions, 21-22
  Scheffé method; see Scheffé method
  standard error of, 30-31
  t tests and; see t tests
  Tukey method for comparison; see Tukey
    method
Measure(s)
  of central tendency, 17-22
    importance of, 17-21
  of variability; see Variability measures
Measurement scales, 7-8
Median, 19-20
  position in distributions, 21-22
Mode, 20-21
  position in distributions, 21-22
Models
  single-factor; see Variance analysis, repeated

Models—cont'd
    observations on same subjects—single-
      factor model
    two-factor; see Variance analysis, repeated
      observations on same subjects—two-
      factor model
Motor ability, tests of, 186
Multiple correlation; see Correlation
Multiple determination coefficient, 164
Multiple regression; see Regression
Multivariate techniques, purpose of, 158-159

N

Negative numbers, 192-193
Nominal scale, 7-8
Nonparametric techniques, 171-173
  contrasted with parametric techniques, 172
  selection of, 173
  when not to use, 173
Normal curve
  areas of, tables of, 218-221
  measures that fit, 15-16
Normal distributions, 15-17
  characteristics of, 16-17
  importance of, 15
Norms and tests, 183-184
Numbers
  negative, 192-193
  positive, 192-193
  random, tables of, 208-217

O

Objectivity of tests, 182
Ordinal scale, 8

P

Paradigms, typical research, 174-180
Parametric techniques contrasted with non-
  parametric techniques, 172
Pearson coefficient, 176
Percent(s), 191-192
Percentage points
  of studentized range, tables of, 223-225
  of t distribution, table of, 229
  of χ² distribution, 226-228
Percentiles, 31-33
Phi coefficient, 86-87
Physical education research; see Research in
  physical education
Point biserial coefficient, 87-89
Positive numbers, 192-193
Posttest and pretest experiments, 175, 178
Presentation of data, 7-14
  graphic, 11-14
Pretest and posttest experiments 175, 178
Probabilities of false conclusions, 47
Problem; see Research problem
Proportions, 191-192

Q

Quartiles, 33

R

r

computing, 64-70
scattergram method, 67-70
formula for, 65
-group designs; *see* Group designs, *r*-inter-
preting, 63-64
values of predictive index for selected values
of, 64
R; *see* Correlation, multiple, *R*
R^2; *see* Correlation, multiple R^2
Random assignment, 54
Random sampling, 52-54
Randomization of interfering variables, 57
Randomized blocks analysis; *see* Variance
analysis, one-way, fixed effects, randomized blocks model
Range, 23-24
studentized, percentage points of, tables
of, 223-225
Rank
-order coefficient, 90-91
scale, 8
Ratio
correlation, 89
scale, 8
Regression
coefficients, estimated partial, 161
linear, simple, 73-79
standard error of estimate, 77-78
multiple, 159-164
assumptions of, 160
prediction equations, 159-164
prediction equations, computational
methods, 161-163
prediction equations, form of, 160
prediction equations, interpretation of,
163-164
Reliability, 57
of tests, 182-183
Repetition maximum (RM), 103
Research design, 50-57
good, characteristics of, 51-57
answering question of scientific hypothesis, 51-55
control groups, 52
question of primary interest, 52
testable hypothesis, 51
practical, 51-52
random assignment, 54
reliability, 57
sampling, 52-54
variance control, 55-57
Research in physical education, 35-44
descriptive, 36-37
experimental, 40-42
hypothesis testing, nonexperimental, 39-40
purposes of, 35-36
scientific, 35
research problem; *see* Research problem
retrospective research, 37-39
true scientific research, definition, 37

Research in physical education—cont'd
types of, 36-42
confidence in results, 42
Research paradigms, typical, 174-180
Research problem, 42-44
choosing a good research problem, 42-44
importance of problem, 43
previous investigations, 43
relationship of data to problem, 43-44
sophistication of, 44
too broad to be practical, 44
Retrospective research, 37-39
RM (repetition maximum), 103
Rounding, 190-191

S

Samples and *t* test; *see t* tests
Sampling, 52-54
Scale(s)
category, 7-8
measurement, 7-8
nominal, 7-8
ordinal, 8
rank, 8
ratio, 8
Scattergram method for computing *r*, 67-70
Scheffé method, 111-112
analytical procedure, 111
example of, 111-112
Scientific research; *see* Research
Scores
continuous, 7
discrete, 7
z, 28-30
Sign test, 178
Significance
of difference between multiple *R*'s, 167
levels of, tables of, 222
test for multiple *R*, 165-166
Single-factor model; *see* Variance analysis,
repeated observations on same subjects
—single-factor model
Single group designs; *see* Group designs, single
Skills
mathematics, review of, 188-196
order of operations, 193
tests of, 185
Spearman coefficient, 176
Spearman Rho coefficient, 90
Square(s)
roots, tables of, 202-207
tables of, 198-201
Standard deviation, 26-28
Standard error
of estimate, 77-78
of mean, 30-31
Statistical error; *see* Error, statistical
Statistical tests, 47
Statistical treatments and typical research
paradigms, 174-180
Statistics
importance of, 1

Statistics—cont'd
 nature of, 1-6
 role of, 1-6
 types of, 2-3
 understanding of, 1-2
 uses of, 3-6
Studentized range, percentage points, tables
  of, 223-225
Symbolic directions, reading of, 188-189

T

t
 distribution of, 93-95
  critical area of rejection under, 94
 percentage points of, table of, 229
 tests, 93-102, 175, 177
 tests, involving one mean, 95-97
  assumptions of, 95-96
  example of, 96-97
  summary of procedures, 97
 tests, involving two means from dependent
   or related samples, 99-101
  assumptions of, 99-100
  example of, 100-101
 tests, involving two means from independent
   samples, 97-99
  assumptions for, 98
  example of, 98-99
Tables, 197-233
 contingency, 82-83
 correlation coefficient, values for different
   levels of significance, 222
 F distribution, 230-233
 normal curve areas, 218-221
 percentage points
  of studentized range, 223-225
  of *t* distribution, 229
  of χ^2 distribution, 226-228
 random numbers, 208-217
 square roots, 202-207
 squares, 198-201
Test(s), 181-187
 of attitudes, 187
 binomial, 175
 of body mechanics, 186-187
 Cochran Q, 179
 evaluation of, 181-184
 F, 117
 feasibility of, 184
 Fisher, 177
 of fitness, 186
 of knowledge, 184-185
 Kolmogorov-Smirnov, 175-177
 Mann-Whitney U, 177
 McNemar, 175, 178
 of motor ability, 186
 norms and, 183-184
 objectivity, 182
 reliability, 182-183
 sign, 178
 significance, for multiple *R,* 165-166
 of skills, 185

Test(s)—cont'd
 statistical, 47
 t; *see t* tests
 validity of, 181-182
 Walsh, 175, 178
 Wilcoxon, 175, 178
Testing; *see* Hypothesis, testing
Tetrachoric coefficient, 86
Tukey method, 109-111
 analytical procedure, 109-110
 differences between sample means, 110
 example of, 110-111
 randomized blocks analysis and, example,
  121
Two-factor model; *see* Variance analysis, repeated observations on same subjects—
   two-factor model
Two-group designs; *see* Group designs, two-

V

Validity of tests, 181-182
Variables
 dependent, and multiple correlation, 166-
  167
 independent, 56-57
  maximum manipulation of, 55-56
  multiple correlation and, 166-167
 interfering
  identifiable, control of, 56-57
  identifiable, elimination of, 56
  randomization of, 57
  matching, 56-57
Variability measures, 23-34
 deciles 33
 deviation, 192
  average, 24-26
  standard, 26-28
 need for, 23
 percentiles, 31-33
 quartiles, 33
 range, 23-24
 standard error of mean, 30-31
 z scores, 28-30
Variance analysis, 103
 contrast between randomized blocks and
   completely randomized models for
   power of *F* test, 117
 covariance; *see* Covariance analysis
 Friedman, 176, 179
 Kruskal-Wallis, 179
 one-way, 103-112
 one-way, fixed effects. completely randomized model, 104-109
  analytical procedure, 105-107
  assumptions of test, 105
  example of, 107-109
  layout of data, 104
  purpose, 104
  summary of results, 106
 one-way, fixed effects, randomized blocks
   model, 113-122
  analytical procedure, 115-118

Variance analysis—cont'd
  one-way, fixed effects, randomized blocks
      model—cont'd
    analytical procedure, example, 119-121
    assumptions of test, 114-115
    example of, 118-121
    illustration of constant treatment and
      blocking effects on population means,
      115
    layout of data, 114
    purpose, 113
    summary of results, 118
    summary of results, example, 121
    Tukey method, 121
  repeated observations on same subjects—
      single-factor model, 133-135
    analytical procedure, 135
    assumptions of test, 134-135
    layout of data, 134
    purpose, 133-134
  repeated observations on same subjects—
      two-factor model, 136-145
    analytical procedure, 138-141
    analytical procedure, example, 141-145
    assumptions of test, 137-138
    example of, 141-145
    layout of data, 136, 137
    purpose, 136-137

Variance analysis—cont'd
  Scheffé method; *see* Scheffé method
  Tukey method; *see* Tukey method
  two-way, 123-145
  two-way, fixed effects, completely ran-
      domized model, 123-133
    analytical procedure, 125-128
    assumptions of test, 125
    example, 128-133
    layout of data, 124-125
    purpose, 123-124
    summary of results, 127
Variance control in research design, 55-57

W

Walsh test, 175, 178
Weights, beta, Doolittle method for, 161, 162
Wilcoxon test, 175, 178

X

χ^2 distribution, percentage points of, tables
  of, 226-228

Z

z scores, 28-30
Zero, 193